STEP-UP to
USMLE Step 2 CK

FOURTH EDITION

STEP-UP to USMLE Step 2 CK

FOURTH EDITION

EDITORS

Brian Jenkins, MD
Family Medicine
President and Chief Educator
Doctors in Training.com, LLC
Fort Worth, Texas

Michael McInnis, MD
Internal Medicine
Chief Educator
Doctors in Training.com, LLC
Fort Worth, Texas

Chris Lewis, MD
Family Medicine
Chief Educator
Doctors in Training.com, LLC
Fort Worth, Texas

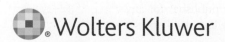
. Wolters Kluwer

Philadelphia · Baltimore · New York · London
Buenos Aires · Hong Kong · Sydney · Tokyo

Publisher: *Lisa McAllister*
Acquisitions Editor: *Shannon Magee*
Product Development Editor: *Amy Weintraub*
Marketing Manager: *Joy Fisher-Williams*
Production Project Manager: *Bridgett Dougherty*
Designer: *Holly Reid McLaughlin*
Compositor: *S4Carlisle Publishing Services*

4th Edition

9 8 7 6 5 4 3 2

Printed in China

Library of Congress Cataloging-in-Publication Data

Jenkins, Brian, 1977- , author.
Step-up to USMLE step 2 CK / Brian Jenkins, Michael McInnis, Chris Lewis. — Fourth edition.
    p. ; cm.
Preceded by Step-up to USMLE step 2 CK / Jonathan P. Van Kleunen, Michael McInnis, Brian Jenkins. 3rd ed. 2014.
Includes bibliographical references and index.
ISBN 978-1-4963-0974-7 (alk. paper)
I. McInnis, Michael, author. II. Lewis, Chris (Physician), author. III. Van Kleunen, Jonathan P. Step-up to USMLE step 2 CK. Preceded by (work): IV. Title.
[DNLM: 1. Clinical Medicine—United States—Outlines. W 18.2]
RC58
616.0076—dc23

2015029040

CONTENTS ● ● ●

1 CARDIOVASCULAR DISORDERS

I	Normal Cardiac Anatomy, Physiology, and Function	1
II	Ischemic Heart Disease	4
III	Arrhythmias	9
IV	Heart Failure	14
V	Valvular Diseases	16
VI	Cardiomyopathies	18
VII	Pericardial Diseases	20
VIII	Myocardial Infections	20
IX	Hypertension (HTN)	22
X	Shock	25
XI	Vascular Diseases	26
XII	Pediatric Cardiology	29

2 PULMONARY DISORDERS

I	Measures of Pulmonary Function	33
II	Respiratory Infections	35
III	Acute Respiratory Distress Syndrome (ARDS)	40
IV	Obstructive Airway Diseases	41
V	Respiratory Neoplasms	43
VI	Interstitial Lung Diseases and Other Lung Diseases	46
VII	Vascular and Thromboembolic Pulmonary Conditions	48
VIII	Pleural Diseases	49
IX	Sleep Apnea	51
X	Pulmonary Surgical Concerns	52
XI	Pediatric Pulmonary Concerns	53

3 GASTROINTESTINAL DISORDERS

I	Gastrointestinal (GI) Infections	56
II	Oral and Esophageal Conditions	61
III	Gastric Conditions	65
IV	Intestinal Conditions	67
V	Pancreatic Disorders	78
VI	Biliary Disorders	80
VII	Hepatic Disorders	84
VIII	Pediatric GI Disorders	86

4 GENITOURINARY DISORDERS

I	Normal Renal Function	90
II	Disorders of the Kidney	92
III	Glomerular Diseases	95
IV	Renal Failure	97
V	Acid-base Disorders	99
VI	Electrolyte Disorders	101

VII   Bladder and Ureteral Disorders *104*
VIII   Male Reproduction *105*
IX   Pediatric Genitourinary Concerns *108*

5   ENDOCRINE DISORDERS

I   Disorders of Glucose Metabolism *109*
II   Thyroid Disorders *114*
III   Parathyroid Disorders *117*
IV   Pituitary and Hypothalamic Disorders *118*
V   Adrenal Disorders *121*
VI   Multiple Endocrine Neoplasia (MEN) *124*
VII   Pediatric Endocrine Concerns *125*

6   HEMATOLOGY AND ONCOLOGY

I   Anemias *126*
II   Genetic Disorders of Hemoglobin *133*
III   Leukocyte Disorders and Hypersensitivity *136*
IV   Clotting Disorders *137*
V   Hematologic Infections *141*
VI   Hematologic Neoplastic Conditions *146*
VII   Oncologic Therapy *150*
VIII   Other Pediatric Hematologic and Oncologic Concerns
      (Not Addressed in Other Sections) *151*

7   SELECTED TOPICS IN EMERGENCY MEDICINE, CRITICAL CARE, AND SURGERY

EMERGENCY MEDICINE *153*
I   Accidents and Injury *153*
II   Toxicology *156*
III   Cardiovascular Emergencies *158*
IV   Traumatology *160*
V   Abuse and Sexual Assault *164*
BASIC CRITICAL CARE *165*
I   Issues in the Intensive Care Unit (ICU) *165*
II   Hemodynamic Stability *166*
BASIC SURGICAL CONCERNS *168*
I   Preoperative and Postoperative Issues *168*
II   Surgical Emergencies *170*
III   Transplantation *172*

8   NEUROLOGIC DISORDERS

I   Normal Neurologic and Neurovascular Function *174*
II   Neurologic Infection *177*
III   Headache *179*
IV   Cerebrovascular and Hemorrhagic Diseases *179*

V   Seizure Disorders *184*
VI   Degenerative Neurologic Disorders *186*
VII Peripheral Motor and Neuromuscular Disorders *188*
VIII Neoplasms *190*
IX   Sleep and Loss of Consciousness *191*
X   Pediatric Neurologic Issues *193*
XI   Ophthalmology *195*
XII Audiovestibular Disorders *200*
XIII Dementia and Delirium *201*

9 MUSCULOSKELETAL DISORDERS

I   Common Adult Orthopedic Conditions *203*
II   Spine *206*
III Metabolic Bone Diseases *209*
IV Infection *211*
V   Osteoarthritis (OA) *213*
VI   Rheumatologic Diseases *214*
VII Neoplasms *218*
VIII Pediatric Orthopedics *219*

10 DERMATOLOGY

I   Infections *224*
II   Inflammatory Skin Conditions *229*
III Bullous Diseases *233*
IV Neoplasms *234*
V   Plastic Surgery *237*

11 GYNECOLOGIC AND BREAST DISORDERS

I   Menstrual Physiology *239*
II   Contraception *243*
III Menstrual Disorders and Issues *245*
IV Common Gynecologic Infections *249*
V   Sexually Transmitted Infections (STIs) *250*
VI   Gynecologic Neoplasms *253*
VII Disorders of the Breast *256*

12 OBSTETRICS

I   Normal Pregnancy Physiology *260*
II   Prenatal Care *261*
III Medical Complications of Pregnancy *264*
IV Obstetric Complications of Pregnancy *270*
V   Labor and Delivery *275*
VI   Gestational Trophoblastic Disease *280*

13 PEDIATRICS

I Development and Health Supervision 282
II Immune Disorders 287
III Genetic Disorders (Chromosomal Pathology) 289

14 PSYCHIATRIC DISORDERS

I Psychotic Disorders 293
II Mood Disorders 294
III Anxiety Disorders 296
IV Obsessive-Compulsive and Related Disorders 298
V Stress- and Trauma-Related Disorders 298
VI Somatic Symptom and Related Disorders 299
VII Eating Disorders 300
VIII Personality Disorders 301
IX Substance Abuse 302
X Pediatric Psychiatric Disorders 302

15 EPIDEMIOLOGY AND ETHICS

I Research Studies 305
II Biostatistics 306
III Ethics 309

Index 313

CARDIOVASCULAR DISORDERS

 I. Normal Cardiac Anatomy, Physiology, and Function

A. **Cardiac and coronary artery anatomy** (*see Figure 1-1*)
B. **Cardiac cycle** (*see Figure 1-2*)

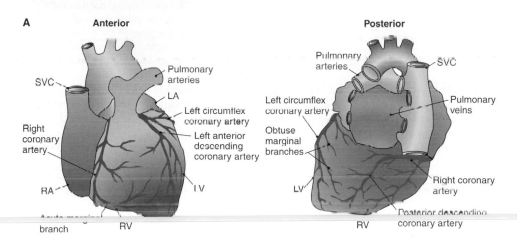

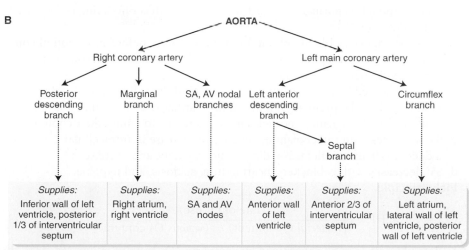

FIGURE 1-1 Coronary artery anatomy.

(**A**) Anterior and posterior views of the heart. (**B**) Coronary artery hierarchy and regions of the heart supplied by branches. AV, atrioventricular; LA, left atrium; LV, left ventricle; RA, right atrium; RV, right ventricle; SA, sinoatrial; SVC, superior vena cava. (Modified from Lilly, L. S. [2011]. *Pathophysiology of Heart Disease.* 5th ed. Baltimore: Lippincott Williams & Wilkins; with permission.)

Quick **HIT**

The **left anterior descending artery** is the most common site of coronary artery occlusion.

Quick **HIT**

In 70% of patients, the posterior descending artery (PDA) derives from the right coronary artery. In 10%, the PDA derives from the circumflex, and in 20%, the PDA derives from an anastomosis of the right coronary and the circumflex.

Quick **HIT**

Coronary arteries fill during **diastole**, whereas systemic arteries fill during **systole**; conditions or drugs that reduce diastolic filling allow less coronary perfusion.

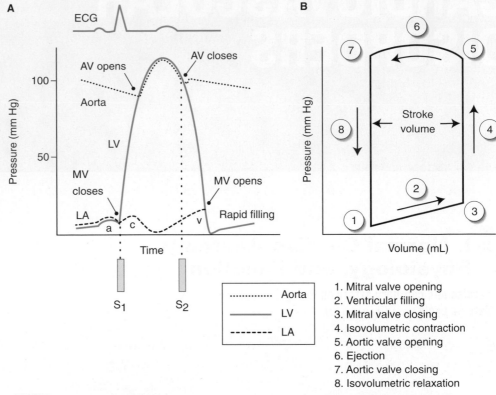

1. Mitral valve opening
2. Ventricular filling
3. Mitral valve closing
4. Isovolumetric contraction
5. Aortic valve opening
6. Ejection
7. Aortic valve closing
8. Isovolumetric relaxation

FIGURE 1-2 **(A) Pressure relationships between left-sided heart chambers and timing with normal heart sounds and the electrocardiogram for one full cardiac cycle. (B) Normal left ventricular pressure-volume loop for one full cardiac cycle.**

AV, aortic valve; ECG, electrocardiogram; LA, left atrium; LV, left ventricle; MV, mitral valve.
(Modified from Lilly, L. S. [2011]. *Pathophysiology of Heart Disease*. 5th ed. Baltimore: Lippincott Williams & Wilkins; with permission.)

C. Cardiac output (CO)

1. Heart rate (HR)
   a. Number of cardiac contractions per unit time; commonly expressed as beats per minute (bpm)
   b. If HR is too high (normal = 60 to 100 bpm), then diastolic filling is decreased.
2. **Stroke volume (SV)**
   a. SV is the **change in blood volume from immediately before initiation of contraction to completion of contraction** (i.e., SV = end diastolic volume to end systolic volume).
   b. It is determined by **contractility** (i.e., SV = [end diastolic volume] − [end systolic volume]), **preload** (amount of myocardial stretch at end of diastole), and **afterload** (resistance ventricles must overcome to empty their contents).
   c. **SV increases** with catecholamine release, an increase in intracellular Ca, a **decrease** in extracellular Na, digoxin use, anxiety, and exercise.
   d. **SV decreases** with β-blockers, heart failure, acidosis, and hypoxia.
3. **Fick principle**

$$CO = SV \times HR = \frac{(\text{rate of } O_2 \text{ use})}{[(\textit{arterial } O_2 \text{ content}) - (\textit{venous } O_2 \text{ content})]}$$

   a. Rate of O_2 use can be determined by comparing O_2 content in expired air to that in inhaled air; arterial and venous O_2 content can be measured directly from the corresponding vasculature.
   b. CO increases during exercise, initially by increasing SV and later by increasing HR.
4. **Mean arterial pressure** = CO × total peripheral resistance (TPR)

   = diastolic arterial pressure + 1/3 pulse pressure
5. **Pulse pressure** = systolic arterial pressure − diastolic arterial pressure

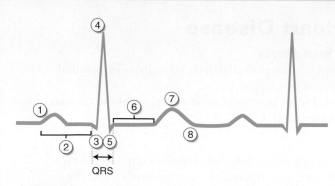

1. P wave–atrial depolarization
2. PR interval–conduction from the atria through the AV node (<0.2 sec)
3. Q wave ⎤ QRS complex–
4. R wave ⎥ ventricular depolarization;
5. S wave ⎦ <0.12 sec
6. ST segment–isoelectric ventricular contraction
7. T wave–ventricular repolarization
8. U wave–relative hypokalemia

FIGURE 1-3 **General structure of the electrocardiogram tracing and significance of specific regions.**
AV, atrioventricular.
(Modified from Lilly, L. S. [2011]. *Pathophysiology of Heart Disease.* 5th ed. Baltimore: Lippincott Williams & Wilkins; with permission.)

D. Electrocardiogram (ECG) (see Figure 1-3)

1. Measures flow of electrical impulses through the heart to provide information regarding **cardiac function**
2. Reviewing an ECG (a consistent order of analysis is useful for picking up abnormalities)
   a. Check calibration on tracing
   b. Rhythm (regular, irregular, pathognomonic signs?)
   c. Rate (normal, tachycardia, bradycardia?)
   d. Intervals (PR, QRS, ST)
   e. QRS axis (normal, deviated?)
   f. P wave (normal, abnormal?)
   g. QRS complex (normal, hypertrophy, widened, infarction?)
   h. ST segment and T wave (normal, depressed, elevated, inverted?)
3. Morphology of action potentials varies with location in the heart (see Figure 1-4).

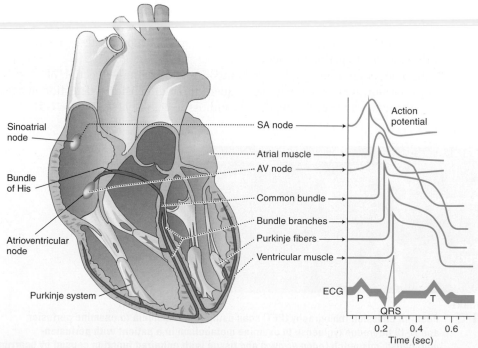

FIGURE 1-4 **Morphology of action potentials at different locations along the conduction pathways of the heart and their relation to the electrocardiogram.**
AV, atrioventricular; ECG, electrocardiogram; SA, sinoatrial.

Cardiovascular Disorders

II. Ischemic Heart Disease

A. Brief introduction to ischemic heart disease

1. Inadequate supply of O_2 for a given myocardial demand leads to **myocardial hypoxia** and an accumulation of waste products.
2. Most cases of ischemic heart disease arise **from atherosclerosis of the coronary arteries (coronary artery disease [CAD])**.

B. Atherosclerosis

1. Gradual narrowing of arteries caused by endothelial dysfunction, progressive formation of plaques (which consist of lipids and smooth muscle), and the associated inflammatory response
2. Plaques can calcify, rupture, and thrombose, which leads to further narrowing of arteries and progressive occlusion of blood flow.
3. **History and physical (H/P)** = asymptomatic for most of disease progression; later sequelae include angina, claudication, progressive hypertension (HTN), retinal changes, extra heart sounds, myocardial infarction (MI), and stroke
4. **Labs** = stress testing, echocardiography, nuclear studies, or angiography can be used to detect coronary ischemia
   a. Exercise stress test—patient exercises on an aerobic fitness machine at increasingly strenuous workloads; heart rate and ECG are constantly monitored; test is continued until patient achieves 85% of predicted maximal heart rate (predicted maximal heart rate = 220 − age) or patient develops angina or signs of ischemia as seen on ECG; ischemic heart disease is diagnosed with signs of **reproducible angina** or obvious signs of **ischemia at low workloads**
   b. Nuclear exercise test—thallium-201 or technetium-99m-sestamibi is injected during exercise testing, and scintigraphy (e.g., planar or single positron emission computed tomography [SPECT]) is performed to assess myocardial perfusion; used in cases of suspected ischemic heart disease in which results of regular exercise stress testing are equivocal
   c. Exercise stress test with echocardiography—exercise stress testing performed in conjunction with echocardiography to increase sensitivity of detecting myocardial ischemia
   d. Pharmacologic stress testing—administration of cardiac inotrope (e.g., dobutamine) in place of exercise to increase myocardial demand; frequently performed in conjunction with SPECT or performed in patients for whom comorbidities interfere with the ability to perform exercise
   e. Positron emission tomography (PET) myocardial imaging—injection of positron-emitting isotopes with subsequent three-dimensional detection imaging to evaluate heart for perfusion defects and tissue viability (see Figure 1-5)

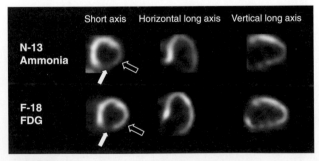

FIGURE
1-5 Positron emission tomography (PET) scan using N-13 ammonia to examine perfusion and Fl-18 fluorodeoxyglucose to examine metabolism in a patient with perfusion-metabolism mismatch (*open arrows*) and tissue with impaired function caused by scarring (*closed arrows*).

(From Topol, E. J. [Ed.]. [2007]. *Textbook of Cardiovascular Medicine* [3rd ed., p. 939]. Philadelphia: Lippincott Williams & Wilkins.)

f. Coronary angiography—gold standard for identifying CAD but more invasive than other techniques

5. **Treatment** = management is primarily intended to minimize risk factors (e.g., tobacco use, HTN, hyperglycemia, hypercholesterolemia); diet low in fats and cholesterol and high in antioxidants (e.g., vitamins E and C, β-carotene) is helpful in preventing disease

C. Dyslipidemia

1. Abnormal serum cholesterol levels (**high** low-density lipoprotein [**LDL**] and/or **low** high-density lipoprotein [**HDL**]) that are associated with increased risk of ischemic heart disease

2. Can result from a congenital disorder (less common) or an acquired condition (most common)

3. **Normal cholesterol physiology**
   a. Cholesterols and triglycerides are carried by lipoproteins.
   b. Increased LDL leads to increased CAD risk; increased HDL is protective.
   c. Increased LDL and decreased HDL result from a diet high in fatty foods, tobacco use, obesity, alcohol use, diabetes mellitus (DM), and certain medications (e.g., oral contraceptive pills [OCP], diuretics).

4. **H/P** = usually asymptomatic; extremely high triglycerides and LDL lead to xanthomas (i.e., lipid deposits in tendons), xanthelasmas (i.e., lipid deposits in eyelids), and cholesterol emboli in retina (visible on funduscopic examination); symptoms are more severe and appear earlier in life in primary disorders compared with acquired conditions

5. **Labs** = increased total cholesterol and LDL; possible decreased HDL; total cholesterol may be >300 to 600 mg/dL in primary disorders; screening for hyperlipidemia is performed in men >35 years of age and women >45 years of age (younger if patient has other risk factors for CAD)

6. **Treatment** = focuses on **prevention** of cardiovascular disease and includes tobacco cessation, exercise, and dietary restrictions (e.g., low fat, low cholesterol); guidelines published in 2013 by the American College of Cardiology (ACC) and American Heart Association (AHA) recommend starting **moderate- or high-intensity statin therapy** in patients who meet specific criteria (see Figure 1-6), without specific target values for LDL, HDL, or other lipid parameters; the guidelines do not specifically recommend other cholesterol-lowering medications due to lack of sufficient evidence, although these other medications are often used in patients who do not tolerate moderate- or high-intensity statin therapy (see Table 1-1)

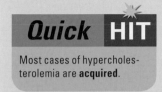

Quick HIT

Most cases of hypercholesterolemia are **acquired**.

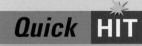

Quick HIT

Blood for serum cholesterol levels should be collected from a **fasting** patient (12–14 hr) to minimize postprandial influence.

In addition to diet and lifestyle modification, individuals should be started on moderate- or high-intensity statin therapy if they fall into one of the following groups:

– Clinical ASCVD
   • Acute Coronary Syndrome
   • MI
   • Stable or Unstable Angina
   • Revascularization Procedures
   • Stroke or TIA
   • Atherosclerotic PAD
– LDL-C > 190 mg/dL
– Diabetes mellitus **and** age 40–75 years
– 10-year ASCVD Risk 7.5% **and** age 40–75

FIGURE 1-6 **Recommendations for statin therapy for ASCVD prevention.**

ASCVD, atherosclerotic cardiovascular disease; LDL-C, low-density lipoprotein cholesterol; MI, myocardial infarction; PAD, peripheral arterial disease; TIA, transient ischemic attack.

TABLE 1-1	Lipid-Lowering Agents				
Drug	**Site of Action**	**Effect on LDL**	**Effect on HDL**	**Effect on Triglycerides**	**Side Effects**
HMG-CoA reductase inhibitors (lovastatin, pravastatin, simvastatin)	Liver	↓↓	↑	↓	Myositis, increased LFT (check before starting medication)
Cholesterol absorption inhibitors (ezetimibe)	Intestines	↓	No change	No change	Myalgias, possible increased LFT
Fibrates (gemfibrozil, fenofibrate)	Blood (all stimulate lipoprotein lipase)	↓	↑	↓↓↓	Myositis, increased LFT (check before starting medication)
Bile acid sequestrants (cholestyramine, colestipol, colesevelam)	GI tract	↓	No change	—/↑	Bad taste, GI upset
Niacin	Liver	↓	↑↑	↓	Facial flushing, nausea, paresthesias, pruritus, increased LFT, insulin resistance, exacerbates gout

GI, gastrointestinal; HDL, high-density lipoprotein; LDL, low-density lipoprotein; LFT, liver function tests; ↑, increased; ↑↑, more increased; ↑↑↑, most increased; —/↑, no change or increased.

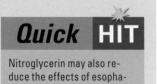

Quick HIT

Nitroglycerin may also reduce the effects of esophageal spasm.

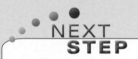

NEXT STEP

Use a formal stress test to rule out a cardiac cause for chest pain before considering alternative diagnoses.

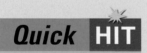

Quick HIT

Myocardial ischemia can be asymptomatic in patients with DM because of **sensory neuropathy**.

D. Angina pectoris

1. Etiology
   a. **Temporary myocardial ischemia** during exertion that causes chest pain
   b. Most commonly caused by **CAD**; also occurs secondary to arterial vasospasm (Prinzmetal angina) and valvular disease
   c. Gastroesophageal reflux disease (GERD) and esophageal spasm can mimic symptoms.
2. **H/P = substernal chest pain** that may radiate to left shoulder, arm, jaw, or back
3. **Labs** = stress testing or nuclear studies used for diagnosis
   a. Important in assessment of chest pain
   b. Seeks to increase cardiac workload to assess myocardial ischemia
   c. Accomplished either through exercise or pharmacologic testing
4. **Treatment = sublingual nitroglycerin** and cessation of intense activity until completion of workup; full workup (including stress testing or nuclear studies) for cause is needed to define long-term treatment

E. Unstable angina

1. **Worsening angina** that occurs at rest
2. Frequently caused by **plaque rupture**, hemorrhage, or thrombosis in coronary arteries
3. One-third of patients have an MI within 3 years.
4. **H/P** = angina with worse pain and increased frequency than in prior episodes; **symptoms occur at rest**; less responsive to prior treatment regimens
5. **ECG = ST depression**, T-wave flattening or inversion
6. Any patient suspected of having an MI must have a workup in a hospital setting with an **ECG** and **serial cardiac enzymes**.
7. **Treatment** = seeks to relieve cause of ischemia and decrease myocardial O_2 demand
   a. **Pharmacotherapy** = IV morphine, supplemental O_2, nitroglycerin, aspirin, β-blockers (to reduce cardiac workload), a statin (preferably before percutaneous coronary intervention [PCI]); if no PCI planned, use clopidogrel or ticagrelor for antiplatelet therapy; if PCI, use glycoprotein (GP) IIb/IIIa inhibitor (abciximab, tirofiban, or eptifibatide) for antiplatelet therapy; anticoagulate with unfractionated heparin (if PCI planned) or low molecular weight heparin (if no PCI planned) to help prevent further thrombus formation; administer potassium and magnesium to keep K^+ levels >4 mEq/L and Mg^{2+} levels >2 mEq/L

b. **Percutaneous transluminal coronary angioplasty (PTCA)**
   (1) Suggested in cases that are nonresponsive to medications
   (2) Catheter inserted through femoral or brachial artery and maneuvered through heart to stenotic vessel
   (3) Balloon on catheter inflated to dilate stenosis
   (4) Catheters can also be used for atherectomy (i.e., plaque is shaved by burr on catheter) or stent placement (i.e., intravascular support structure).
c. **Coronary artery bypass graft (CABG)**
   (1) Considered for left main stenosis >50%, three-vessel disease, or history of CAD and DM
   (2) Donor vessel grafted to coronary artery to bypass obstruction
   (3) Saphenous vein and internal mammary artery are most commonly used.

F. Myocardial infarction (MI)

1. **Tissue death** resulting from ischemia caused by **occlusion of coronary vessels** or **vasospasm**; often secondary to thrombus formation following plaque rupture
2. **Risk factors** = increased age, HTN, hypercholesterolemia, family history of CAD, DM, and tobacco use; males > females; postmenopausal females > premenopausal females
3. **H/P** = chest pain ("**elephant on chest**") in distribution similar to episodes of angina; possible shortness of breath, diaphoresis, nausea, and vomiting; examination findings can include tachycardia, decreased blood pressure, pulmonary rales, new S_4, and new systolic murmur
4. **ECG** = **ST elevation** and T-wave changes; possible new arrhythmia, left bundle branch block (LBBB), or Q-wave changes (see Figure 1-7; Table 1-2)
5. **Labs** = serial cardiac enzymes
   a. Changes in enzymes in the initial **24 hr** after MI are helpful for making a diagnosis of acute infarction, so enzymes are measured every 8 hr in the first 24 hr after presentation (three sets total).
   b. Creatine kinase myocardial fraction (CK-MB) increases 2 to 12 hr post-MI, peaks in 12 to 40 hr, and decreases in 24 to 72 hr.
   c. Lactase dehydrogenase (LDH) increases in 6 to 24 hr and peaks in 3 to 6 days (rarely used for diagnosis).
   d. Troponin-I increases in 2 to 3 hr, peaks in 6 hr, and gradually decreases over 7 days.

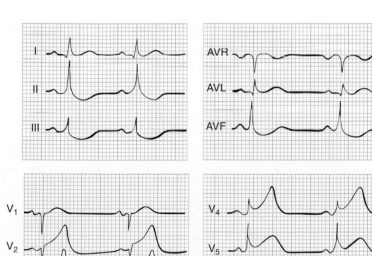

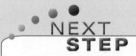

NEXT STEP

Reversible myocardial ischemia is an indication for cardiac catheterization to assess the need for percutaneous transluminal coronary angioplasty (PTCA) or coronary artery bypass graft (CABG).

Quick HIT

Because general CK will be increased with significant muscular trauma or degradation, CK-MB is a better indicator of cardiac muscle damage.

NEXT STEP

Troponin is the best choice to detect MI. **CK-MB** is less sensitive and less specific.

Cardiovascular Disorders

FIGURE 1-7 **Acute myocardial infarction shown on electrocardiogram.**
Note the ST elevation in leads V_2 to V_5, suggesting anterior wall involvement. (From Thaler, M. S. [2015]. *The Only EKG Book You'll Ever Need* [8th ed., p. 260]. Philadelphia: Wolters Kluwer; with permission.)

Cardiovascular Disorders

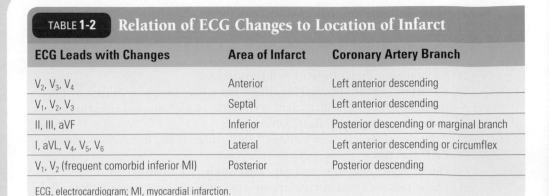

ECG Leads with Changes	Area of Infarct	Coronary Artery Branch
V_2, V_3, V_4	Anterior	Left anterior descending
V_1, V_2, V_3	Septal	Left anterior descending
II, III, aVF	Inferior	Posterior descending or marginal branch
I, aVL, V_4, V_5, V_6	Lateral	Left anterior descending or circumflex
V_1, V_2 (frequent comorbid inferior MI)	Posterior	Posterior descending

ECG, electrocardiogram; MI, myocardial infarction.

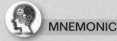

MNEMONIC

For acute treatment of MI, remember the mnemonic "**MONA** had **Hep B**":
- **M**orphine
- **O**$_2$
- **N**itroglycerin
- **A**SA
- **Hep**arin (or LMWH)
- **B**eta-blocker.

6. Treatment
   a. Acutely, give IV morphine, supplemental O_2, nitroglycerin, aspirin, heparin (unfractionated heparin for patients undergoing percutaneous coronary intervention [PCI], low molecular weight heparin for patients not managed with PCI), β-blocker, a statin, and antiplatelet therapy (clopidogrel or ticagrelor).

TABLE 1-3 **Common Medications Used in Ischemic Disease**

Drug	Indications	Cardiovascular Benefits	Contraindications
ASA	MI prevention; during and after MI	Decreases thrombosis risk	High risk of GI bleeding
Clopidogrel	During angina and MI; after PTCA	Decreases thrombosis risk	High risk of GI bleeding
GP IIb/IIIa inhibitor (abciximab, eptifibatide)	During angina or NSTEMI; after PTCA or thrombolysis	Decreases thrombosis risk	High risk of GI bleeding, thrombocytopenia
Nitroglycerin	During angina and MI	Decreases venous pressure, causing decrease in preload and end-diastolic volume; as a result, blood pressure, ejection time, and O_2 consumption decrease while contractility and heart rate increase	Significant hypotension
β-Blocker	MI prevention; during angina; during and post-MI	Decreases blood pressure, contractility, heart rate, and O_2 consumption; increases end-diastolic volume and ejection time; **decreases mortality** following MI	Long-term use with PVD, asthma, COPD, DM (can mask hypoglycemia), and depression (can worsen symptoms)
ACE-I (or ARB)	Post-MI	Decreases afterload, leading to decreased O_2 consumption and blood pressure; **decreases mortality** following MI; particularly helpful with comorbid CHF or DM	Pregnancy
HMG-CoA reductase inhibitors (e.g., statins)	Post-MI	Decreases risk of atherosclerosis progression by lowering LDL level	Use of multiple lipid-lowering medications
Heparin	Immediately post-MI, inpatient setting	Decreases risk of thrombus formation	Active hemorrhage
Morphine	During and immediately post-MI	No direct cardiac benefit but decreases pain during MI, leading to decreased heart rate, blood pressure, and O_2 consumption	Respiratory distress
Thrombolytics (tPA, urokinase)	Immediately post-STEMI, inpatient setting	Breaks up thrombus; **decreases mortality** if used within 12 hr post-MI	High bleeding risk

ACE-I, angiotensin-converting enzyme inhibitors; ASA, acetylsalicylic acid; CHF, congestive heart failure; COPD, chronic obstructive pulmonary disease; DM, diabetes mellitus; ECG, electrocardiogram; GI, gastrointestinal; MI, myocardial infarction; PTCA, percutaneous transluminal coronary angioplasty; PVD, peripheral vascular disease.

b. For ST-elevation MI (STEMI), perform PCI if possible; patients undergoing PCI should also receive a GP IIb/IIIa inhibitor (abciximab, tirofiban, or eptifibatide). If PCI is not available within 12 hours of presentation, consider fibrinolysis with tPA.

c. Administer potassium and magnesium to keep levels >4 mEq/L and >2 mEq/L; if patient is hypotensive, stop nitroglycerin and give intravenous (IV) fluids; give amiodarone for patients with ventricular tachycardia (Vtach).

d. If emergent cardiac catheterization was not performed, perform cardiac catheterization to measure vessel patency and consider possible PTCA or CABG if significant stenosis is found.

e. Long-term treatment = risk reduction medications should include **low-dose acetylsalicylic acid (ASA) or clopidogrel, a β-blocker, an angiotensin-converting enzyme inhibitor (ACE-I), an aldosterone antagonist, and a statin (HMG-CoA reductase inhibitor)**; exercise, smoking cessation, and dietary modifications are also important for risk reduction (see Table 1-3).

7. **Complications** = infarct extension, arrhythmias, myocardial dysfunction, papillary muscle necrosis, wall rupture, aneurysm, mural thrombus, pericarditis, **Dressler syndrome** (fever, pericarditis, and increased erythrocyte sedimentation rate [ESR] 2 to 4 weeks post-MI)

III. Arrhythmias

A. Heart block

1. Impaired myocardial conduction that occurs when electrical impulses encounter tissue that is electronically inexcitable, resulting in an arrhythmia

2. First degree
   a. **Caused** by increased vagal tone or functional conduction impairment
   b. H/P = asymptomatic
   c. ECG = PR >0.2 sec (see Figure 1-8A)
   d. **Treatment** = none necessary

3. Second degree—Mobitz I (Wenckebach)
   a. Caused by **intranodal** or His bundle conduction defect, drug effects (e.g., β blockers, digoxin, calcium channel blockers), or increased vagal tone
   b. H/P = asymptomatic
   c. ECG = progressive PR lengthening until skipped QRS, PR progression, then resets and begins again (see Figure 1-8B)
   d. **Treatment** = adjust doses of medications associated with heart block; treatment usually not necessary unless symptomatic bradycardia is present (pacemaker indicated)

4. Second degree—Mobitz II
   a. Caused by an **infranodal** conduction problem (bundle of His, Purkinje fibers)
   b. H/P = usually asymptomatic
   c. ECG = **randomly skipped QRS** without changes in PR interval (see Figure 1-8C)
   d. **Treatment** = ventricular pacemaker
   e. **Complications** = can progress to third-degree heart block

5. Complete or third-degree heart block
   a. Cause is **absence** of conduction between atria and ventricles
   b. H/P = syncope, dizziness, hypotension
   c. ECG = no relationship between P waves and QRS (see Figure 1-8D)
   d. Treatment = avoid medications affecting atrioventricular (AV) conduction; ventricular pacemaker

B. Paroxysmal supraventricular tachycardia (PSVT)

1. Tachycardia (HR >100 bpm) arising in atria or AV junction
2. Occurs mostly in **young patients** with **healthy hearts**
3. Cause frequently is reentry anomaly
   a. **AV nodal reentry**—presence of both slow and fast conduction pathways in AV node; conduction proceeds quickly through fast pathway and progresses up slow pathway in retrograde fashion; conduction loop is created, resulting in reentrant tachycardia (see Figure 1-9)

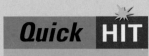

Quick HIT

The greatest risk of sudden cardiac death is in the first few hours post-MI from **Vtach, ventricular fibrillation (Vfib)**, or **cardiogenic shock**.

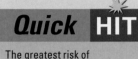

Quick HIT

The greatest risk of ventricular wall rupture is 4–8 days post-MI.

Cardiovascular Disorders

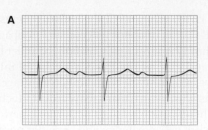

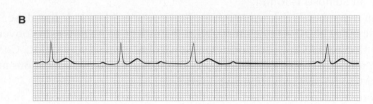

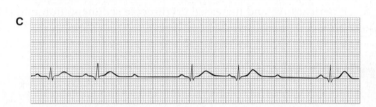

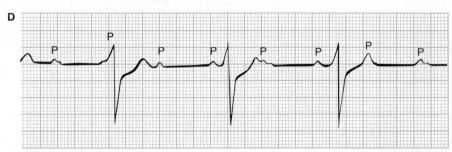

FIGURE 1-8 **(A) Primary heart block: regular PR prolongation without skipped QRS. (B) Secondary-Mobitz I heart block: progressive lengthening of PR until QRS is skipped. (C) Secondary-Mobitz II heart block: regular PR with random skipped QRS. (D) Tertiary heart block: no relationship between P and QRS.**

(From Thaler, M. S. [2015]. *The Only EKG Book You'll Ever Need* [8th ed., pp. 170, 171, 172, and 176]. Philadelphia: Wolters Kluwer; with permission.)

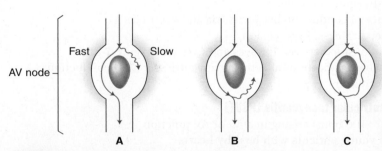

FIGURE 1-9 **Mechanism of atrioventricular nodal reentry tachycardia.**

AV, atrioventricular. **(A)** Action potential reaches division in conduction pathway with both fast and slow fibers. **(B)** Conduction proceeds quickly down fast pathway to reach distal fibers and also proceeds up slow pathway in retrograde fashion. **(C)** Impulse returns to original division point after fibers have repolarized, allowing a reentry conduction loop and resultant tachycardia.

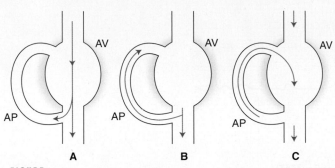

FIGURE
1-10 **Mechanism of atrioventricular reentry tachycardia as seen for Wolff-Parkinson-White syndrome.**

AV, atrioventricular node; AP, accessory pathway. (**A**) Action potential passes through AV node and encounters accessory pathway during conduction to ventricles. (**B**) Accessory pathway conducts action potential back to AV node. (**C**) Return of secondary action potential to AV node completes reentry loop and results in tachycardia.

   b. **AV reentry** as found in **Wolff-Parkinson-White (WPW) syndrome**—similar to AV nodal reentry, but instead of fast and slow pathways existing in the AV node, a separate accessory conduction pathway exists between the atria and ventricles that returns a conduction impulse to the AV node to set up a reentry loop; ECG shows a delta wave (i.e., slurred upstroke of the QRS) and shortened PR (see Figure 1-10)
4. H/P = sudden tachycardia, possible chest pain, shortness of breath, palpitations, syncope
5. ECG = P waves hidden in T waves; 150 to 250 bpm HR; normal QRS (see Figure 1-11)
6. Treatment = carotid massage, Valsalva maneuver, or IV adenosine may halt an acute arrhythmia, but cardioversion or calcium channel blocker is required in cases of hemodynamic instability; pharmacologic therapy (e.g., β-blocker or calcium channel blocker for AV nodal reentrant tachycardia and type IA or IC antiarrhythmic for WPW syndrome) or **catheter ablation** of accessory conduction pathways is frequently used for long-term control in symptomatic patients

C. Multifocal atrial tachycardia (MAT)
1. Caused by several ectopic foci in the atria that discharge automatic impulses (multiple pacemakers), resulting in tachycardia
2. H/P = usually asymptomatic
3. ECG = **variable morphology of P waves**; HR >100 bpm (see Figure 1-12)
4. Treatment = calcium channel blockers or β-blockers acutely; catheter ablation or surgery to eliminate abnormal pacemakers

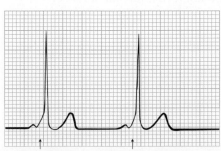

Delta wave   Delta wave

FIGURE
1-11 **Wolff-Parkinson-White syndrome on electrocardiogram.**

Note the presence of delta waves, slurred upstrokes preceding each QRS that are characteristic of the condition. (From Thaler, M. S. [2015]. *The Only EKG Book You'll Ever Need* [8th ed., p. 212]. Philadelphia: Wolters Kluwer; with permission.)

Cardiovascular Disorders

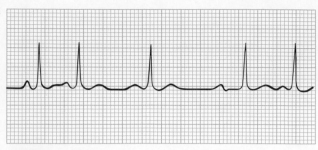

FIGURE 1-12 **Multifocal atrial tachycardia (MAT).**

Note the variety in shape of P waves and PR intervals and the irregular ventricular rate.
(From Thaler, M. S. [2015]. *The Only EKG Book You'll Ever Need* [8th ed., p. 312]. Philadelphia: Wolters Kluwer; with permission.)

D. Bradycardia

1. HR <60 bpm
2. Caused by increased vagal tone or nodal disease
3. **Risk factors** = elderly, history of CAD
4. **H/P** = frequently asymptomatic; possible weakness, syncope
5. Predisposition to development of ectopic beats
6. **Treatment** = stop precipitating medications; pacemaker if severe

E. Atrial fibrillation (Afib)

1. Lack of coordinated atrial contractions with independent sporadic ventricular contractions
2. Caused by rapid, disorderly firing from a second atrial focus
3. **Risk factors** = pulmonary disease, CAD, HTN, anemia, valvular disease, pericarditis, hyperthyroidism, rheumatic heart disease (RHD), sepsis, alcohol use
4. **H/P** = possibly asymptomatic; shortness of breath, chest pain, palpitations, irregularly irregular pulse
5. **ECG** = **no discernible P waves**, irregular QRS rate (see Figure 1-13)
6. **Treatment** = **anticoagulation; rate control** via calcium channel blockers, β-blockers, or digoxin; electric or chemical (i.e., class IA, IC, or III antiarrhythmics) cardioversion if presenting within initial 2 days; cardioversion can be performed in delayed presentation if absence of thrombi is confirmed by transesophageal echocardiogram; if presenting after 2 days or if thrombus is seen on echocardiogram, then anticoagulate and wait 3 to 4 weeks before cardioversion; AV nodal ablation can be considered for recurrent cases
7. **Complications** = increased risk of MI, heart failure; poor atrial contraction causes blood stasis, which leads to mural thrombi formation and a risk of embolization

> **NEXT STEP**
>
> In a patient with Afib >2 days, TEE should be performed **before** cardioversion to rule out mural thrombus formation.

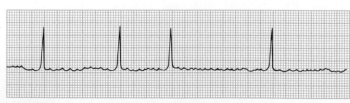

FIGURE 1-13 **Atrial fibrillation—irregular QRS rate and no discernable P waves.**

(From Thaler, M. S. [2015]. *The Only EKG Book You'll Ever Need* [8th ed., p. 133]. Philadelphia: Wolters Kluwer; with permission.)

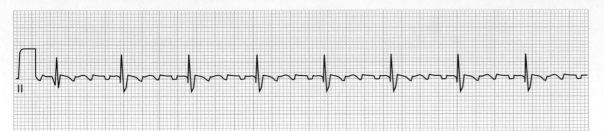

1-14 Atrial flutter—rapid sawtooth P waves preceding QRS.

(From Thaler, M. S. [2015]. *The Only EKG Book You'll Ever Need* [8th ed., p. 331]. Philadelphia: Wolters Kluwer; with permission.)

F. Atrial flutter (Aflutter)
1. Caused by rapid firing of an ectopic focus in the atria
2. **Risk factors** = CAD, congestive heart failure (CHF), chronic obstructive pulmonary disease (COPD), valvular disease, pericarditis
3. H/P = possibly asymptomatic; palpitations, syncope
4. ECG = regular tachycardia >150 bpm with occasionally set ratio of P waves to QRS; **sawtooth pattern of P waves** (see Figure 1-14)
5. **Treatment** = rate control with calcium channel blockers, β-blockers; electrical or chemical (class IA, IC, or III antiarrhythmics) cardioversion if unable to be controlled with medication; catheter ablation to remove ectopic focus may be possible in some cases
6. **Complications** = may degenerate into Afib

G. Premature ventricular contraction (PVC)
1. Caused by ectopic beats from a ventricular origin
2. Common, frequently benign; can also be caused by hypoxia, abnormal serum electrolyte levels, hyperthyroidism, caffeine use
3. H/P = usually asymptomatic; possible palpitations, syncope
4. ECG = early and wide QRS without preceding P wave followed by brief pause in conduction
5. **Treatment** = none if patient is healthy; β-blockers in patients with CAD
6. **Complications** = associated with increased risk of sudden death in patients with CAD

H. Ventricular tachycardia (Vtach)
1. Series of **3+ PVCs** with HR 160 to 240 bpm
2. **Risk factors** = CAD, history of MI
3. H/P = possibly asymptomatic if brief; palpitations, syncope, hypotension
4. ECG = series of regular, wide QRS complexes independent of P waves (see Figure 1-15)

> **Quick HIT**
>
> PVCs become concerning for the development of other ventricular arrhythmias if there are >3 PVCs/min.

> **Quick HIT**
>
> Torsades de pointes is Vtach with a sine wave morphology; it carries a poor prognosis and can rapidly convert to Vfib; Mg may be useful in treatment.

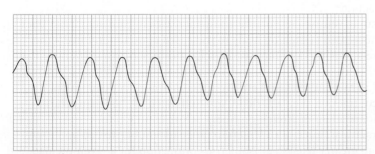

1-15 Ventricular tachycardia—wide, rapid QRS with no discernable P waves.

(From Thaler, M. S. [2015]. *The Only EKG Book You'll Ever Need* [8th ed., p. 141]. Philadelphia: Wolters Kluwer; with permission.)

TABLE **1-4**	Classes of Antiarrhythmic Medications		
Class	**General Mechanism of Action**	**Examples**	**Potential Uses**
IA	Na$^+$ channel blockers (prolong action potential)	Quinidine, procainamide	PSVT, Afib, Aflutter, Vtach
IB	Na$^+$ channel blockers (shorten action potential)	Lidocaine, tocainide	Vtach
IC	Na$^+$ channel blockers (no effect on action potential)	Flecainide, propafenone	PSVT, Afib, Aflutter, PSVT
II	β-Blockers	Propanolol, esmolol, metoprolol	PVC, PSVT, Afib, Aflutter, Vtach
III	K$^+$ channel blockers	Amiodarone, sotalol, bretylium	Afib, Aflutter, Vtach (not bretylium)
IV	Ca^{2+} channel blockers	Verapamil, diltiazem	PSVT, MAT, Afib, Aflutter
Other	K$^+$ channel activation, decrease in intracellular cAMP	Adenosine	PSVT

Afib, atrial fibrillation; Aflutter, atrial flutter; cAMP, cyclic adenosine monophosphate; MAT, multifocal atrial tachycardia; PSVT, paroxysmal supraventricular tachycardia; PVC, premature ventricular contraction; Vtach, ventricular tachycardia.

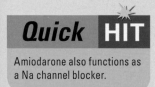

Quick HIT

Amiodarone also functions as a Na channel blocker.

5. **Treatment** = electrical cardioversion followed by antiarrhythmic medications (class IA, IB, II, or III); for recurrent Vtach, internal defibrillator may be necessary (senses ventricular arrhythmia and automatically releases electric pulse to restore normal rhythm)
6. **Complications** = sustained Vtach can quickly deteriorate into Vfib if not corrected

I. Ventricular fibrillation (Vfib)
1. Lack of ordered ventricular contraction leads to **no CO** and is rapidly fatal.
2. Frequently occurs after severe MI, post-Vtach
3. **Risk factors** = CAD, MI
4. **H/P** = syncope, hypotension, pulselessness
5. **ECG** = **totally erratic tracing**; no P waves or QRS
6. **Treatment** = CPR, immediate electric (± chemical) cardioversion

J. Antiarrhythmic medications (see Table 1-4)

 # IV. Heart Failure

A. Heart physiology
1. Principles of contraction
   a. Increases in diastolic ventricular volume cause increases in cardiac muscle fiber stretching; this increased stretching leads to increased contraction force—the Frank-Starling relationship (i.e., increased **preload** causes increased ventricular output).
   b. Pressure generated by ventricles and end-systolic volume is dependent on load-opposing contraction (i.e., **afterload**, approximated at the mean arterial pressure) but independent of stretch on fibers before contraction.
   c. Increasing **contractility** (force of contraction independent of preload and afterload) leads to greater tension at isometric contraction for a given preload.
2. Ejection fraction (EF) $= \dfrac{SV}{\text{end diastolic volume}}$ (**normal EF** = 55% to 75%)

3. Changes in volume—pressure relationship determines compliance of heart
4. Insufficient CO for systemic demand results from progressive heart dysfunction (i.e., CHF).

B. Systolic dysfunction

1. Inadequate CO for systemic demand
2. Caused by decreased contractility, increased preload, increased afterload, HR abnormalities, or high output conditions (e.g., anemia, hyperthyroidism)

C. Diastolic dysfunction

1. Decreased ventricular compliance leads to decreased ventricular filling, increased diastolic pressure, and decreased CO.
2. Caused by hypertrophy or restrictive cardiomyopathy

D. Congestive heart failure (CHF)

1. Left side of heart
   a. Left ventricle **unable to produce adequate CO**
   b. Blood backs up, leading to pulmonary edema, which eventually causes pulmonary HTN
   c. Progressive **left ventricular hypertrophy (LVH)** to compensate for poor output causes eventual failure because the heart is unable to keep pace with systemic need for CO.
2. Right side of heart
   a. Increased pulmonary vascular resistance leads to **right ventricular hypertrophy (RVH)** and systemic venous stasis.
   b. **Most commonly caused by left-sided failure**; also can result from unrelated pulmonary HTN, valvular disease, or congenital defects
3. **Risk factors** = CAD, HTN, valvular disease, cardiomyopathy, COPD, drug toxicity, alcohol use
4. **H/P** = fatigue, dyspnea on exertion, orthopnea, paroxysmal nocturnal dyspnea, cough; displaced point of maximal impulse, S_3, jugular vein distention (JVD), rales, peripheral edema, hepatomegaly; symptoms and signs are more severe during exacerbations
5. **Labs** = plasma brain natriuretic peptide (BNP) and N-terminal pro-BNP will be increased with left ventricle dysfunction
6. **Radiology** = chest X-ray (CXR) shows cardiac enlargement, **Kerley B lines** (i.e., increased marking of lung interlobular septa caused by pulmonary edema), **cephalization of pulmonary vessels** (i.e., increased marking of superior pulmonary vessels caused by congestion and stasis); echocardiogram can assess chamber size and function
7. **ECG** = possible findings consistent with ischemic disease, possible LVH
8. **Treatment**
   a. Systolic dysfunction—start pharmacologic therapy with **loop diuretics** (decrease preload) and **ACE-I** or angiotensin receptor blockers (ARB) (decrease preload and afterload and increase CO); add β-blocker once patient is stable on ACE-I; add aldosterone antagonist (spironolactone or eplerenone) in select patients; digoxin (increases contractility) can be added to improve symptoms; vasodilators (hydralazine plus a nitrate) can relieve symptoms in some patients (especially blacks) (see Figure 1-16)
   b. Diastolic dysfunction—use calcium channel blocker, ARB, or ACE-I to control blood pressure; β-blockers are useful for controlling HR and decreasing cardiac workload
   c. Treat underlying conditions that cause dysfunction (e.g., HTN, valvular pathology); salt-restricted diet helps avoid excessive intravascular fluid volume; assistive devices or cardiac transplant may be required in progressive cases.

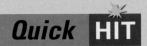

Quick HIT

The heart does well in adjusting to changes in blood volume and work demands, but persistently high demands placed on it will cause it to gradually fail.

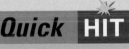

Quick HIT

COPD leads to right-side hypertrophy that ends in right-sided failure (i.e., **cor pulmonale**).

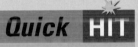

Quick HIT

S_3 is the most frequent sign of CHF.

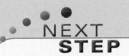

NEXT STEP

ACE-I, **β-blockers** (bisoprolol, carvedilol, or extended-release metoprolol) and **aldosterone antagonists** have been shown to decrease mortality in CHF; consider incorporating these drugs in the treatment plans, when appropriate, because other medications have not been proved to reduce mortality.

Cardiovascular Disorders

Cardiovascular Disorders

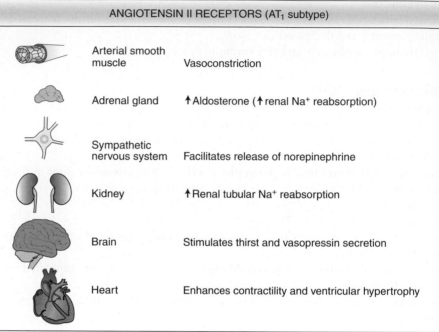

ANGIOTENSINOGEN
(secreted by liver)

Renin (secreted by kidney)

ANGIOTENSIN I

Angiotensin-
converting enzyme

ANGIOTENSIN II

ANGIOTENSIN II RECEPTORS (AT₁ subtype)	
Arterial smooth muscle	Vasoconstriction
Adrenal gland	↑Aldosterone (↑renal Na⁺ reabsorption)
Sympathetic nervous system	Facilitates release of norepinephrine
Kidney	↑Renal tubular Na⁺ reabsorption
Brain	Stimulates thirst and vasopressin secretion
Heart	Enhances contractility and ventricular hypertrophy

FIGURE
1-16 **Renin-angiotensin-aldosterone system and its end effects, which contribute to hypertension.**
ACE-I, angiotensin-converting enzyme inhibitor; ARB, angiotensin receptor blockers. ACE-I act to inhibit the conversion of angiotensin I to angiotensin II, and ARB block angiotensin II activity at the receptor level.
(Modified from Lilly, L. S. [2011]. *Pathophysiology of Heart Disease* [5th ed.]. Baltimore: Lippincott Williams & Wilkins; with permission.)

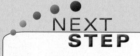

NEXT STEP

Perform an echocardiogram to diagnose any suspected valvular lesion.

 V. Valvular Diseases (*see Figure 1-17; Table 1-5*)

Diagram	S₁ S₂	S₁ S₂	S₁ S₂	S₂ S₁	S₂ S₁
Murmur Type	Systolic ejection	Holosystolic	Late systolic	Early diastolic	Mid/late diastolic
Examples (Location/ Radiation)	Aortic stenosis (2nd right interspace → neck but may radiate widely)	Mitral regurgitation (Apex → axilla)	Mitral valve prolapse (Apex → axilla)	Aortic regurgitation (Along left side of sternum)	Mitral stenosis (Apex)
	Pulmonic stenosis (2nd–3rd left interspace)	Tricuspid regurgitation (LLSB → RLSB)		Pulmonic regurgitation (Upper left side of sternum)	

FIGURE
1-17 **Common murmurs associated with valvular diseases.**
LLSB, left lower sternal border; RLSB, right lower sternal border.
(Modified from Lilly, L. S. [2011]. *Pathophysiology of Heart Disease* [5th ed.]. Baltimore: Lippincott Williams & Wilkins; with permission.)

TABLE 1-5   Valvular Diseases

Valvular Disease (Description)	Causes	Symptoms	Exam	Radiology	Treatment
Aortic stenosis (narrowing of aortic valve causes obstructed blood flow from LV)	• **Congenital defect** • RHD • Calcification in elderly patients • Tertiary syphilis	• Chest pain • Dyspnea on exertion • **Syncope**	• Weak, prolonged pulse • **Crescendo-decrescendo systolic murmur** radiating from right upper sternal border to carotids • Weak S_2 • Valsalva decreases murmur	• Calcified aortic valve, dilated aorta on CXR • Echo and cardiac catheterization helpful for diagnosis	• Valve replacement
Mitral regurgitation (mitral valve incompetency causes blood backflow to LA)	• Mitral valve prolapse (floppy valve) • **RHD** • Papillary muscle dysfunction • Endocarditis • LV dilation	• Asymptomatic in early/mild cases • Palpitations • Dyspnea on exertion • Orthopnea • Paroxysmal nocturnal dyspnea	• Harsh blowing **holosystolic murmur** radiating from apex to axilla • S_3 • Widely split S_2 • Midsystolic click	• LVH; LA enlargement on CXR • Echo helpful for diagnosis	• Vasodilators if symptomatic • Prophylactic anticoagulation with history of embolism or atrial fibrillation • Surgical repair in severe or acute cases
Aortic regurgitation (aortic valve incompetency causes blood backflow to LV)	• Congenital defect • Endocarditis • RHD • Tertiary syphilis • Aortic root dilatation (possibly from aortic dissection)	• Initially asymptomatic • Dyspnea on exertion • Chest pain • Orthopnea	• Bounding pulses • Widened pulse pressure • **Diastolic decrescendo murmur** at right second intercostal space • Late diastolic rumble (**Austin Flint murmur**) • Capillary pulsations in nail bed, more visible when pressure is applied (**Quincke sign**)	• Dilated aorta; LV enlargement on CXR • Echo helpful for diagnosis	• ACE-I, calcium channel blockers, or nitrates (decrease afterload) • Valve replacement
Mitral stenosis (obstructed blood flow to LV causes increased LA volume)	• RHD	• Initially asymptomatic (~10 y) • Dyspnea on exertion • Orthopnea • Paroxysmal nocturnal dyspnea • Peripheral edema • Hepatomegaly	• Opening snap after S_2 • Diastolic rumble • Loud S_1	• RVH; LA enlargement; mitral valve calcification on CXR • Echo helpful for diagnosis	• Diuretics (reduce preload) • Antiarrhythmics for Afib secondary to atrial enlargement • Surgical repair prior to symptomatic progression

ACE-I, angiotensin-converting enzyme inhibitors; Afib, atrial fibrillation; CXR, chest X-ray; Echo, echocardiogram; LA, left atrium; LV, left ventricle; LVH, left ventricular hypertrophy; RHD, rheumatic heart disease; RVH, right ventricular hypertrophy.

Cardiovascular Disorders

VI. Cardiomyopathies *(see Figure 1-18; Table 1-6)*

NEXT STEP

Differentiate restrictive cardiomyopathy from constrictive pericarditis with CT or MRI.

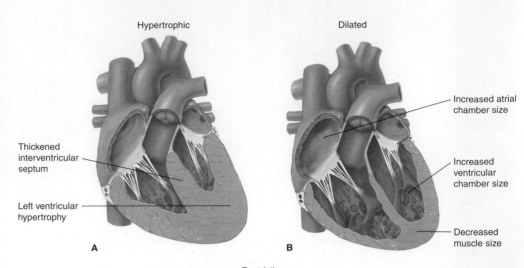

Hypertrophic

Dilated

Thickened interventricular septum

Left ventricular hypertrophy

Increased atrial chamber size

Increased ventricular chamber size

Decreased muscle size

A

B

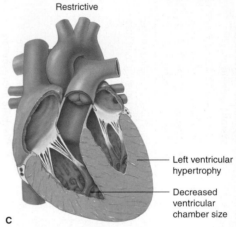

Restrictive

Left ventricular hypertrophy

Decreased ventricular chamber size

C

FIGURE 1-18 **Diagrams of most common variations of cardiomyopathy.**
(**A**) Hypertrophic: note ventricular wall and septal thickening leading to outlet obstruction. (**B**) Dilated: note decreased wall thickness and increased ventricular size. (**C**) Restrictive: note increased ventricular wall thickness and decreased chamber size.
(From Anatomical Chart Company. [2010]. *Atlas of Pathophysiology* [3rd ed., p. 45]. Philadelphia: Wolters Kluwer/ Lippincott Williams & Wilkins.)

TABLE 1-6 Cardiomyopathies

Cardiomyopathy (Description)	Causes	Symptoms	Exam	Radiology	Treatment
Hypertrophic (Ventricular hypertrophy; thickened septum causes decreased filling; LV outflow obstruction; both systolic and diastolic dysfunction)	• Congenital (**autosomal dominant**)	• Syncope • Dyspnea • Palpitations • Chest pain • **Symptoms worse with exertion**	• S_4 • Systolic murmur, louder with Valsalva, softer with squatting • Diffuse, forceful apical impulse • ECG may show arrhythmia, LVH, abnormal Q waves	• Boot-shaped heart on CXR • Echo helpful for diagnosis	• β-Blockers • Calcium channel blockers • Pacemaker • Partial septal excision • Avoid volume depletion and intense physical exertion
Dilated (Ventricular dilation causes systolic dysfunction)	• **Idiopathic** • Alcohol use • Beriberi • Coxsackievirus B myocarditis • Cocaine use • Doxorubicin • HIV • Pregnancy • Hemochromatosis • Ischemic heart disease • Chagas disease	• Similar to CHF and bi-valvular regurgitation	• S_3 • **Systolic and diastolic murmurs** • ECG may show ST and T wave changes, weak QRS, tachycardia, LBBB	• Balloon-like heart on CXR • Echo helpful in diagnosis	• Stop alcohol or cocaine use • Diuretics • ACE-I • β-Blockers • Anticoagulation
Restrictive (Decreased heart compliance causes impaired diastolic filling)	• Sarcoidosis • Amyloidosis	• Similar to CHF with right-sided symptoms worse	• Ascites • JVD • Biopsy is diagnostic	• Often normal	• Treat underlying cause • Palliative treatment for heart failure

ACE-I, angiotensin-converting enzyme inhibitors; CHF, congestive heart failure; CXR, chest X-ray; ECG, electrocardiogram; Echo, echocardiogram; JVD, jugular vein distention; LBBB, left bundle branch block; LV, left ventricle; LVH, left ventricular hypertrophy.

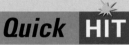

Quick HIT

Squatting relieves symptoms in hypertrophic cardiomyopathy.

Quick HIT

Hypertrophic cardiomyopathy is the most common cause of sudden death in **young athletes**.

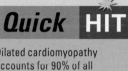

Quick HIT

Dilated cardiomyopathy accounts for 90% of all cardiomyopathies.

Cardiovascular Disorders

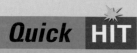

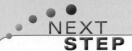

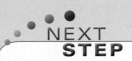

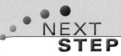

VII. Pericardial Diseases

A. Acute pericarditis
1. Acute inflammation of the pericardial sac accompanied by pericardial effusion
2. Caused by **viral infection**, tuberculosis, systemic lupus erythematosus (SLE), uremia, neoplasm, drug toxicity (e.g., isoniazid, hydralazine), post-MI inflammation (**Dressler syndrome**), **radiation**, **recent heart surgery**
3. H/P = anterior chest pain with inspiration (i.e., **pleuritic chest pain**), dyspnea, cough; **pain lessens with leaning forward**; fever, **friction rub** (best heard when leaning forward); pulsus paradoxus (i.e., fall in systolic blood pressure >10 mm Hg with inspiration) occurs because increased physiologic right ventricle (RV) filling during inspiration combined with pathologic left ventricle (LV) compression by pericardial effusion causes impaired LV filling, decreased stroke volume, and decreased inspiratory systolic blood pressure
4. ECG = global **ST elevation**, PR depression
5. **Radiology** = CXR is helpful in ruling out other systemic causes; effusion frequently seen on echocardiogram
6. **Treatment** = treat underlying cause; pericardiocentesis for large effusions; nonsteroidal anti-inflammatory drugs (NSAIDs) for pain and inflammation; colchicine may be useful for preventing recurrence owing to viral or idiopathic causes
7. **Complications** = chronic constrictive pericarditis if untreated

B. Chronic constrictive pericarditis
1. Sequela of chronic untreated pericardial irritation
2. Diffuse thickening of pericardium with possible calcifications leads to decreased diastolic filling and decreased CO.
3. Most commonly caused by **radiation** or **heart surgery**
4. H/P = symptoms consistent with heart failure (JVD, dyspnea on exertion, orthopnea, peripheral edema), increasing JVD with inspiration (**Kussmaul sign**); Afib common
5. **Labs** = cardiac catheterization shows **equal pressure in all chambers**
6. **Radiology** = possible pericardial calcifications on CXR; echocardiogram, computed tomography (CT), and magnetic resonance imaging (MRI) show pericardial thickening
7. Treatment = NSAIDs, colchicine, corticosteroids; surgical excision of pericardium (high mortality)

C. Cardiac tamponade
1. Large pericardial effusion causes compression of heart and **greatly decreased CO**; can result from progressive, **acute pericarditis**, **chest trauma**, LV rupture following MI, or dissecting aortic aneurysm
2. High mortality
3. H/P = dyspnea, tachycardia, tachypnea; JVD, pulsus paradoxus
4. **Radiology** = enlarged cardiac silhouette on CXR; large effusion seen on echocardiogram
5. **ECG** = low voltage, sinus tachycardia; electrical alternans is relatively specific but not sensitive
6. **Treatment** = **immediate pericardiocentesis**

VIII. Myocardial Infections

A. Myocarditis
1. Inflammatory reaction in heart limited to cardiac muscle involvement
2. Most commonly caused by infection (e.g., viruses [**Coxsackie virus**, parvovirus B-19, HHV-6, adenovirus, echovirus, Epstein-Barr virus (EBV), cytomegalovirus (CMV), influenza virus], bacteria, rickettsiae, fungi, parasites)
3. Occasionally caused by **drug toxicity** (e.g., doxorubicin, chloroquine, penicillins, sulfonamides, cocaine, radiation), toxins, or endocrine abnormalities

4. H/P = patient may report history of recent upper respiratory infection; pleuritic chest pain, dyspnea, S_3 or S_4 heart sound, possible diastolic murmur, possible friction rub
5. ECG = ST- and T-wave changes, conduction abnormalities
6. **Radiology** = possible cardiomegaly on CXR; echocardiogram useful in assessing heart function
7. **Labs** = difficult to diagnose because of variations in laboratory findings; viral titers and serology may help suggest a particular infectious agent; myocardial biopsy frequently shows myocyte inflammation with primarily monocytes and macrophages and focal areas of necrosis
8. **Treatment** = treat infection; stop offending medications; avoid exertional activity; treat heart failure symptoms as for acute exacerbation of heart failure

B. Acute rheumatic fever

1. Uncommon sequela of **untreated group A streptococcus** infection
2. Streptococcus infection can provoke autoantibodies that attack joints and heart valves (mitral > aortic > tricuspid).
3. Incidence is low in the United States because of antibiotic treatment.
4. The term "**rheumatic heart disease**" describes both the acute carditis (pericarditis, myocarditis, valvulitis) and chronic valvular damage.
5. **H/P** = migratory arthritis, hot and swollen joints, fever, subcutaneous nodules on extensor surfaces, Sydenham chorea (i.e., purposeless involuntary movement), erythema marginatum (i.e., painless rash)
6. Diagnosis made using Jones criteria (see Figure 1-19)
7. **Labs** = increased erythrocyte sedimentation rate (ESR), C-reactive protein (CRP), and white blood cell (WBC) count; 90% of patients have antistreptococcal antibodies
8. **ECG** = increased PR interval
9. **Treatment** = NSAIDs for joint inflammation; use corticosteroids, if carditis is severe; β-lactam (penicillin family) antibiotic for infection
10. **Complications** = progressive valve damage if untreated

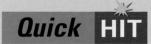

Quick HIT

Several of the drugs that cause myocarditis are used in **cancer** therapy (cyclophosphamide, doxorubicin, daunorubicin).

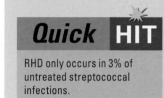

Quick HIT

RHD only occurs in 3% of untreated streptococcal infections.

Cardiovascular Disorders

JONES CRITERIA for Acute Rheumatic Fever — THINK J♥NES PEACE

Major Criteria	Minor Criteria
J: **J**oints (polyarthritis, hot/swollen joints)	P: **P**revious rheumatic fever
♥: **H**eart (carditis, valve damage)	E: **E**CG with PR prolongation
N: **N**odules (subcutaneous, extensor surfaces)	A: **A**rthralgias
E: **E**rythema marginatum (painless rash)	C: **C**RP and ESR elevated
S: **S**ydenham chorea (flinching movement disorder)	E: **E**levated temperature

Diagnosis of RHD is made with a history of recent streptococcal infection and either the presence of 2 major criteria or 1 major with 2 minor criteria.

FIGURE 1-19 JONES criteria mnemonic for diagnosis of rheumatic heart disease (RHD).
CRP, C-reactive protein; ECG, electrocardiogram; ESR, erythrocyte sedimentation rate; RHD, rheumatic heart disease.

C. Endocarditis

1. Bacterial infection of endocardium (i.e., inner lining of heart), with or without valve involvement
2. More common in patients with **congenital heart defects**, **intravenous drug abuse**, or prosthetic valves
3. Patients with SLE may present in a similar manner with noninfective endocarditis (**Libman-Sacks endocarditis**).

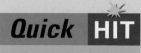

Quick HIT

Prosthetic valves are particularly susceptible to *Staphylococcus epidermidis* and *Staphylococcus aureus* infection.

| TABLE **1-7** | Duke Criteria for Diagnosis of Infective Endocarditis |

Definitive diagnosis of infective endocarditis requires:	• Direct histologic evidence of infective endocarditis **OR** • Positive Gram stain or culture from surgical debridement of cardiac abscess or autopsy specimen **OR** • 2 major criteria **OR** • 1 major and 3 minor criteria **OR** • 5 minor criteria

Major Criteria	Minor Criteria
• Serial blood cultures positive for organisms associated with infective endocarditis • Presence of vegetations or cardiac abscess seen on echocardiogram • Evidence of new onset valvular regurgitation • Blood culture positive for *Coxiella burnetii*	• Predisposing heart condition or intravenous drug use • Fever ≥38°C • Vascular phenomenon (e.g., arterial emboli, septic pulmonary infarcts, mycotic aneurysm, intracranial hemorrhage, conjunctival hemorrhage, Janeway lesions) • Immunologic phenomenon (e.g., glomerulonephritis, Osler nodes, Roth spots, positive rheumatoid factor) • Positive cultures not meeting requirements for major criteria **OR** • Serologic evidence of infection without positive culture

4. Both acute (sudden presentation) and subacute (insidious progression) forms
   a. **Acute endocarditis** is caused by *Staphylococcus aureus, Streptococcus pneumoniae, Streptococcus pyogenes, Neisseria gonorrhoeae*
   b. **Subacute endocarditis** caused by viridans streptococci, *Enterococcus*, fungi, and *Staphylococcus epidermidis*
5. **Duke criteria** are used as guide for making diagnosis (see Table 1-7)
6. **H/P** = fever (very high in acute form), chills, night sweats, fatigue, arthralgias; possible new murmur; small, tender nodules on finger and toe pads (i.e., **Osler nodes**); peripheral petechiae (i.e., **Janeway lesions**), subungual petechiae (i.e., **splinter hemorrhages**), retinal hemorrhages (i.e., **Roth spots**)
7. **Labs** = serial blood cultures will grow same pathogen; increased ESR; increased CRP
8. **Radiology** = echocardiogram (preferably transesophageal echocardiogram [TEE]) may show vegetations on valves; CXR may reveal congestion consistent with septic emboli and right-sided heart failure
9. **Treatment** = **long-term (4 to 6 weeks) IV antibiotics** (initially broad spectrum, then bug specific); β-lactam plus an aminoglycoside is the most commonly used regimen (adjusted for resistance and particular pathogen); antibiotic prophylaxis before surgery or dental work if valves are damaged; valve replacement may be necessary for severely damaged valves
10. **Complications** = severe damage to endocardium and valves, **septic embolization**, or abscess formation, if untreated

IX. Hypertension (HTN)

A. Primary (essential) HTN
1. Cause is idiopathic
2. Accounts for >95% all cases of HTN
3. Diagnosed when systolic blood pressure ≥140 mm Hg and/or diastolic blood pressure ≥90 mm Hg, as measured in three readings taken at three separate appointments
4. **Risk factors** = family history of HTN, high-salt diet (especially if salt sensitive), tobacco use, obesity, increased age; blacks > whites
5. **H/P** = asymptomatic until progression, then headache may be the only symptom until complications develop; blood pressure ≥140/90 mm Hg; arteriovenous

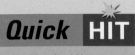

Quick **HIT**

The patient should be sitting quietly for 5 minutes before blood pressure is measured to minimize **false high readings**.

TABLE 1-8 Common Antihypertensive Agents

Class of Medication	Examples	Mechanism of Action	Prescription Strategy	Side Effects
Diuretics	Thiazides (HCTZ, etc.); K$^+$-sparing (spironolactone, etc.); loop diuretics too potent for regular anti-HTN use	Reduce circulatory volume to decrease CO and mean arterial pressure	Early; particularly effective in blacks and salt-sensitive patients	Increased serum glucose, cholesterol, or triglycerides; hypokalemia (thiazides), hyponatremia
Ca^{2+} channel blockers	Dihydropyridines (nifedipine, amlodipine)	Reduce influx of calcium in vascular smooth muscle to cause vasodilation	Second line; dihydropyridines mainly affect vascular smooth muscle and are utilized more often for HTN	Hypotension, headache, constipation, increased GI reflux, peripheral edema
	Nondihydropyridines (diltiazem, verapamil)	Reduce influx of calcium in coronary arteries, slows automaticity and conduction of AV node	Nondihydropyridine are less frequently used for HTN	Bradycardia, hypotension, headache, increased GI reflux, peripheral edema
ACE-I	Lisinopril, captopril, enalapril	Block conversion of angiotensin I to angiotensin II and increase circulating bradykinin to decrease angiotensin II vasopressor activity and aldosterone secretion, causing decrease in total peripheral resistance	First or second line; important cardiac and renal uses; more effective in young white patients	Dry cough, angioedema, azotemia, hyperkalemia, teratogenicity
ARB	Losartan, valsartan, irbesartan	Block binding of angiotensin II to second-line receptors to inhibit vasopressor activity and decrease aldosterone secretion	First or second line	Azotemia, hyperkalemia, teratogenicity
β-Blockers	Nonselective (propranolol, timolol); β$_1$-selective (metoprolol, atenolol, esmolol)	Decrease HR, contractility, CO, and decrease renin secretion to decrease total peripheral resistance	Early; many important cardiac uses (e.g., CAD, CHF); more effective in white patients	Bronchoconstriction if non-β$_1$ selective, HDL reduction, increased triglycerides
α-Blockers	Prazosin, doxazosin, terazosin	Block α adrenergic receptors (prevent constriction of vascular tone) to decrease total peripheral resistance	Adjunct to other medications, less commonly used	Postural hypotension, headache, rebound HTN if stopped
Vasodilators	Hydralazine, minoxidil, nitroprusside	Direct relaxation of vascular smooth muscle	Adjunct to other medications; less commonly used	Reflex tachycardia, possible adverse cardiovascular incidents

ACE-I, angiotensin-converting enzyme inhibitors; ARB, angiotensin receptor blockers; CO, cardiac output; GI, gastrointestinal; HCTZ, hydrochlorothiazide; HDL, high-density lipoprotein; HA, heart rate; HTN, hypertension; CAD, coronary artery disease; CHF, congestive heart failure.

nicking (i.e., apparent retinal-vein narrowing secondary to arterial wall thickening), cotton-wool spots, or retinal hemorrhages (i.e., **flame hemorrhages**) on funduscopic examination; loud S$_2$, possible S$_4$

6. **Treatment** = do not start medications until three consecutive high readings have been recorded
    a. Initially, prescribe weight loss, exercise, salt restriction, smoking cessation, and alcohol reduction.
    b. A thiazide diuretic, calcium channel blocker, ACE-I, or ARB is typically the first drug prescribed unless comorbid condition indicates otherwise (see Table 1-8, Table 1-9)
7. **Complications** = untreated or poorly treated disease increases risk of CAD, stroke, aortic aneurysm, aortic dissection, CHF, kidney disease, and ophthalmologic disease

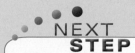

NEXT STEP

If patient has been normotensive in the past and now systolic blood pressure is >140 mm Hg or diastolic blood pressure >90 mm Hg, recheck in 2 months.

Cardiovascular Disorders

TABLE 1-9	Recommendations and Contraindications for Antihypertensive Drug Selection			
Comorbid Condition	**Recommended Antihypertensive**	**Reason for Recommendation**	**Contraindicated Antihypertensive**	**Reason for Contraindication**
DM	ACE-I	Delays renal damage	±Thiazide diuretic	Impaired glucose tolerance
			±β-Blocker	Can mask signs of hypoglycemia
CHF	ACE-I/ARB Aldosterone antagonist β-Blocker	Improves mortality Improves mortality Improves mortality	Ca^{2+} channel blocker	Reduced rate/ contractility can exacerbate heart failure
Post-MI	β-Blocker ACE-I/ARB Aldosterone antagonist	Improves mortality Improves mortality Improves mortality		
Benign prostatic hypertrophy	Selective α_1-blocker	Reduces symptoms		
Migraine headache	Verapamil, β-blocker	May reduce symptoms		
Osteoporosis	Thiazide diuretic	Maintains normal/ high serum calcium		
Asthma/ COPD			Nonselective β-blocker	Exacerbates bronchoconstriction
Pregnancy	Hydralazine Methyldopa Labetalol Nifedipine		±Thiazide diuretic	Increased blood volume during pregnancy should be maintained
			ACE-I ARB	Teratogenic Teratogenic
Gout			Diuretic	Increase serum uric acid
Depression			β-Blocker	May worsen symptoms

ACE-I, angiotensin-converting enzyme inhibitors; ARB, angiotensin receptor blocker; CHF, congestive heart failure; COPD, chronic obstructive pulmonary disease; DM, diabetes mellitus; MI, myocardial infarction.

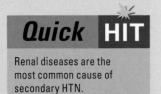

Quick HIT

Renal diseases are the most common cause of secondary HTN.

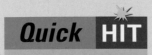

Quick HIT

ACE inhibitors are contraindicated in cases of **bilateral renal artery stenosis** because they can accelerate renal failure by impeding sufficient renal perfusion and lowering glomerular filtration rate.

B. Secondary HTN
1. HTN due to an identifiable cause (see Table 1-10)
2. Some causes can be reversible, whereas others are progressive.

C. Hypertensive urgency
1. Blood pressure ≥180/120 mm Hg (nonpregnant patient) without symptoms and without evidence of end-organ damage
2. H/P = by definition, hypertensive urgency is asymptomatic; no signs of end-organ damage
3. **Hypertensive emergency** (malignant HTN) = BP ≥180/120 mm Hg with evidence of end-organ damage (e.g., progressive renal failure, pulmonary edema, aortic dissection, encephalopathy, papilledema)

TABLE **1-10**	Causes of Secondary HTN			
Condition	**Common Patient Group**	**Signs/Symptoms**	**Diagnosis**	**Treatment**
Renal diseases (various)		Depends on disease identity	Depends on disease identity	ACE-I (delays progression)
Renal artery stenosis	<25 yr of age (fibro-muscular dysplasia) or >50 yr of age (atherosclerosis)	Renal artery bruit, hypokalemia	Arteriography, MRA, CT, renal artery duplex scan	Angioplasty, stent placement, ACE-I if one-sided, surgical repair
OCP (combination pill)	Women >35 yr of age, obese women, long-term OCP use		History	Stop use, change to progestin-only pill or intramuscular medroxyprogesterone
Pheochromocytoma	Young patients; patients with history of endocrine tumors	Episodic HTN, diaphoresis, headaches; symptoms occur suddenly	Increased 24-hr urinary fractionated metanephrines; CT, MRI	Surgical removal of tumor with pharmacologic control of HTN up until time of surgery
Primary hyper-aldosteronism (Conn syndrome)		Headache, hypokalemia, metabolic alkalosis	High ratio of plasma aldosterone to plasma renin activity (high PAC:PRA ratio)	Surgical removal of tumor; aldosterone antagonists
Excess glucocor-ticoids (Cushing syndrome)		Central obesity, hirsutism, buffalo hump, striae, and glucose intolerance	Serum cortisol, dexametha-sone suppression test	Treat underlying cause, reduce exogenous steroids
Coarctation of the aorta	Male > female; Turner syndrome, aortic valve pathology, PDA	HTN in arm but not in legs, weak femoral pulse	Possible LVH on ECG; echocardiogram can localize defect	Surgical repair
Hyperparathyroidism (hypercalcemia)		Confusion, nephrolithiasis, constipation	Increased serum calcium and PTH level, decreased serum phosphates	Hydration
Hyperthyroidism		Tachycardia, diaphoresis, tremor, weight loss, heat intolerance	Decreased TSH, high free T_4	Radioiodine thyroid ablation, thionamides

ACE-I, angiotensin-converting enzyme inhibitors; CT, computed tomography; ECG, electrocardiogram; HTN, hypertension; LVH, left ventricular hypertrophy; MRI, magnetic resonance imaging; OCP, oral contraceptive pill; PDA, patent ductus arteriosus; TSH, thyroid stimulating hormone.

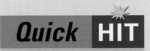

Cardiovascular Disorders

4. **Treatment** = for hypertensive emergency, the goal blood pressure varies by the systemic effects seen; drugs used may include IV nitroprusside, nitroglycerin, labetalol, nicardipine; once blood pressure is controlled, convert to oral drugs for further blood pressure reduction and maintenance therapy

 X. Shock *(See Table 1-11)*

A. Circulatory collapse in which blood delivery is inadequate for tissue demands

B. High mortality without timely treatment

C. H/P = history should consider allergies, changes in medications, recent medication use, infection history, or recent cardiac/neurologic events; hypotension, cool/clammy skin, changes in mental status, decreased urine output

D. Labs = complete blood count (CBC), electrolyte panel, arterial blood gases (ABG), cardiac enzymes, liver function tests, lactic acid, prothrombin time or partial thromboplastin time (PT/PTT), toxicology screen; urinalysis should be included in workup

Quick HIT

In a hypertensive emergency, the **initial decrease** (first 2 hours) in mean arterial pressure **should not exceed 25%** of the presenting pressure to avoid triggering an ischemic event.

TABLE 1-11	Common Types of Shock		
Type of Shock	**Mechanism**	**Cause**	**Treatment**
Cardiogenic	Failure of myocardial pump	MI, arrhythmias, cardiac contusion/ tamponade, pulmonary embolism	Inotropes (dobutamine), intra-aortic balloon pump, PTCA (for MI)
Septic	Decreased total peripheral resistance	Gram-negative bacteria, DIC, possibly endotoxin mediated	Treat underlying infection, pressor agents (norepinephrine), IV fluids
Hypovolemic	Inadequate blood or plasma volume	Hemorrhage, severe burns, trauma	IV fluids, transfusions, surgery may be required to stop volume loss; specialized dressings, skin grafts may be required with severe burns to prevent ongoing fluid loss
Anaphylactic	Generalized type I hypersensitivity reaction	Massive degranulation of mast cells and basophils in response to allergic reaction	Maintain airway, epinephrine, diphenhydramine, IV fluids
Neurogenic	Widespread peripheral vasodilation and bradycardia	Brain or spinal cord injury	IV fluids, pressor agents, atropine for bradycardia

CNS, central nervous system; DIC, disseminated intravascular coagulation; IV, intravenous; MI, myocardial infarction; PTCA, percutaneous transluminal coronary angioplasty.

XI. Vascular Diseases

A. Aortic conditions

1. **Abdominal aortic aneurysm (AAA)**
   a. Localized dilation of aorta, most commonly inferior to the renal arteries
   b. **Risk factors** = tobacco use, age >55 years, atherosclerosis, HTN, family history
   c. **H/P** = frequently **asymptomatic** until later progression; possible lower back pain; **pulsating abdominal mass, abdominal bruits**; hypotension and severe pain occur with any rupture
   d. **Radiology** = ultrasound (US) can detect location and size quickly; CT or MRI are used for more accurate localization and size determination
   e. **Screening** = United States Preventive Services Task Force (USPSTF) recommends a one-time screening US for men ages 65 to 75 years with a history of smoking
   f. **Treatment** = monitor with periodic US if <5.5 cm diameter in men or <5.0 cm in women; surgical repair (open or using endovascular stenting) if symptomatic or ≥5.5 cm diameter in men or ≥5.0 cm in women
   g. **Complications** = untreated aortic aneurysms can rupture with >90% mortality
2. **Aortic dissection**
   a. Intimal tear leads to blood entering media, causing formation of false lumen
   b. Stanford classification—**Stanford A** aortic dissection involves ascending aorta; **Stanford B** is distal to left subclavian artery
   c. **Risk factors** = HTN, coarctation of the aorta, syphilis, Ehlers-Danlos syndrome, Marfan syndrome, trauma (rare)
   d. **H/P** = acute, "ripping" chest pain, syncope; decreased peripheral pulses, normal or increased blood pressure
   e. **ECG** = normal or LVH
   f. **Radiology** = widening of aorta and superior mediastinum on CXR; CT with contrast, echocardiogram, MRI, magnetic resonance angiography (MRA), or angiography good for definite diagnosis

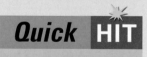

Quick HIT

Normal aortic diameter is 1.5–2.5 cm; an increase to twice this size or more is considered aneurysmal.

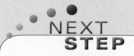

Quick HIT

Rupture of an aortic aneurysm is usually fatal.

NEXT STEP

If a patient presents with new severe chest pain, an immediate ECG may help to differentiate an aortic dissection from an acute MI (ECG will be normal or will show mild LV hypertrophy in aortic dissection and will be abnormal in MI, except during early evolution).

    g. **Treatment** = stabilize blood pressure (e.g., β-blocker, nitroprusside) if unstable; Stanford A dissections need emergency surgery; Stanford B dissections can be treated medically unless rupture or occlusion develops

    h. **Complications** = possible MI, renal insufficiency, ischemic colitis, stroke, or paraplegia

B. Peripheral vascular disease (PVD)

1. Occlusion of peripheral blood supply secondary to atherosclerosis
2. **Risk factors** = HTN, DM, CAD, smoking
3. **H/P** = leg pain with activity that improves with rest (i.e., **intermittent claudication**), resting leg pain in severe disease; dry skin, skin ulcers, decreased hair growth in affected area; male erectile dysfunction with aortoiliac disease
4. **Labs** = ankle-brachial index (ABI) is ratio of systolic blood pressure at ankle to that at brachial artery; ABI ≤0.9 indicates vascular insufficiency at ankle; ABI <0.4 indicates severe disease (frequently seen with resting pain)
5. **Radiology** = US is useful for locating stenosis and variations in blood pressure; CT or MR angiography or traditional angiography will map narrowing in the arterial distribution of interest
6. **Treatment** = exercise (increases collateral circulation); instruction in foot examination (early detection of ulcers from vascular insufficiency); treatment of underlying diseases; ASA, **pentoxifylline**, or **cilostazol** to help to slow occlusion; percutaneous transluminal angioplasty (PTA) indicated for failed nonoperative treatment, significant disability caused by claudication, or predictable benefit and improvement in prognosis; bypass grafting if incapacitating claudication, resting pain, or necrotic foot lesions develop; prolonged ischemia may require limb amputation

C. Venous conditions

1. **Varicosities**
   a. Incompetent venous valves that cause elongation, dilation, and tortuosity of veins
   b. **H/P** = usually asymptomatic; pain and fatigue that lessens with leg elevation; possible visible or palpable veins, increased local pigmentation, edema, or ulceration
   c. **Treatment** = exercise, compression hosiery, leg elevation; surgical removal or injection sclerotherapy for cosmetic improvement or symptomatic varicosities

2. **Arteriovenous malformations (AVM)**
   a. Abnormal communications between arteries and veins
   b. Congenital or acquired
   c. **H/P** = palpable, warm, pulsating masses, if superficial; painful if mass compresses adjacent structures
   d. Large AVM can cause local ischemia and increase the risk of thrombus formation.
   e. **Treatment** = surgical removal or sclerosis, if symptomatic, or if located in brain or bowel

3. **Deep vein thrombosis (DVT)**
   a. Development of thrombosis in large vein; most common in lower extremity
   b. Location, in order of decreasing frequency: **calf**, femoral, popliteal, and iliac veins
   c. Can cause inflammation of affected vein (i.e., **thrombophlebitis**)
   d. **Risk factors** = **prolonged inactivity** (travel, immobilization), heart failure, hypercoagulable states, neoplasm, **pregnancy**, oral contraceptive pill (OCP) use, **tobacco use**, vascular trauma
   e. **H/P** = possibly asymptomatic; deep leg pain, swelling, warmth
   f. **Labs** = D-dimer will be elevated with DVT formation, but test is more useful in using a normal result to rule out DVT
   g. **Radiology** = compressive venous US is used for detection
   h. **Treatment** = leg elevation; low molecular weight heparin or unfractionated heparin initially, warfarin for long-term management; inferior vena cava (IVC) filter should be placed in a patient with contraindications to anticoagulation
   i. **Complications** = clot can embolize to lungs (i.e., **pulmonary embolus**) with 40% mortality; chronic DVT can cause chronic venous insufficiency

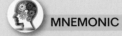

MNEMONIC

Remember the six Ps to grade PVD severity: **P**ain, **P**allor, **P**oikilothermia, **P**ulselessness, **P**aresthesia, and **P**aralysis.

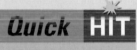

Quick HIT

Removal or sclerotherapy of the saphenous vein is discouraged because of its potential use in bypass grafting.

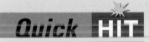

Quick HIT

Virchow triad = blood stasis, hypercoagulability, and vascular damage increase patients' risk of DVT.

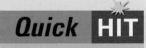

Quick HIT

Homan sign (calf pain with passive foot dorsiflexion) is unreliable for DVT detection.

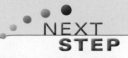

NEXT STEP

Patients with recent surgery or who are at increased risk for hemorrhage should receive an **IVC filter** instead of anticoagulation to reduce the risk of pulmonary embolism.

D. Vasculitis

1. **Temporal (giant cell) arteritis**
   a. Commonly caused by subacute granulomatous inflammation of the external carotid and vertebral arteries
   b. **Risk factors = women > men, 50 years of age and older**
   c. Half of patients also have **polymyalgia rheumatica.**
   d. **H/P = new onset of headache** (unilateral or bilateral) with scalp pain, **temporal region tenderness**, jaw claudication, **transient or permanent monocular blindness**, weight loss, myalgias, arthralgias, fever; funduscopic examination should be performed to address vision loss (may show thrombosis of ophthalmic or ciliary arteries)
   e. **Labs = increased ESR**; temporal artery biopsy shows inflammation in vessel media and lymphocytes, plasma cells, or giant cells in vessel adventitia
   f. **Radiology** = US may show stenosis or occlusion of temporal or occipital arteries
   g. **Treatment** = prednisone for 1 to 2 months followed by taper; low-dose ASA to reduce risk of vision loss or stroke from vessel occlusion; vitamin D and calcium supplementation to reduce risk of osteoporosis from prolonged high-dose corticosteroid use; ophthalmology follow-up

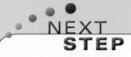

NEXT STEP

If temporal arteritis is suggested from the H/P, do not wait for temporal artery biopsy to start prednisone.

2. **Takayasu arteritis**
   a. Inflammation of aortic arch and its branches
   b. Can cause cerebrovascular and myocardial ischemia
   c. **Risk factors** = Asian heritage, women 10 to 40 years of age
   d. **H/P** = malaise, vertigo, syncope; fever, decreased carotid and limb pulses
   e. **Labs** = biopsy of affected vessel shows plasma cells and lymphocytes in media and adventitia, giant cells, and vascular fibrosis
   f. **Radiology** = arteriography may detect abnormal vessels and stenoses; CT or MRI is useful for detecting vessel wall abnormalities
   g. **Treatment** = corticosteroids, immunosuppressive agents; bypass grafting of obstructed vessels

3. **Kawasaki disease**
   a. Necrotizing inflammation of large, medium, and small vessels
   b. Most commonly seen in **young children**
   c. Coronary vasculitis develops in 25% of patients, leading to possible aneurysm, MI, or sudden death.
   d. **H/P** = fever, lymphadenopathy, conjunctival lesions, maculopapular rash, edema, eventual desquamation of hands and feet
   e. **Labs** = possible autoantibodies to endothelial cells
   f. **Radiology** = echocardiogram can detect coronary artery aneurysms (particularly useful when performed with dobutamine stress test); angiography can detect coronary vessel irregularities
   g. **Treatment** = ASA, IV gamma globulin; frequently self-limited

4. **Polyarteritis nodosa**
   a. Inflammation of small or medium arteries leads to ischemia.
   b. Affects kidneys, heart, gastrointestinal (GI) tract, muscles, nerves, joints; **spares the lungs**
   c. **Risk factors = hepatitis B or C**; young > elderly; men > women
   d. **H/P** = fever, HTN, hematuria, anemia, neuropathy, weight loss, joint pain, palpable purpura, or ulcers on skin
   e. **Labs** = increased WBC, decreased hemoglobin (Hgb) and hematocrit, increased ESR, proteinuria, hematuria; negative perinuclear antineutrophil cytoplasmic antibodies (**p-ANCA**); arterial biopsy may help in diagnosis
   f. **Radiology** = angiography may show numerous aneurysms
   g. **Treatment** = corticosteroids, immunosuppressive agents

5. **Eosinophilic granulomatosis with polyangiitis (Churg-Strauss syndrome)**
   a. Inflammation of small or medium arteries
   b. **H/P = asthmatic symptoms**, fatigue, malaise, mononeuropathy (pain, paresthesia, or weakness); erythematous or papular rash
   c. **Labs** = increased serum eosinophils, increased ESR, p-ANCA; lung biopsy may show eosinophilic granulomas
   d. **Treatment** = corticosteroids, immunosuppressive agents

6. **Henoch-Schönlein purpura**
   a. IgA immune complex–mediated vasculitis affecting arterioles, capillaries, and venules
   b. More frequently in **children** than adults
   c. **H/P** = **recent upper respiratory infection**; **palpable purpura** on the buttocks and lower extremities, abdominal pain and GI bleeding, polyarticular arthritis/arthralgias, hematuria
   d. **Labs** = biopsy of purpura demonstrates **IgA deposition**; similar findings in renal biopsy
   e. **Treatment** = frequently self-limited; use corticosteroids for severe GI symptoms

XII. Pediatric Cardiology

A. Fetal circulation (*see Figure 1-20*)
1. Gas exchange occurs in uteroplacental circulation.
2. Fetal Hgb has greater O_2 affinity than adult Hgb and pulls O_2 from maternal blood.

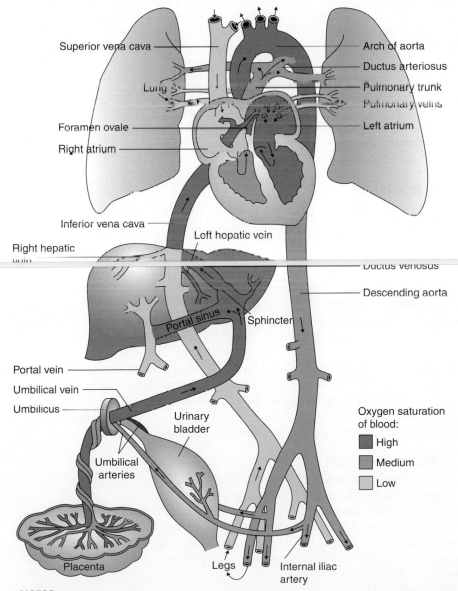

FIGURE
1-20 Diagram of fetal circulation—*arrows* indicate the direction of blood flow; three shunts (ductus venosus, foramen ovale, ductus arteriosus) exist in utero but close shortly after birth.

(From Lilly, L. S. [2011]. *Pathophysilogy of Heart Disease* [5th ed.]. Baltimore: Lippincott Williams & Wilkins; with permission.)

3. Umbilical arteries carry deoxygenated blood to placenta; umbilical veins carry oxygenated blood from placenta to portal system.
4. Changes occurring after birth
   a. Lung expansion causes increased pulmonary blood flow, leading to an increase in relative blood oxygenation.
   b. A decreasing serum level of prostaglandin E_2 results in **ductus arteriosus closure**; umbilical cord clamping results in end of placental circulation and an increase in systemic vascular resistance.
   c. This increased vascular resistance, in turn, induces **ductus venosus closure** and umbilical artery and vein constriction.
   d. Left atrial pressure increases (because of increased pulmonary blood flow) and umbilical circulation decreases, causing a decrease in IVC pressure.
   e. Decrease in IVC and right atrial pressures leads to **foramen ovale closure**.

B. Ventricular septal defect (VSD)

1. Opening in ventricular septum allowing shunting of blood (see Figure 1-21A)
2. **Most common** congenital heart defect
3. H/P = asymptomatic if small; frequent respiratory infections, failure to thrive, dyspnea, shortness of breath, heart failure symptoms with larger defects; pansystolic murmur at lower left sternal border, loud pulmonic S_2, systolic thrill
4. **ECG** = left ventricular hypertrophy, right ventricular hypertrophy; frequently normal
5. **Radiology** = echocardiogram shows shunt
6. **Treatment** = clinically, follow small defects; diuretics or ACE-I are useful for decreasing fluid volume and vascular resistance in patients with large shunts; repair large defects soon (before Eisenmenger syndrome develops)
7. **Complications** = if untreated, Eisenmenger syndrome develops (irreversible); increased risk of endocarditis

C. Atrial septal defect (ASD)

1. Opening in atrial septum allowing movement of blood between atria (see Figure 1-21B)
2. Initially, blood flow is left-to-right across defect.
3. H/P = possibly asymptomatic; large defects can cause cyanosis, heart failure symptoms, dyspnea, fatigue, or failure to thrive; strong impulse at lower left sternal border, **wide fixed split** S_2, systolic ejection murmur at upper left sternal border
4. **ECG** = right axis deviation
5. **Radiology** = echocardiogram shows blood flow between atria, dilated RV, and large heart; CXR shows increased pulmonary vascular markings caused by pulmonary HTN
6. **Treatment** = small defects do not need repair but require **antibiotic prophylaxis** before surgery or dental work; surgical closure for symptomatic infants or when pulmonary blood flow is twice that of systemic blood flow
7. **Complications** = untreated ASD leads to right-to-left shunt (i.e., **Eisenmenger syndrome**), RV dysfunction, pulmonary HTN, arrhythmias

D. Patent ductus arteriosus (PDA)

1. Failure of ductus arteriosus to close after birth (see Figure 1-21C)
2. Left-to-right shunt (aorta to pulmonary artery)
3. **Risk factors** = **prematurity**, high altitude, first-trimester maternal rubella, maternal prostaglandin administration; females > males
4. H/P = possibly asymptomatic; heart failure symptoms, dyspnea; wide pulse pressure, continuous "machinery" murmur at second left intercostal space, loud S_2, bounding pulses
5. **ECG** = possible LVH
6. **Radiology** = possible cardiomegaly on CXR; echocardiogram shows large left atrium (LA) and LV; angiography confirms diagnosis
7. **Treatment** = **indomethacin** induces closure; surgical closure if unresponsive

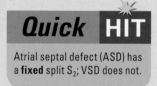

Quick HIT

Atrial septal defect (ASD) has a **fixed** split S_2; VSD does not.

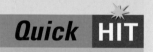

Quick HIT

Patients with ASD are more susceptible to oxygen desaturation at **high altitudes** and decompression sickness during **deep sea diving**.

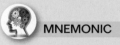

MNEMONIC

Treatment for a PDA may be remembered with the mnemonic Come **In** and **Close** the Door: (indomethacin **closes** a PDA).

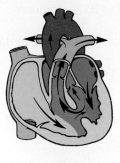

A   VSD

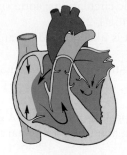

B   ASD

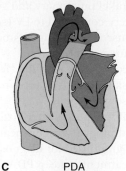

C   PDA

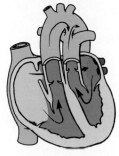

D   Transposition of
great vessels

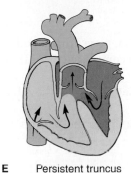

E   Persistent truncus
arteriosus

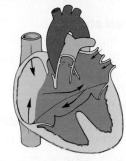

F   Complete endocardial
cushion defect

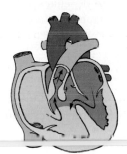

G   Tetralogy of
Fallot

FIGURE 1-21 **Common congenital heart defects.**

(**A**) Ventricular septal defect (VSD)—the *arrows* depict shunting of blood predominantly from the left to right ventricle. (**B**) Atrial septal defect (ASD)—the *arrow* depicts shunting of blood from the left to right atrium. (**C**) Patent ductus arteriosus (PDA)—the *arrow* depicts shunting of blood from the aorta to pulmonary arteries. (**D**) Transposition of the great vessels—the aorta arises from the right ventricle, and the pulmonary artery arises from the left ventricle. Shunting can occur between the great vessels via a PDA. (**E**) Persistent truncus arteriosus—single vessel exits both ventricles (with VSD) and gives rise to both systemic and pulmonary circulation. (**F**) Complete endocardial cushion defect—ASD, VSD, and single atrioventricular canal. (**G**) Tetralogy of Fallot—combination of ventricular septal defect, right ventricular outflow obstruction, aorta overriding the ventricular septum, and right ventricular hypertrophy.

MNEMONIC

To remember cyanotic con-genital heart diseases, use the **5 Ts** mnemonic:
- **T**runcus arteriosus
- **T**ransposition of the great vessels
- **T**ricuspid atresia
- **T**etralogy of Fallot
- **T**otal anomalous pulmonary venous return

E. Persistent truncus arteriosus

1. Failure of aorta and pulmonary artery to separate during development results in a single vessel that supplies systemic and pulmonary circulation (see Figure 1-21E)
2. **H/P** = cyanosis after birth; dyspnea, fatigue, failure to thrive; heart failure symptoms soon develop; harsh systolic murmur at lower left sternal border, loud S_1 and S_2, bounding pulses
3. **ECG** = likely LVH, RVH
4. **Radiology** = angiography or echocardiogram used for diagnosis; CXR may show boot-shaped heart, no pulmonary artery, and large aorta arching to right side
5. **Treatment** = surgical correction

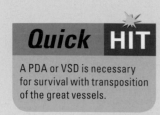

Quick HIT

A PDA or VSD is necessary for survival with transposition of the great vessels.

MNEMONIC

To remember the characteristics of tetralogy of Fallot, use the mnemonic "IHOP":
- **I**nterventricular septal defect (VSD)
- **H**ypertrophy of the right ventricle
- **O**verriding aorta
- **P**ulmonic stenosis

F. Transposition of the great vessels
1. Parallel pulmonary and systemic circulations; aorta connected to RV; pulmonary artery connected to LV (see Figure 1-21D)
2. Cause is poorly understood but is likely linked to cardiac septal development in the truncus arteriosus.
3. Incompatible with life (fetus is stillborn) unless comorbid PDA or VSD
4. **Risk factors** = Apert syndrome, Down syndrome, cri-du-chat syndrome, trisomy 13 or 18
5. **H/P** = cyanosis after birth; cyanosis worsens as PDA closes; loud S_2
6. **Radiology** = narrow heart base, abnormal pulmonary markings on CXR; echocardiogram used for diagnosis
7. **Treatment** = **keep PDA open with prostaglandin E**; balloon atrial septostomy to widen VSD; prompt surgical correction

G. Tricuspid atresia
1. Failure of tricuspid valve to form, preventing blood flow from the right atrium to the right ventricle; usually accompanied by ASD, VSD, and right ventricular hypoplasia
2. **H/P** = usually presents immediately after birth with cyanosis, holosystolic murmur from the VSD
3. **Radiology** = Echocardiography shows the defect(s)
4. **Treatment** = surgical correction

H. Tetralogy of Fallot
1. VSD, RVH, overriding aorta, RV outflow obstruction (see Figure 1-21G)
2. **Risk factors** = Down syndrome, cri-du-chat syndrome, trisomy 13 and 18
3. **H/P** = early cyanosis, dyspnea, fatigue; children squat for relief during hypoxemic episodes; systolic ejection murmur at left sternal border, RV lift, single S_2
4. **ECG** = right axis deviation
5. **Radiology** = echocardiogram or cardiac catheterization used for diagnosis; boot-shaped heart seen on CXR
6. **Treatment** = prostaglandin E to maintain PDA; O_2, propranolol, IV fluids, morphine, knee-to-chest positioning during cyanotic episodes; surgical correction

I. Total anomalous pulmonary venous return
1. Pulmonary veins fail to empty into the left atrium and instead empty into the systemic venous circulation (most commonly the left brachiocephalic vein); incompatible with life unless the foramen ovale or ductus arteriosus remains patent
2. **H/P** = presents as neonate with cyanosis, respiratory failure, shock; may have systolic and diastolic murmur, hepatomegaly from right ventricular heart failure
3. **Radiology** = echocardiogram or angiography used for diagnosis
4. **Treatment** = surgical correction

J. Endocardial cushion defect
1. Malformation of atrioventricular valves, atrial septum, and/or ventricular septum during fetal development causes a variety of valvular and septal defects (see Figure 1-21F).
2. **Complete defect** has ASD, VSD, and a single atrioventricular canal.
3. **Incomplete defect** has ASD and minor atrioventricular valve abnormalities.
4. Found in **20% of children with Down syndrome**
5. **H/P** = incomplete form resembles presentation for ASD; complete form causes heart failure symptoms, pneumonitis; murmurs consistent with particular defect
6. **ECG** = left axis deviation
7. **Radiology** = echocardiogram or cardiac catheterization used for diagnosis
8. **Treatment** = surgical correction

PULMONARY DISORDERS

I. Measures of Pulmonary Function

A. Pulmonary function tests (PFTs)

1. Uses for PFTs
   a. Categorizing various types of lung processes and changes in lung air volumes
   b. Assessing severity of pulmonary disease
   c. Evaluating success of treatment
2. Specific measurements
   a. **Lung volumes** (see Figure 2-1, Table 2-1, Table 2-2)
   b. **Airflow** (see Figure 2-2)
      (1) FEV_1/FVC is ratio of air volume expired in 1 second to functional vital capacity (FEV = forced expiratory volume).
      (2) $FEF_{25\%-75\%}$ is forced expiratory flow rate between 25% and 75% of FVC.
   c. **Alveolar membrane permeability**
      (1) Diffusing capacity of lungs, or D_{Lco}, is a relative measurement of the lungs' ability to transfer gases from alveoli to pulmonary capillaries.
      (2) PFTs usually list D_{Lco} as a percentage of the normal expected value.

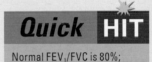

Quick HIT

Normal FEV_1/FVC is 80%; <80% suggests obstructive pathology; >110% suggests a restrictive pattern.

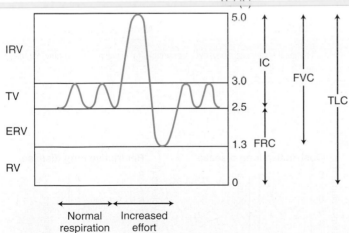

FIGURE 2-1 **Healthy lung volumes and variation with effort of breathing.**

ERV, expiratory reserve volume; FRC, functional reserve capacity; FVC, functional vital capacity; IC, inspiratory capacity; IRV, inspiratory reserve volume; RV, residual volume; TLC, total lung capacity; TV, tidal volume.

TABLE 2-1	Definitions of Lung Volume Terms and Formulas
Lung Volume	**Definition**
Tidal volume (TV)	Inspiratory volume during normal respiration
Inspiratory reserve volume (IRV)	Air volume beyond normal tidal volume that is filled during maximal inspiration
Inspiratory capacity (IC)	Total inspiratory air volume considering both tidal volume and inspiratory reserve volume **(IC = TV + IRV)**
Expiratory reserve volume (ERV)	Air volume beyond tidal volume that can be expired during normal respiration
Residual volume (RV)	Remaining air volume left in lungs following maximal expiration
Functional reserve capacity (FRC)	Air volume remaining in lungs after expiration of tidal volume **(FRC = RV + ERV)**
Functional vital capacity (FVC)	Maximal air volume that can be inspired and expired **(FVC = IC + ERV)**
Total lung capacity (TLC)	Total air volume of lungs **(TLC = FVC + RV)**

TABLE 2-2	Changes in Pulmonary Function Tests from Normal Lung to Obstructive and Restrictive Disease States	
Measurement	**Obstructive**	**Restrictive**
TLC	↑	↓
FVC	↓	↓
RV	↑	↓
FRC	↑	↓
FEV_1	↓	↓
FEV_1/FVC	↓ (70%)	Normal or ↑

FEV_1, 1-second forced expiratory volume; FRC, functional reserve capacity; FVC, functional vital capacity; RV, residual volume; TLC, total lung capacity; ↑, increase; ↓, decrease.

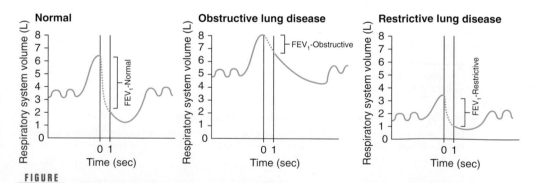

FIGURE
2-2   **Spirometry tracings for normal respiration compared with obstructive and restrictive pulmonary diseases.**
FEV_1, 1-second forced expiratory volume.
(Modified from Mehta, S., Milder, E. A., Mirachi, A. J., & Milder, E. [2006]. *Step-Up: A High-Yield, Systems-Based Review for the USMLE Step 1* [3rd ed., p. 96]. Philadelphia: Lippincott Williams & Wilkins; with permission.)

B. Alveolar-arterial (A-a) gradient (*see Table 2-3*)
  1. This measurement compares the oxygenation status of alveoli (PAo_2) to arterial blood (Pao_2).
  2. **Normal A-a gradient = 5 to 15 mm Hg**
  3. Increased A-a gradient is seen in pulmonary embolism (PE), pulmonary edema, and right-to-left vascular shunts.
  4. False-normal A-a gradient may be seen in cases of hypoventilation or at high altitudes.

TABLE 2-3	Calculation of the Alveolar-arterial (A-a) Gradient	
Variable	**Definition**	**Value**
Pao_2	Arterial O_2 content	Measured directly from arterial blood gas sample; normal value is roughly **90–100 mm Hg**
PAo_2	Alveolar O_2 content	Calculated as: $$= \text{(Atmospheric air pressure)} \times (Fio_2) - \frac{Paco_2}{0.c}$$ for **room air,** this becomes: $$= 713 \text{ mm Hg} \times 0.21 - \frac{Paco_2}{0.8}$$ $$= 150 \text{ mm Hg} - \frac{Paco_2}{0.8}$$
$Paco_2$	Arterial CO_2 content	Measured directly from arterial blood gas sample; normal value is roughly **40 mm Hg**
Fio_2	Fraction of O_2 in inspired air	For room air, this fraction is typically **0.21**
A-a gradient	Difference between alveolar and arterial oxygenation status	$$\mathbf{PAo_2 - Pao_2} = 713 \text{ mm Hg} \times 0.21 - \frac{Paco_2}{0.8} - Pao_2; \mathbf{5\text{–}15}$$ **mm Hg is considered a normal A-a gradient**

II. Respiratory Infections

A. Upper respiratory infections (URIs) (*see Figure 2-3*)
  1. **Common cold (viral rhinitis)**
    a. Inflammation of the upper airways most commonly caused by rhinovirus, coronavirus, or adenovirus
    b. **History and physical (H/P)** = nasal and throat irritation, sneezing, **rhinorrhea** (i.e., nasal congestion and increased secretions), **nonproductive cough**; possible fever, no exudates or productive cough
    c. **Labs** = negative throat culture
    d. **Treatment** = rest, analgesia, treat symptoms; antibiotics are **not** helpful
  2. **Pharyngitis**
    a. Pharyngeal infection caused by group A β-hemolytic streptococci ("strep throat") or common cold virus
    b. **H/P = sore throat,** lymphadenopathy, possible nasal congestion; fever, red and swollen pharynx, **tonsillar exudates** (more common with bacterial infection)
    c. **Labs** = throat culture grows streptococcal species, and rapid streptococcal antigen test is positive for strep throat; negative culture suggests viral etiology
    d. **Treatment** = self-limited; β-lactam antibiotics (e.g., penicillin, amoxicillin, etc.) reduce infection time
    e. **Complications** = untreated infection can cause acute rheumatic fever and **rheumatic heart disease**; treatment does not affect the development of poststreptococcal glomerulonephritis (characterized by a high antistreptolysin O titer)

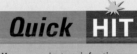

Quick HIT

Upper respiratory infections are those that occur in the **sinuses** or **pharynx**; lower respiratory infections are those that occur in the **lungs** or **bronchi**.

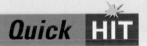

Quick HIT

Prescribing antibiotics for viral rhinitis is a contributing factor to the development of resistant strains of bacteria.

Quick HIT

It is important to complete the full prescribed course of an antibiotic to achieve cure and prevent relapse and complications as well as to prevent development of **antibiotic-resistant strains**.

Quick HIT

Approximately **3%** of untreated streptococcal infections will result in rheumatic heart disease.

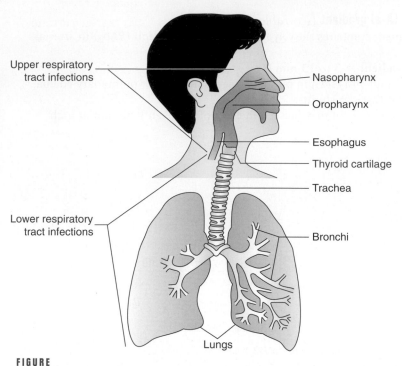

FIGURE
2-3 Diagram of the upper and lower respiratory regions and appropriate sites of infection.

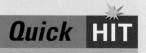

Quick HIT

Signs of a peritonsillar abscess include difficulty opening the mouth, asymmetric tonsils, and displacement of the uvula away from the abscess.

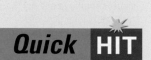

Quick HIT

Acute sinusitis can spread to the central nervous system (CNS) and cause **meningitis** if untreated.

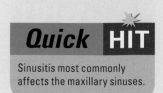

Quick HIT

Sinusitis most commonly affects the maxillary sinuses.

3. Tonsillar infections
   a. Spread of streptococcal pharyngitis to palatine tonsils, leading to tonsillar inflammation (i.e., **tonsillitis**)
   b. H/P = similar to streptococcal pharyngitis; ear pain, difficulty swallowing, possible high fever, **tonsillar exudates**
   c. **Treatment** = same as streptococcal pharyngitis
   d. **Complications** = airway compromise; abscess (requires intravenous [IV] antibiotics and surgical incision and drainage followed by tonsillectomy after resolution to prevent recurrence)

4. Viral influenza
   a. Generalized infection with URI symptoms caused by one of several influenza viruses
   b. H/P = arthralgias, **myalgias**, sore throat, nasal congestion, nonproductive cough, nausea, **vomiting, diarrhea; high fevers** (typically >100°F/37.8°C and can reach up to 106°F/41°C), lymphadenopathy
   c. **Labs** = rapid antigen immunoassay of respiratory secretions (nasal swab); polymerase chain reaction (PCR) has better sensitivity but takes several hours
   d. **Treatment** = treat symptoms; **fluid intake important** to replace losses from vomiting and diarrhea; self-limited (several days), but **oseltamivir** or **zanamivir** may shorten course of disease; annual vaccination is recommended for all persons >6 months old

5. Sinusitis
   a. Sinus infection associated with allergic rhinitis, barotrauma, viral infection, prolonged nasogastric tube placement, or asthma
   b. **Acute sinusitis** is usually caused by *Streptococcus pneumoniae, Haemophilus influenzae, Moraxella catarrhalis,* or viral infection.
   c. **Chronic sinusitis** (lasting >3 months) is usually caused by sinus obstruction, anaerobic infection; patients with diabetes mellitus (DM) are predisposed to mucormycosis.
   d. H/P = **pain over infected sinuses**, purulent nasal discharge, maxillary toothache pain, pain on palpation of affected sinuses; transillumination test (i.e., light held close to sinuses) may detect congestion in frontal of maxillary sinuses but is **unreliable**

e. **Radiology** = radiograph shows opacification and fluid levels in affected sinuses; computed tomography (CT) is diagnostic; frequently, radiologic tests are not needed because of clinical diagnosis

f. **Treatment** = treat symptoms; amoxicillin for 2 weeks in acute cases and for 6 to 12 weeks in chronic cases; surgical drainage or correction of anatomic obstruction may be required for full cure

B. Lower respiratory infections (*see Figure 2-3*)

1. **Acute bronchitis**

   a. Inflammation of trachea and bronchi caused by spread of URI or exposure to inhaled irritants

   b. **H/P** = **productive cough**, sore throat; fever, wheezing, tight breath sounds

   c. **Labs** = sputum culture is only performed in persistent cases and is most commonly negative

   d. **Radiology** = chest X-ray (CXR) may show only mild congestion

   e. **Treatment** = self-limited if viral (**most** cases); patient groups with an increased risk of bacterial infection (e.g., smokers, elderly, patients with other lung disease) may be given antibiotics (e.g., fluoroquinolones, tetracycline, erythromycin)

2. **Pneumonia**

   a. Infection of the bronchoalveolar tree can be caused by common nasopharyngeal bacteria or bacteria, viruses, or fungi from the surrounding environment; common causes vary by age group (see Table 2-4, Table 2-5).

   b. **H/P** = productive or nonproductive cough, dyspnea, chills, night sweats, **pleuritic chest pain**; **decreased breath sounds**, rales, wheezing, **dullness to percussion**, egophony (i.e., change in voice quality heard during auscultation over a consolidated region of lung), tactile fremitus, **tachypnea**

   c. **Labs** = increased white blood cell count (WBC) (slight increase with viral cause, significant increase with bacterial or fungal cause) with left shift (more immature forms); positive sputum culture and possible positive blood culture with bacterial or fungal cause (see Figure 2-4)

   d. **Radiology** = CXR shows **lobar consolidation**, infiltrates, or general increased density of lung fields

   e. **Treatment** = viral pneumonia is self-limited and only requires supportive care; bacterial and fungal pneumonias require antibiotics (started as broad coverage and changed to pathogen-specific therapy as culture results become available); healthier patients may be able to be treated as outpatients; admission criteria include elderly patients, multiple medical comorbidity, significant laboratory abnormalities, multilobar involvement, and signs of sepsis

3. **Tuberculosis (TB)**

   a. Pulmonary infection caused by *Mycobacterium tuberculosis*

   b. Following primary infection, disease enters inactive state; untreated infections can become reactivated (most active cases) and extend to extrapulmonary sites (i.e., miliary TB).

   c. Although the number of yearly cases in the United States decreased with the advent of pharmacologic treatment in the 1950s, the incidence of cases has slowly **increased** since 1985 (now approximately 10 new cases per 100,000 people each year), in large part because of the human immunodeficiency virus (**HIV**) **epidemic.**

   d. **Risk factors** = immunosuppression, alcoholism, lung disease, DM, advanced age, homelessness, malnourishment, crowded living conditions, and close proximity to infected patients (e.g., **health care workers**); TB is significantly more common in **developing nations** than in the United States

   e. **H/P** = cough, hemoptysis, dyspnea, weight loss, night sweats; fever, rales

   f. **Labs** = positive purified protein derivative (PPD) tuberculin skin test is screening test for exposure (see Table 2-6); positive sputum acid-fast stain, positive culture (may take weeks, so not useful in planning therapy); one bronchoscopy is considered equal to three sputum samples for specimen collection (see Figure 2-5)

   g. **Radiology** = CXR may show apical fibronodular infiltrates (reactivated disease), lower-lobe infiltrates (primary lesion), and calcified granulomas/lymph nodes (Ghon complexes)

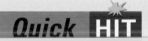

Symptoms and signs of tuberculosis are more common in **reactivated** disease, and primary disease may be asymptomatic.

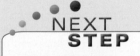

A positive PPD should be followed by a CXR to look for signs of TB.

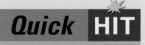

Recipients of the Bacillus Calmette-Guérin (BCG) vaccine (commonly used in other countries) will show a false-positive PPD.

Pulmonary Disorders

Pulmonary Disorders

TABLE 2-4 Overview of Etiologies of Pneumonia

Pathogen	Patients Affected	Characteristic Symptoms	Treatment
Viral pneumonia Viral (influenza, parainfluenza, adenovirus, cytomegalovirus, respiratory syncytial virus)	**Most common pneumonia in children**; common in adults	Classic symptoms[a]; **nonproductive cough**	**Self-limited**
Typical bacterial pneumonia *Streptococcus pneumoniae*	**Most common pneumonia in adults**; higher risk of infection in patients with sickle cell disease	Classic symptoms; high fevers, pleuritic pain, **productive cough**	β-Lactams, macrolides
Haemophilus influenzae	Patients with COPD; higher risk of infection in patients with sickle cell disease	Classic symptoms; **slower onset**	β-Lactams, TMP-SMX
Staphylococcus aureus	Nosocomial pneumonia, immunocompromised patients	Classic symptoms; abscess formation	β-Lactams
Klebsiella pneumoniae	Alcoholics, patients with high risk of aspiration, patients staying in the hospital for extended amounts of time, patients with sickle cell disease	Classic symptoms; **"currant-jelly"** sputum	Both cephalosporins and aminoglycosides (gentamicin, tobramycin)
Pseudomonas aeruginosa	Chronically ill and immunocompromised patients, **patients with cystic fibrosis**, nosocomial pneumonia	Classic symptoms; rapid onset	Fluoroquinolones (ciprofloxacin), aminoglycosides, 3rd-generation cephalosporins
Group B *Streptococcus*	Neonates and infants	Respiratory distress, lethargy	β-Lactams
Enterobacter sp.	Nosocomial pneumonia, elderly patients	Classic symptoms	TMP-SMX
Atypical bacterial pneumonia *Mycoplasma pneumoniae*	**Young adults**	Less severe symptoms; possible rash; **positive cold agglutinin test**	Macrolides (azithromycin, clarithromycin, erythromycin)
Legionella pneumophila	Associated with **aerosolized water** (air conditioners)	Slow onset of classic symptoms; nausea, diarrhea, confusion, or ataxia	Macrolides, fluoroquinolones
Chlamydophila pneumoniae	More common in very young and elderly	Slow onset of classic symptoms; frequent sinusitis	Doxycycline, macrolides
Fungal pneumonia Fungi	Travelers to **southwest United States** (coccidioidomycosis), **caves** (histoplasmosis), or Central America (blastomycosis)	Less severe symptoms; subacute disease for initial history	Antifungal agents (amphotericin B, fluconazole [*Coccidioides*], itraconazole [*Histoplasma, Blastomyces*])
Pneumocystis jirovecii	Immunocompromised patients (HIV) (CD4 count <200)	Slow onset of classic symptoms; GI symptoms	TMP-SMX

[a]Classic symptoms = productive or nonproductive cough, dyspnea, chills, night sweats, pleuritic chest pain.
COPD, chronic obstructive pulmonary disease; GI, gastrointestinal; HIV, human immunodeficiency virus; TMP-SMX, trimethoprim-sulfamethoxazole.

h. **Treatment = respiratory isolation** for any inpatient; report all diagnosed cases to local and state health agencies; **multidrug treatment** initially with isoniazid (INH), rifampin, pyrazinamide, and ethambutol followed by INH and rifampin only for a total of 6 months; give vitamin B$_6$ with INH to prevent peripheral neuritis (INH competes with vitamin B$_6$ as a cofactor in neurotransmitter synthesis, so supplemental vitamin B$_6$ helps offset this competition); monthly sputum acid-fast tests should be performed during therapy to confirm adequate treatment; treat all patients with an asymptomatic positive PPD with INH for 9 months (or various alternate regimens)

i. **Complications** = meningitis, bone involvement (i.e., Pott disease), widespread dissemination to multiple organs (i.e., miliary TB)

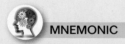

MNEMONIC

Remember the multidrug regimen for TB as **RIPE** (**R**ifampin, **I**soniazid, **P**yrazinamide, **E**thambutol).

TABLE 2-5	Most Common Etiologies of Pneumonia by Age Group	
Age Group	**Community Acquired**	**Nosocomial**
Neonatal	Group B streptococcus *Escherichia coli* *Klebsiella pneumoniae* *Staphylococcus aureus* *Streptococcus pneumoniae*	*Staphylococcus aureus* Group B streptococcus *Klebsiella pneumoniae* Respiratory syncytial virus
Infant–5 yr of age	Respiratory syncytial virus *Streptococcus pneumoniae* *Staphylococcus aureus* *Mycoplasma pneumoniae* *Chlamydophila pneumoniae*	*Staphylococcus aureus* *Klebsiella pneumoniae* Respiratory syncytial virus
5–20 yr of age	*Streptococcus pneumoniae* *Mycoplasma pneumoniae* *Chlamydophila pneumoniae* Respiratory syncytial virus	*Staphylococcus aureus* *Klebsiella pneumoniae* Respiratory syncytial virus
20–40 yr of age	*Mycoplasma pneumoniae* *Streptococcus pneumoniae* Viruses (various) *Chlamydophila pneumoniae*	*Streptococcus pneumoniae* Viruses (various) *Staphylococcus aureus*
40–60 yr of age	*Streptococcus pneumoniae* *Mycoplasma pneumoniae*	*Streptococcus pneumoniae* *Haemophilus influenzae* *Staphylococcus aureus* *Enterobacter* spp
60+ yr of age	*Streptococcus pneumoniae* *Haemophilus influenzae* *Chlamydophila pneumoniae* *Staphylococcus aureus* *Escherichia coli* Respiratory syncytial virus	*Streptococcus pneumoniae* *Haemophilus influenzae* *Staphylococcus aureus* *Enterobacter* spp.

Modified from Mehta, S., Milder, E. A., Mirachi, A. J., & Milder, F. (2006). *Step-Up: A High-Yield, Systems-Based Review for the USMLE Step 1* (3rd ed., p. 105). Philadelphia: Lippincott Williams & Wilkins; with permission.

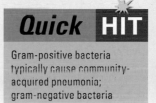

Quick HIT

Gram-positive bacteria typically cause community-acquired pneumonia; gram-negative bacteria typically cause nosocomial pneumonia.

Pulmonary Disorders

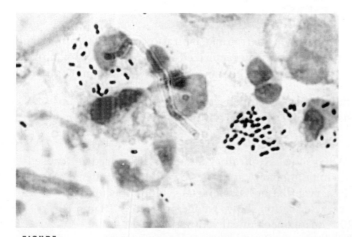

FIGURE 2-4 Paired gram-positive cocci seen in sputum consistent with *Streptococcus pneumoniae* pneumonia.

(From Washington, W., Allen, S., & Janda, W., et al. [2006]. *Koneman's Color Atlas and Textbook of Diagnostic Microbiology* [6th ed., p. 304] Philadelphia: Lippincott Williams & Wilkins; with permission.)

Pulmonary Disorders

TABLE **2-6**	Criteria Used to Determine Positive PPD for Tuberculosis
Size of Induration[a]	**When Considered Positive**
5 mm	HIV positive, close contact with TB-infected patient, signs of TB seen on CXR
10 mm	Homeless patients, immigrants from developing nations, IVDA patients, chronically ill patients, health care workers, patients with recent incarceration
15 mm	Always considered positive

[a]Induration is considered the firm cutaneous region and not the region of erythema.
CXR, chest X-ray; HIV, human immunodeficiency virus; IVDA, intravenous drug abuse; PPD, purified protein derivative; TB, tuberculosis.

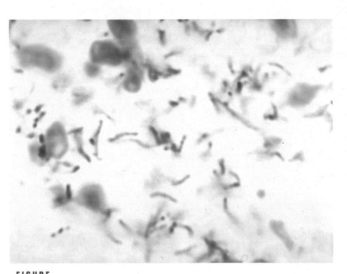

FIGURE
2-5 Numerous acid-fast bacilli seen in pulmonary histologic section consistent with *Mycobacterium tuberculosis* infection.

(From Rubin, R., & Strayer, D. S. [2012]. *Pathology* [6th ed., p. 386]. Philadelphia: Wolters Kluwer/Lippincott Williams & Wilkins; with permission.)

III. Acute Respiratory Distress Syndrome (ARDS)

A. Acute respiratory failure caused by sepsis, trauma, aspiration, near drowning, drug overdose, shock, or lung infection that is characterized by **refractory hypoxemia**, decreased lung compliance, and pulmonary edema, and carries a **high mortality**

B. H/P = acute dyspnea and pulmonary decompensation in setting of serious underlying condition; cyanosis, tachypnea (begins within 48 hours of initial insult), wheezing, rales, rhonchi

C. Labs = arterial blood gas (ABG) shows **respiratory alkalosis**, decreased O_2 (caused by impairment of O_2 transfer to pulmonary capillaries by pulmonary edema), decreased CO_2 (caused by hyperventilation); other tests should reflect underlying pathology; Swan-Ganz catheterization shows **wedge pressure <18 mm Hg**; **$Pao_2:Fio_2$ ratio will be <200 during mechanical ventilation**

D. Radiology = bilateral pulmonary edema and infiltrates

E. Treatment = treatment in **intensive care unit** with mechanical ventilation frequently required; mechanical ventilation should include positive end-expiratory pressure

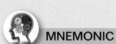
MNEMONIC

Remember the common causes of ARDS by the acronym ARDS: **A**spiration/**A**cute pancreatitis/**A**ir or **A**mniotic embolism, **R**adiation, **D**rug overdose/**D**iffuse lung disease/**D**IC/**D**rowning, **S**hock/**S**epsis/**S**moke inhalation.

(PEEP), increased inspiratory times, and Fio_2 adjusted to maintain O_2 saturation (Sao_2) >90%; **underlying cause must be treated**; keep fluid volumes low to prevent pulmonary edema; use of extracorporeal membrane oxygenation (ECMO) may improve outcome in severe cases

IV. Obstructive Airway Diseases

A. Asthma

1. **Reversible** airway obstruction secondary to bronchial hyperactivity, acute airway inflammation, mucus plugging, and smooth muscle hypertrophy
2. **Exacerbations** (i.e., sudden bronchoconstriction and airway inflammation) are triggered by allergens (e.g., dust, smoke, pollen, fumes, pet dander), URI, exercise, stress, β-blockers, aspirin (rare), and sulfites (rare).
3. Although the prevalence of asthma in the United States has increased in the past 20 years, the reasons for this trend are poorly understood.
4. **Risk factors** = family history of asthma, allergies, atopic dermatitis, low socioeconomic status
5. Disease can be worse in childhood and improve with age.
6. **H/P** = cough, dyspnea, wheezing, chest tightness; tachypnea, tachycardia, **prolonged expiratory duration**, decreased breath sounds, wheezing, **accessory muscle use**, possible pulsus paradoxus; cyanosis, decreased arterial O_2 saturation (Sao_2) on pulse oximetry, or difficulty talking in severe attacks
7. **Labs** = **peak expiratory flow rate (PEFR)** decreased and used along with clinical symptoms and frequency of medication use to classify disease as **mild intermittent, mild persistent, moderate persistent, or severe** (see Table 2-8); PFT shows decreased FEV_1, normal/elevated D_{Lco}; ABG may show mild hypoxia and respiratory alkalosis but is less useful except during severe exacerbations
8. **Radiology** = CXR shows hyperinflation
9. **Treatment** = algorithm of medications depends on classification of disease severity (see Table 2-7, Table 2-8); patient education for avoidance of exacerbating factors and recognition of impending respiratory collapse is important to long-term control

B. Chronic bronchitis

1. Chronic bronchial inflammation **associated with tobacco use** (common) or chronic asthma (uncommon); occurs in continuum with emphysema as **chronic obstructive pulmonary disease (COPD)**
2. **H/P** = productive cough, recurrent respiratory infections, dyspnea; wheezing, rhonchi
3. Diagnosis made with history of **productive cough for 3 months of the year for >2 years**
4. **Labs** = PFTs show gradually worsening signs of obstructive disease as condition progresses
5. **Treatment** = **tobacco cessation**, antibiotics given for URI because of the greater incidence of a bacterial etiology; bronchodilators during exacerbations
6. **Complications** = emphysema frequently results without smoking cessation

C. Emphysema (later stage—COPD)

1. Long-term tobacco use leads to chronic bronchoalveolar inflammation associated with release of proteolytic enzymes by neutrophils and macrophages; **destruction of alveoli and bronchioles** results with panacinar airspace enlargement and a decreased capillary bed.
2. Less common form (appears at younger age) caused by α_1-antitrypsin deficiency
3. **H/P** = **dyspnea**, possible productive cough, morning headache; barrel chested, **pursed-lip breathing**, prolonged expiratory duration, decreased heart sounds, decreased breath sounds, wheezing, rhonchi, accessory muscle use, jugular venous distension (JVD); exacerbations present with worsening symptoms

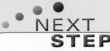

NEXT STEP

Status asthmaticus is a prolonged, nonresponsive asthma attack that can be fatal and should be treated with **aggressive** bronchodilator therapy, corticosteroids, O_2, and, possibly, intubation.

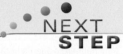

NEXT STEP

A normal CO_2 during an exacerbation signals impending respiratory failure and requires additional β_2-agonists, supplemental O_2, and, possibly, ventilation.

MNEMONIC

Patients with **chronic bronchitis** are "blue bloaters" because secondary development of cor pulmonale causes cyanosis and peripheral edema; patients with **emphysema** are "pink puffers" because of their pursed-lip breathing, dyspnea, and barrel chests.

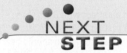

NEXT STEP

To differentiate between emphysema and chronic bronchitis, check the D_{Lco}; it is normal in chronic bronchitis but decreased in emphysema.

Quick HIT

The common form of emphysema has a centrilobular distribution, whereas the form associated with α_1-antitrypsin deficiency has a panlobular distribution.

Pulmonary Disorders

TABLE 2-7	Commonly Used Medications for Treatment of Asthma	
Medication	**Mechanism of Action**	**Role**
Rapid-acting β_2-agonists (albuterol, pirbuterol, bitolterol)	Bronchodilators that relax airway smooth muscle; have rapid onset of action	First-line therapy in mild intermittent cases and during exacerbations
Long-acting β_2-agonists (salmeterol, formoterol, sustained-release albuterol)	Bronchodilators that relax airway smooth muscle; have gradual onset and sustained activity	Regular use in patients with moderate persistent or severe asthma
Inhaled corticosteroids (beclomethasone, flunisolide)	Decrease number and activity of cells involved with airway inflammation	Mild persistent or worse cases; frequently combined with β_2-agonist use
Leukotriene inhibitors (montelukast, zafirlukast, zileuton)	Block activity or production of leukotrienes that are involved in inflammation and bronchospasm	Oral agents; adjunctive therapy in mild persistent or worse cases
Theophylline	Bronchodilator	Former first-line therapy, but now replaced by β_2-agonists because of side effects (tachycardia, seizures) and interactions with other drugs; may be useful as adjunct in mild persistent or worse cases
Anticholinergic agents (ipratropium)	Blocks vagal-mediated smooth muscle contraction	Adjunctive therapy in moderate to severe cases
Systemic steroids (methylprednisolone, prednisone)	Similar action to inhaled steroids; stronger effect than inhaled preparation	Adjunctive therapy in severe, refractory cases

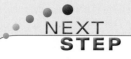

NEXT STEP

If a patient with COPD has a resting Sao$_2$ ≤88%, a home O$_2$ program should be initiated.

4. **Labs** = PFT shows decreased FEV_1, **decreased FEV_1/FVC**, increased total lung capacity (TLC), decreased PEFR; ABG during acute exacerbations shows decreased O_2 and increased CO_2 (beyond a baseline increase already seen in these patients)
5. **Radiology** = CXR shows **flat diaphragm, hyperinflated lungs**, subpleural blebs and bullae (i.e., small fluid-filled sacs), and decreased vascular markings
6. **Treatment** = **smoking cessation**; supplemental O_2; inhaled, short-acting β_2-agonists; inhaled anticholinergics; inhaled corticosteroids and long-acting β_2-agonists may be useful in severe cases; antibiotics given for respiratory infections; pneumococcal and influenza vaccines important to reduce infection risk; enzyme replacement may have a role in α_1-antitrypsin deficiency therapy; lung transplant may be an option in late severe disease
7. **Complications** = chronic respiratory decompensation, cor pulmonale, frequent respiratory infections, frequent comorbid lung cancer

D. Bronchiectasis

1. **Permanent dilation** of small and medium bronchi because of destruction of bronchial elastic components
2. Occurs secondary to **chronic airway obstruction**, chronic tobacco use, TB, fungal infections, severe pneumonia, or cystic fibrosis
3. **H/P** = persistent, productive cough; hemoptysis, frequent respiratory infections, dyspnea; **copious sputum**, wheezing, rales, and hypoxemia
4. **Radiology** = multiple cysts and bronchial crowding seen on CXR; CT shows dilation of bronchi, bronchial wall thickening, and bronchial wall cysts
5. **Treatment** = pulmonary hygiene (e.g., hydration, sputum removal), chest physical therapy; antibiotics given when sputum production increases; inhaled β_2-agonists and corticosteroids may reduce symptoms; resection of severely diseased regions of lung indicated for hemorrhage, substantial sputum production, or inviability
6. **Complications** = cor pulmonale, massive hemoptysis, abscess formation

TABLE 2-8	Classification of Asthma Severity and Treatment Algorithms			
Type	Symptoms	PEFR	Treatment of Exacerbations	Long-term Control
Mild intermittent	• ≤2 times/wk • Nocturnal awakening ≤2 times/month • May only occur during exercise	• When asymptomatic, >80% predicted value	• Inhaled short-acting β_2-agonist as needed • IV corticosteroids if persistent symptoms	• No daily medications needed • May use mast cell stabilizers if known trigger
Mild persistent	• Bronchodilator use >2 times/wk • Nocturnal awakening >every 2 wk	• >20% fluctuations over time	• Inhaled short-acting β_2-agonist as needed • IV corticosteroids if persistent symptoms	• Inhaled low-dose corticosteroid • Consider mast cell stabilizer, leukotriene inhibitor, or theophylline
Moderate persistent	• Daily symptoms • Daily bronchodilator use • Symptoms interfere with activity • Nocturnal awakening >1 time/wk	• 60%–80% predicted value	• Inhaled short-acting β_2-agonist as needed • IV corticosteroids if persistent symptoms	• Inhaled low to medium dose corticosteroids and long-acting β_2-agonist • Consider leukotriene inhibitor or theophylline
Severe	• Symptoms with minimal activity • Awake multiple times/night • Require multiple medications on daily basis	• Wide variations • Rarely >70% predicted value • Associated FEV_1 <60% predicted value	• Inhaled short-acting β_2-agonist as needed • IV corticosteroids if persistent symptoms	• Inhaled high-dose corticosteroids and long-acting β_2-agonist • Consider systemic corticosteroids

FEV_1, 1-second forced expiratory volume; IV, intravenous; PFFR, peak expiratory flow rate.

V. Respiratory Neoplasms

A. Solitary pulmonary nodule

1. A lung nodule <5 cm diameter may be discovered incidentally on CXR or CT (see Figure 2-6, Figure 2-7).
2. Can be granuloma, hamartoma, cancer (primary or metastasis), carcinoid tumor, or pneumonia

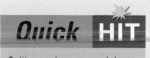

Solitary pulmonary nodules are cancerous in 40% of cases.

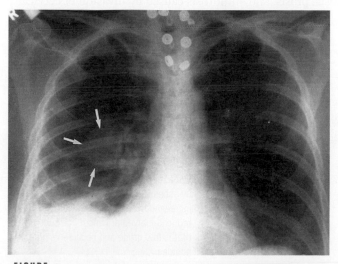

FIGURE
2-6 **Chest X-ray demonstrating a solitary pulmonary nodule (*arrows*); in this patient, the finding was determined to be a loculated pleural effusion.**

(From Daffner, R. H. & Hartman, M. [2013]. *Clinical Radiology: The Essentials* [4th ed., p. 116]. Philadelphia: Wolters Kluwer/ Lippincott Williams & Wilkins; with permission.)

Pulmonary Disorders

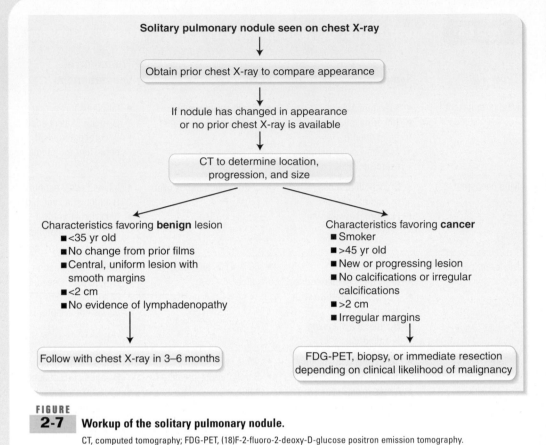

FIGURE 2-7 **Workup of the solitary pulmonary nodule.**

CT, computed tomography; FDG-PET, (18)F-2-fluoro-2-deoxy-D-glucose positron emission tomography.

B. Lung cancer

1. Most frequently associated with tobacco use (roughly 90% of cases); can also be caused by occupational exposures (e.g., smoke, asbestos, radon)
2. Classified according to cell lineage and histologic appearance (see Table 2-9)
3. H/P = possibly asymptomatic; hemoptysis, cough, dyspnea, pleuritic chest pain, fatigue, weight loss, frequent pulmonary infections; additional symptoms may accompany **paraneoplastic syndromes** (see Table 2-10); local extension of tumors may result in the following:
   a. **Horner syndrome**: miosis, ptosis, and anhidrosis caused by invasion of cervical ganglia

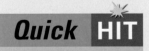

Quick HIT

Smoking cessation is the only action shown to prevent lung cancer in active smokers (**never smoking** also prevents lung cancer).

Quick HIT

Metastases make up 10% of solitary cancerous lesions and are most commonly associated with breast, colon, prostate, endometrial, and cervical cancers.

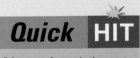

Quick HIT

Adenocarcinoma is the most common type of lung cancer seen in **nonsmokers**.

TABLE 2-9	Common Types of Primary Lung Cancer		
Primary Lung Cancer Type	**Primary Malignancies (%)**	**Location**	**Characteristics**
Squamous cell carcinoma	25–35	Central	Cavitary lesions; direct extension to hilar lymph nodes
Adenocarcinoma	25–35	Peripheral	Wide metastases; can be caused by asbestos; pleural effusions show increased hyaluronidase levels; bronchioloalveolar cancer is a subtype that is low grade and occurs in single nodules
Small cell carcinoma	20–25	Central	Rapidly growing; early distant metastases; several paraneoplastic syndromes
Large cell carcinoma	5–15	Peripheral	Late distant metastases, early cavitation

TABLE 2-10 Common Paraneoplastic Syndromes Associated with Primary Lung Cancers

Primary Lung Cancer Type	Associated Paraneoplastic Syndromes
Squamous cell	Hypercalcemia Dermatomyositis
Adenocarcinoma	Disseminated intravascular coagulation (DIC) Thrombophlebitis Microangiopathic hemolytic anemia Dermatomyositis
Small cell	Cushing syndrome Syndrome of inappropriate ADH secretion (SIADH) Ectopic growth hormone and ACTH secretion Peripheral neuropathy Subacute cerebellar degeneration Lambert-Eaton syndrome (similar presentation to myasthenia gravis) Subacute sensory neuropathy Limbic encephalitis Dermatomyositis
Large cell	Gynecomastia Dermatomyositis

ACTH, adrenocorticotropic hormone; ADH, antidiuretic hormone.

    b. **Pancoast syndrome**: Horner syndrome plus brachial plexus involvement
    c. **Superior vena cava syndrome**: obstruction of venous drainage through superior vena cava and associated head swelling and CNS symptoms
  4. **Radiology** = initially seen on CXR or CT as pulmonary nodule; bronchoscopy with biopsy and brushings or fine needle aspiration of lesion are diagnostic
  5. **Treatment** = use of **surgical resection, chemotherapy,** and/or **radiation therapy** based on **type** of lung cancer (large cell, squamous cell, or adenocarcinoma vs. small cell) and **staging** of disease (based on local extension, lymph node involvement, and presence of metastases) (see Table 2-11)

TABLE 2-11 Treatment for Lung Cancer Based on Staging Algorithm

Neoplasm Type	Staging	Surgery	Chemotherapy	Radiation Therapy
Non–small cell (squamous cell, adenocarcinoma, large cell)	No mediastinal invasion, **no lymph node involvement beyond ipsilateral hilar nodes**, no metastases	**Surgical resection** (lobectomy, video-assisted thorascopic surgery)	Adjuvant therapy to surgery	Primary therapy (medically inappropriate for surgery) or postoperative adjuvant therapy to surgery
	No mediastinal invasion or metastases, **has extension to ipsilateral mediastinal nodes**	Consider if significant decrease in tumor size following radiation	Induction therapy if considering surgery or adjuvant to radiation	Primary therapy, continue postoperatively if surgery performed
	Mediastinal invasion, distant nodes, and/or metastases	None	Palliative	Palliative
Small cell	Small lesion, no nodal spread, no metastases	Consider for very small lesions	**Primary therapy**	Adjuvant therapy to chemotherapy
	All other lesions	None	**Primary therapy**	Adjuvant therapy after chemotherapy

6. **Complications** = **poor prognosis** (approximately 10% 5-year survival); recurrence common for primary tumors

C. Laryngeal cancer

1. Squamous cell cancer of the larynx **associated with tobacco and alcohol use**
2. **H/P** = **hoarseness that worsens with time** (over several weeks), dysphagia, ear pain, hemoptysis; laryngoscopy may visualize mass and airway obstruction
3. **Labs** = biopsy is diagnostic
4. **Radiology** = magnetic resonance imaging (MRI) or CT with contrast detects soft tissue mass; positron emission tomography (PET) may be useful for detecting lesions earlier in disease course
5. **Treatment** = partial or total laryngectomy used to remove lesions confined to larynx; radiation therapy can be used in conjunction with surgery or as sole therapy in extensive lesions; advanced cases may require combination of surgery, radiation, and chemotherapy to resect lesion while preserving surrounding structures

VI. Interstitial Lung Diseases and Other Lung Diseases

A. Idiopathic pulmonary fibrosis (IPF)

1. Inflammatory lung disease causing lung fibrosis; it is of unknown cause and generally affects patients >50 years of age
2. **H/P** = progressive exercise intolerance, dyspnea; dry crackles, JVD, tachypnea, and possible digital clubbing
3. **Labs** = PFT will show **restrictive lung disease** characteristics (e.g., FEV_1/FVC normal, decreased FVC, decreased TLC, decreased compliance); bronchioalveolar lavage shows increased polymorphonuclear (PMN) cells; lung biopsy demonstrates extensive fibrosis and loss of parenchymal architecture
4. **Radiology** = CXR shows reticulonodular pattern and "**honeycomb**" lung in advanced cases; CT will show lung fields with "**ground glass**" appearance
5. **Treatment** = corticosteroids combined with either azathioprine or cyclophosphamide are helpful in some patients (follow PFTs to evaluate effectiveness); worsening PFTs should indicate need to change drug regimen; lung transplant is frequently indicated
6. **Complications** = progressive lung fibrosis with frequent mortality within 5 years; most patients do not survive sufficiently long to receive a lung transplant

B. Sarcoidosis

1. Systemic disease characterized by **noncaseating granulomas**, hilar adenopathy, pulmonary infiltrates, and skin lesions; unknown etiology
2. **Risk factors** = blacks > whites; females > males; most frequently occurs between 10 and 40 years of age
3. **H/P** = cough, malaise, weight loss, dyspnea, arthritis (knees, ankles), chest pain; fever, erythema nodosum (i.e., tender red nodules on shins and arms), lymphadenopathy, vision loss, cranial nerve palsies
4. **Labs** = increased serum angiotensin-converting enzyme (ACE), increased calcium, hypercalciuria, increased alkaline phosphatase, decreased WBC, increased erythrocyte sedimentation rate (ESR); PFT shows decreased FVC and decreased D_{Lco}
5. **Radiology** = CXR shows **bilateral hilar lymphadenopathy** and pulmonary infiltrates (ground glass appearance)
6. **Treatment** = occasionally self-resolving; corticosteroids in chronic cases; cytotoxic drugs can be used with failure of steroid therapy; lung transplantation is rarely required (only in severe cases)

C. Pneumoconioses

1. Interstitial lung diseases that result from long-term **occupational exposure** to substances that cause pulmonary inflammation (see Table 2-12)

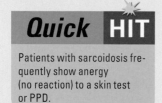

Quick HIT

Patients with sarcoidosis frequently show anergy (no reaction) to a skin test or PPD.

TABLE 2-12	Common Pneumoconioses and How to Diagnose Them			
Disease	**Exposure**	**Labs**	**Radiology**	**Complications**
Asbestosis	Working with insulation, construction, demolition, building maintenance, automobiles	PFT shows restrictive pattern; asbestos fibers seen in **pleural biopsy**[a]	Multinodular opacities, pleural effusions, blurring of heart/diaphragm; chest CT shows linear pleural/parenchymal fibrosis	Increased risk of **malignant mesothelioma** and lung cancer; synergistic effect with tobacco
Silicosis	Mining, pottery making, sandblasting, cutting granite	PFT shows restrictive pattern	Small apical nodular opacities; hilar adenopathy	**Increased risk of TB infection**; progressive fibrosis
Coal worker disease	**Coal mining**	PFT shows restrictive pattern	Small apical nodular opacities	Progressive fibrosis
Berylliosis	**Electronics**, ceramics, tool, die manufacturing	Pulmonary edema, diffuse granuloma formation	Diffuse infiltrates; hilar adenopathy	Increased risk of lung cancer; may need chronic corticosteroid treatment to maintain respiratory function

[a]Not needed for diagnosis with known exposure to asbestos and suggestive radiographic workup.
CT, computed tomography; PFT, pulmonary function test; TB, tuberculosis.

2. **H/P** = symptoms begin when significant pulmonary fibrosis has occurred (several years between exposure and onset of symptoms is common); cough, dyspnea on exertion, heavy sputum production; rales and wheezing are heard on auscultation, digital clubbing
3. **Labs** = PFT shows a restrictive pattern
4. **Radiology** = CXR shows multinodular opacities; CT shows signs of pulmonary fibrosis
5. **Treatment** = usually, no successful treatments are available for these conditions; **prevention** (e.g., proper air filters, following safe-handling recommendations) **is vital to avoiding disease**

D. Goodpasture syndrome

1. Progressive autoimmune disease of lungs and kidneys caused by **antiglomerular basement membrane (anti-GBM) antibodies** and characterized by intra-alveolar hemorrhage and glomerulonephritis
2. **H/P** = **hemoptysis**, dyspnea, recent respiratory infection
3. **Labs** = positive **anti-GBM antibodies**; PFT shows restrictive pattern but increased D_{Lco} (caused by the presence of Hgb in alveoli); urinalysis shows proteinuria and granular casts; renal biopsy shows crescentic glomerulonephritis and IgG deposition along glomerular capillaries
4. **Radiology** = CXR shows bilateral alveolar infiltration
5. **Treatment** = plasmapheresis to remove autoantibodies; corticosteroids and immunosuppressive agents

E. Granulomatosis with polyangiitis (Wegener's)

1. Rare disease with granulomatous inflammation and necrosis of lung and other organ systems; previously called Wegener's granulomatosis
2. Caused by systemic vasculitis that mainly affects lung and kidney, causing formation of noncaseating granulomas and destruction of lung parenchyma
3. **H/P** = hemoptysis, dyspnea, myalgias, chronic sinusitis; **ulcerations of nasopharynx**, fever; additional symptoms from renal (e.g., mild hematuria), CNS (e.g., hearing loss, sensory neuropathy, cranial nerve dysfunction), ophthalmologic (e.g., conjunctivitis, proptosis, corneal ulceration, diplopia), and cardiac (e.g., arrhythmia) involvement

4. **Labs** = positive cytoplasmic antineutrophil cytoplasmic antibody (c-ANCA); biopsy shows **noncaseating granulomas**; renal biopsy detects vasculitic process
5. **Treatment** = cytotoxic therapy (e.g., cyclophosphamide), corticosteroids
6. **Complications** = rapidly fatal if untreated

VII. Vascular and Thromboembolic Pulmonary Conditions

A. Pulmonary embolism (PE)

1. Occlusion of pulmonary vasculature by a dislodged thrombus
2. Increasing pulmonary artery pressure caused by occlusion leads to right-sided heart failure, hypoxia, and pulmonary infarction
3. **Risk factors** = **immobilization, cancer**, prolonged travel, recent surgery, pregnancy, oral contraceptive use, hypercoagulability, obesity, fractures, prior DVT, or severe burns
4. **H/P** = **sudden dyspnea**, pleuritic chest pain, cough, syncope, feeling of impending doom; fever, tachypnea, tachycardia, cyanosis, loud S_2, decreased breath sounds over regions of effusion
5. **Labs** = increased D-dimer; ABG shows decreased O_2 (<80 mm Hg), **increased A-a gradient**; ventilation-perfusion (**V/Q**) **scan** may show areas of mismatch
6. **Electrocardiogram (ECG)** = tachycardia, may show S wave in lead I and T-wave inversion in lead III
7. **Radiology** = CXR may be normal or may show pleural effusion or wedge-shaped infarct; pulmonary angiography is diagnostic but a higher risk study; **spiral CT** may detect proximal PE; V/Q scan can detect areas of V/Q mismatch
8. **Treatment** = **supplemental O_2** to maximize saturation; IV fluids or cardiac pressors as needed for hypotension; **anticoagulate** initially with either low molecular weight heparin (LMWH) or unfractionated heparin (titrated for PTT 1.5 to 2.5 times normal); patients treated with unfractionated heparin need to be converted to either LMWH or warfarin (given to achieve goal international normalized ratio [INR] 2 to 3) for **3 to 6 months**; inferior vena cava filter can be placed if anticoagulation is contraindicated; thrombolysis may be considered for patients with massive PE or those with no cardiac contraindications, recent trauma, or surgery

B. Pulmonary hypertension

1. Increased pulmonary artery pressure caused by **PE, valvular disease**, left-to-right shunts, COPD, or idiopathic causes
2. Idiopathic pulmonary hypertension has a high mortality rate within a few years of diagnosis.
3. **H/P** = dyspnea, fatigue, deep chest pain, cough, syncope, cyanosis; digital clubbing, **loud S_2**, JVD, hepatomegaly
4. **Labs** = increased red blood cell count (RBC) and WBC
5. **ECG** = right ventricular hypertrophy
6. **Radiology** = CXR shows large pulmonary artery and large right ventricle; echocardiogram is useful for measuring pulmonary artery pressure noninvasively and detecting valvular disease; cardiac catheterization is the gold standard test for measuring pressures but carries greater risks than other studies; PFTs may be useful in diagnosing underlying pulmonary disease
7. **Treatment** = treat underlying condition; supplemental O_2 helps maintain blood oxygenation; vasodilators indicated for idiopathic and pulmonary causes to decrease pulmonary vascular resistance; anticoagulants indicated in patients with idiopathic, embolic, or cardiac causes to decrease risk of pulmonary thrombus formation

C. Pulmonary edema

1. Increased fluid in lungs caused by increased pulmonary venous pressure and hydrostatic leak of fluid from vessels

Quick HIT

95% of PEs arise from a deep venous thrombosis (DVT) in the leg.

MNEMONIC

Risk factors for PE may be remembered as the 7 **H**s: **H**eredity (genetic hypocoagulability), **H**istory (prior DVT or PE), **H**ypomobility (fracture, prolonged travel, surgery, obesity), **H**ypovolemia (dehydration), **H**ypercoagulability (cancer, smoking), **H**ormones (pregnancy, oral contraceptive pill [OCP] use), and **H**yperhomocysteinemia.

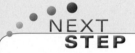

NEXT STEP

A positive or negative V/Q scan is diagnostic or rules out PE, but an equivocal scan indicates need for angiography.

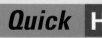

Quick HIT

LMWH is an acceptable alternative to heparin and does not require partial thromboplastin time (PTT) monitoring (but may be assessed by measuring antifactor Xa levels).

2. Caused by **left-sided heart failure**, myocardial infarction (MI), **valvular disease**, arrhythmias, ARDS
3. **H/P** = dyspnea, **orthopnea, paroxysmal nocturnal dyspnea**; tachycardia, frothy sputum, wheezing, rhonchi, rales, dullness to percussion, peripheral edema, S_3 or S_4 heart sound, hypertension
4. **Labs** = increased brain natriuretic peptide (BNP) or abnormal cardiac enzymes help elucidate a cardiac cause
5. **ECG** = T-wave abnormalities or QT prolongation are common changes and can occur suddenly with acute onset
6. **Radiology** = CXR shows fluid throughout lungs, cephalization of vessels (i.e., increased vascular markings in upper lung fields), and Kerley B lines (i.e., prominent horizontal interstitial markings in lower lung fields)
7. **Treatment** = treat underlying condition; diuretics, salt restriction, O_2, vasodilators; nitrates promote redistribution of fluid in peripheral (rather than pulmonary) vasculature; pressors may be required to improve cardiac output if perfusion is inadequate

> **Quick HIT**
>
> A pulmonary wedge pressure measured with a Swan-Ganz catheter is suggestive of a cardiac cause for pulmonary edema if >18 mm Hg and is suggestive of ARDS if <18 mm Hg.

VIII. Pleural Diseases

A. Pleural effusion

1. Serous or lymphatic fluid collection in pleural space is classified according to protein and lactate dehydrogenase (LDH) content and is caused by changes in hydrostatic and oncotic pressure (transudative), **inflammation** (exudative), or lymphatic duct rupture (lymphatic).
2. **H/P** = possibly asymptomatic; dyspnea, pleuritic chest pain, weakness; decreased breath sounds, dullness to percussion, decreased tactile fremitus
3. **Labs** = pleural fluid analysis used for protein and LDH levels (i.e., transudate vs. exudates), glucose (low in TB, malignancy, autoimmune diseases), pH (acidic in malignancy, TB, empyema), amylase (high in pancreatitis, esophageal rupture, some malignancies), triglycerides (high in thoracic duct rupture), complete blood cell count (CBC), Gram stain, and cytology (see Table 2-13)
4. **Radiology** = CXR shows blunting of costophrenic angles; decubitus CXR can demonstrate whether fluid is loculated or free-flowing; CT is useful for measuring pleural thickness or distinguishing a discrete collection from a diffuse one (e.g., abscess vs. empyema)
5. **Treatment** = **treat underlying condition**; relieve pressure on lung with thoracocentesis and chest tube placement; for cases with empyema (i.e., effusion of pus due to infection), a chest tube is required; if recurrent malignant effusion occurs, use pleurodesis (talc or other irritant) to scar the pleural layers together

> **Quick HIT**
>
> 25% of pleural effusions are associated with neoplasm.

Pulmonary Disorders

TABLE 2-13	Distinctive Characteristics and Causes of Types of Pleural Effusions			
Effusion	**Pleural: Serum Protein Ratio**	**Pleural: Serum LDH Ratio**	**Total Pleural LDH**	**Causes**
Transudate	<0.5	<0.6	<2/3 the upper limit of normal serum LDH	CHF, cirrhosis, kidney diseases (nephrotic syndrome)
Exudate	>0.5	>0.6	>2/3 the upper limit of normal serum LDH	Infection, cancer, vasculitis

CHF, congestive heart failure; LDH, lactate dehydrogenase.

TABLE 2-14	Types of Pneumothorax and Their Causes	
Type of Pneumothorax	**Mechanism**	**Causes**
Closed	Internal rupture of respiratory system; chest wall intact	Spontaneous, COPD, TB, blunt trauma
Open	Passage of air through opening in chest wall	Penetrating trauma, iatrogenic (central line placement, thoracocentesis, biopsy)
Tension	Open pneumothorax; "ball-valve" condition allows air to enter but not leave pleural space	Trauma

COPD, chronic obstructive pulmonary disease; TB, tuberculosis.

MNEMONIC

Remember the common causes of PTX by the acronym **A CHEST IN**: **A**sthma, **C**ystic fibrosis, **H**IV (acquired immunodeficiency syndrome [AIDS]), **E**mphysema, **S**pontaneous **T**rauma, **I**atrogenic, **N**eoplasm.

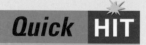

The classic patient for a spontaneous closed pneumothorax is a young, thin, and tall male.

B. Pneumothorax (PTX)

1. Collection of air in pleural space that predisposes patient to pulmonary collapse
2. Can occur spontaneously (less common) or secondary to trauma or a pulmonary medical condition (more common) (see Table 2-14)
3. **H/P = unilateral chest pain**, dyspnea; **decreased chest wall movement**, unilateral decreased breath sounds, increased resonance to percussion, decreased tactile fremitus; respiratory distress, decreased Sao$_2$, hypotension, JVD, or tracheal deviation suggest tension pneumothorax
4. **Radiology** = CXR shows lung retraction and mediastinal shift away from affected side; tension PTX will demonstrate tracheal deviation (see Figure 2-8)
5. **Treatment**
   a. Small (<15% lung field) PTX may resolve with supplemental O$_2$ only.
   b. Larger (>15%) PTX requires **chest tube placement**.

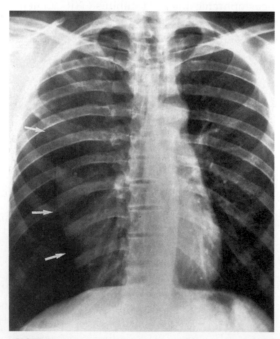

FIGURE
2-8 Chest X-ray demonstrating tension pneumothorax. Note compressed visceral pleural edge (*arrows*) caused by intrapleural air and tracheal deviation and mediastinal shift toward the left.

(From Daffner, R. H. & Hartman, M. [2013]. *Clinical Radiology: The Essentials* [4th ed., p. 138]. Philadelphia: Wolters Kluwer/ Lippincott Williams & Wilkins; with permission.)

   c. Open PTX with small wound is treated with chest tube and occlusive dressing.

   d. Open PTX with larger wounds should be treated with attempted closure and should carry a low threshold for intubation.

   e. Tension pneumothorax requires **immediate needle decompression** (fourth or fifth intercostal space at the midaxillary line, or the second or third intercostal space at the midclavicular line) and chest tube placement.

   f. Recurrent pneumothorax may require pleurodesis.

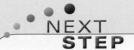

NEXT STEP

With clinical suspicion for tension pneumothorax, do not wait for a CXR—perform **immediate needle decompression**.

C. Hemothorax

1. Collection of blood in pleural space caused by trauma, malignancy, TB, or pulmonary infarction
2. **H/P** = dyspnea, pleuritic chest pain, weakness; decreased breath sounds, dullness to percussion, decreased tactile fremitus
3. **Labs** = thoracocentesis shows bloody effusion
4. **Radiology** = CXR resembles that for pleural effusion (i.e., blunting of costophrenic angles)
5. **Treatment** = supplemental O_2, chest tube placement; treat underlying cause
6. **Complications** = thrombi formation; fibrosis can occur if blood is not drained from pleural space

D. Malignant mesothelioma

1. Uncommon tumor occurring on visceral pleura or pericardium with very poor prognosis
2. **Increased incidence with asbestos exposure** (occurs 20 years after exposure), especially in smokers
3. **H/P** = nonpleuritic chest pain, dyspnea; dullness to percussion over lung bases, palpable chest wall mass, scoliosis toward lesion
4. **Labs** = pleural biopsy is usually diagnostic; thoracocentesis of an associated pleural effusion can be used for cytology studies
5. **Radiology** = CXR shows pleural thickening, pleural effusion; chest CT can display extent of local disease; PET scan can be used to detect extrathoracic disease
6. **Treatment** = extrapleural pneumonectomy with adjuvant chemotherapy and radiation therapy; chemotherapy alone used for unresectable disease

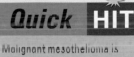

Quick **HIT**

Malignant mesothelioma is usually secondary to asbestos exposure, but **non-small cell lung cancer** (such as adenocarcinoma) is far more common than mesothelioma in individuals exposed to asbestos.

Pulmonary Disorders

IX. Sleep Apnea

A. Episodic cessation of airflow during sleep leading to desaturations and frequent arousals

B. Types

1. **Obstructive:** obstruction of upper airway during sleep with continued respiratory effort; most often associated with obesity or abnormal pharyngeal anatomy
2. **Central:** loss of central respiratory drive leads to cessation of airflow **and** respiratory effort
3. **Mixed:** combines both obstructive and central characteristics

C. **Risk factors** = obesity, sedative use; males more than females

D. Etiology is unknown but may be linked to abnormal feedback control during sleep or decreased sensitivity of upper airway muscles to stimulation.

E. **H/P** = fatigue, excessive daytime sleepiness, snoring, gasping or choking during sleep, morning headaches or confusion, impaired daytime function because of sleepiness; obesity common, anatomic abnormalities of palate or pharynx may be visible

F. **Labs** = Epworth sleepiness scale is useful for predicting likelihood of sleep apnea as cause for daytime somnolence (score >10 common in sleep apnea); polysomnography is definitive test that measures apnea index (AI; average apneic episodes per hour), Sao_2, and number of arousals

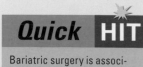

Bariatric surgery is associated with resolution of sleep apnea in 86% of cases.

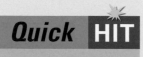

Atelectasis is frequently blamed for postoperative fever, but the relationship is more likely coincidental than causal.

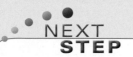

If atelectasis lasts >72 hr, pneumonia is likely to develop.

NEXT STEP

It is important to **visualize** insertion of the endotracheal tube between the vocal cords to reduce the risk of **esophageal** placement.

G. Treatment

1. **Obstructive** = consider weight loss (possibly bariatric surgery) and stop sedative use; **continuous positive airway pressure (CPAP)** is helpful in chronic cases to maintain airway patency; surgical correction of tonsillar hypertrophy, polyp removal, correction of congenital upper airway deformities, or tracheostomy may be necessary in severe or refractory cases
2. **Central** = respiratory stimulants; phrenic nerve pacemaking may be needed in severe cases

X. Pulmonary Surgical Concerns

A. Atelectasis

1. Localized alveolar collapse; **common after surgery** (especially abdominal) **and anesthesia** (generally not clinically serious); can also occur in asthmatics, after foreign body aspiration, or from mass effect (e.g., tumors, pulmonary lesions, or lymphadenopathy)
2. **H/P** = asymptomatic if mild or slow development; pleuritic chest pain, dyspnea; fever, decreased breath sounds, dullness to percussion over affected area
3. **Radiology** = CXR will show fluffy infiltrates in mild cases and lobar collapse in cases of airway obstruction
4. **Treatment** = **incentive spirometry**, ambulation, and inpatient physical therapy are important for prevention in the hospital and postoperatively; severe cases require upper airway suctioning or bronchoscopy with deeper suctioning

B. Intubation

1. Placement of tube into trachea to maintain airway patency and allow mechanical ventilation during anesthesia and times of respiratory distress
2. Almost all intubations are performed **orally** (nasal intubation performed for oral surgery, jaw surgery, and in cases when a laryngoscope cannot help to visualize the vocal cords).
3. **Placement**
   a. Appropriate anesthesia ± muscle relaxants administered
   b. Patient positioned with moderate cervical flexion
   c. Laryngoscope inserted into mouth and used to lift jaw and visualize lower pharynx (pressure applied to **cricoid** may aid in visualization)
   d. Endotracheal tube inserted past vocal cords (**direct visualization is important**) to depth of 21 to 23 cm (measured at lips)
   e. Proper placement is checked by measuring **end tidal CO_2** (rise should follow expiration) and confirming bilateral lung expansion with **auscultation**.
   f. Endotracheal tube cuff is inflated, and tube is secured.
4. **Complications** = dental injury during placement, placement of tube in esophagus, increased risk of infection
5. If intubation is required for >3 weeks, convert to a **tracheostomy** (i.e., surgical insertion of breathing tube through anterior neck into trachea)

C. Ventilation

1. Ventilation is assisted respiration that is required during surgery under anesthesia; it may also be required to maintain patent airway or in cases where the patient is not able to breathe without assistance (e.g., neurologic injury, respiratory decompensation, oxygenation failure, decreased respiratory drive).
2. Inspiration is ventilator driven; expiration occurs through natural recoil of the lungs.
3. Tidal volume (TV), respiratory rate, Fio_2, and inspiratory pressure (i.e., pressure forcing each inspiration) may be adjusted depending on patient's respiratory drive, pulmonary compliance, and oxygenation status.
4. Patients are weaned from the ventilator by changing from more patient-independent modes to more patient-dependent modes.
5. **Extubation** (removal of the tube) can be performed when the patient is capable of breathing independently.

XI. Pediatric Pulmonary Concerns

A. Croup

1. Acute inflammation of larynx caused by **parainfluenza virus types 1 and 2**; less commonly by parainfluenza virus type 3, respiratory syncytial virus (RSV), influenza virus, rubeola, adenovirus, or *Mycoplasma pneumoniae*
2. Most common between 3 months and 5 years of age
3. **H/P** = nasal congestion, **barking cough**, dyspnea, **inspiratory stridor**; fever, mild pharyngeal erythema, lymphadenopathy; respiratory distress in severe cases
4. **Radiology** = neck radiographs may show subglottic narrowing of airway (i.e., **steeple sign**) (see Figure 2-9)
5. **Treatment** = supportive care (e.g., hydration, humidified air, rest, analgesia); aerosolized epinephrine and glucocorticoids (oral, intramuscular, or inhaled) can be used in severe cases to decrease pharyngeal inflammation; with concerns for respiratory distress, the child should be admitted for observation

MNEMONIC

Remember the symptoms of severe cases of croup by the 3 Ss: **S**eal-bark cough, **S**ubglottic swelling, and **S**tridor.

NEXT STEP

If child develops stridor at rest, hospitalization and respiratory monitoring is needed.

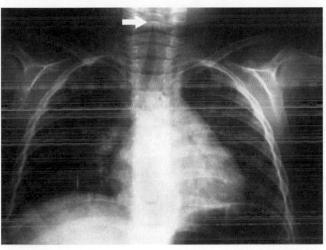

FIGURE 2-9 Chest X-ray of a child with croup demonstrating subglottic narrowing of the airway (*arrow*), which is reminiscent of the shape of a steeple (steeple sign).

(From Wolfson AB, Cloutier RL, Hendey GW, Ling LJ; Schaider JJ, & Rosen CL. [2015]. *Harwood-Nuss' Clinical Practice of Emergency Medicine* [6th ed., p. 1220]. Philadelphia: Wolters Kluwer; with permission.)

B. Epiglottitis

1. Rapidly progressive infection of epiglottis and surrounding tissues that can cause airway obstruction
2. Most common in children from 2 to 7 years of age
3. Caused by *Haemophilus influenzae type B* (Hib) infection; can also be caused by streptococcal or other *H. influenzae* bacteria
4. **H/P** = **dysphagia**, drooling, soft stridor, **muffled voice**, anxiety from symptoms; sudden high fever, inspiratory retractions; child may lean forward with hands on knees to aid breathing; erythematous and swollen epiglottis
5. **Labs** = culture from swab of epiglottis can determine causative bacteria (should only be performed if patient is intubated)
6. **Radiology** = neck radiographs show swollen, opacified epiglottis that partially obstructs the airway (i.e., **thumbprint sign**); laryngoscope (only used in controlled situations) can visualize red and swollen epiglottis (see Figure 2-10)
7. **Treatment** = keep child calm; admit for close observation and respiratory monitoring; unless airway obstruction is mild, **intubate** (nasotracheal) to maintain airway patency; antibiotics for 7 to 10 days; airway obstruction preventing intubation requires emergent tracheostomy

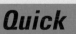
Quick HIT

In cases of suspected epiglottitis, examine the patient's throat **only** in a setting in which prompt intubation is possible because examination of the patient's throat can lead to additional throat irritation and resulting occlusion.

Quick HIT

Widespread use of the **Hib vaccine** has greatly decreased the incidence of epiglottitis.

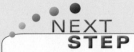
Pulmonary Disorders

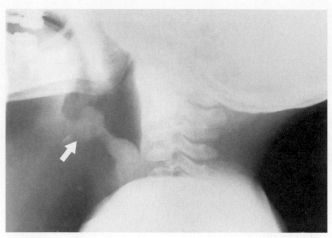

FIGURE
2-10 Lateral chest X-ray of a child with epiglottitis demonstrating a swollen epiglottis (*arrow*) that resembles a thumbprint (thumbprint sign).

(From Wolfson AB, Cloutier RL, Hendey GW, Ling LJ; Schaider JJ, & Rosen CL. [2015]. *Harwood-Nuss' Clinical Practice of Emergency Medicine* [6th ed., p. 1219]. Philadelphia: Wolters Kluwer; with permission.)

C. Bronchiolitis

1. Viral infection of bronchioles caused by **RSV** (most cases) or parainfluenza virus type 3 (less common)
2. Most commonly occurs in winter and spring; usually found in children <2 years of age
3. H/P = nasal congestion, cough, **respiratory distress; wheezing**, fever, tachypnea, crackles, prolonged expiration, hyperresonance to percussion
4. **Radiology** = CXR shows hyperinflation of lungs and patchy infiltrates
5. **Treatment** = adequate hydration, humidified air; inhaled bronchodilators (e.g., β_2-agonists, epinephrine) and systemic glucocorticoids are contraindicated; children with respiratory distress or hypoxemia should be admitted for observation and respiratory monitoring
6. **Complications** = increased risk of developing asthma

D. Respiratory distress syndrome of the newborn

1. Preterm infants (e.g., 24 to 37 weeks' gestation and especially before 30 weeks' gestation) have **surfactant deficiency** because of lung immaturity that leads to decreased lung compliance, atelectasis, and respiratory failure.
2. H/P = **presentation within 2 days of birth**; cyanosis, nasal flaring, expiratory grunting, intercostal retractions, respiratory rate >60 breaths/min, crackles, decreased breath sounds
3. **Labs** = ABG shows increased CO_2, decreased O_2; amniotic fluid analysis (see Figure 2-11) not usually helpful but may guide treatment between 34 and 37 weeks' gestation by determining fetal lung maturity with the amniotic lecithin:sphingomyelin ratio (always treat for <34 weeks, treatment typically unnecessary for >37 weeks)
4. **Radiology** = CXR shows bilateral atelectasis with **ground glass** appearance and decreased lung volumes
5. **Treatment** = maternal administration of corticosteroids before initiation of labor helps to speed fetal lung maturation; neonatal intensive care unit (NICU) admission appropriate for close observation; supplemental O_2 and **surfactant replacement** therapy mainstays of therapy; intubation should be performed for any neonate not responding to treatment or requiring high levels of O_2 to maintain adequate Sao_2
6. **Complications** = increased risk of developing **asthma** in childhood compared with other children

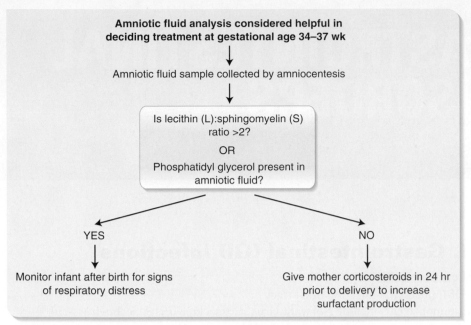

FIGURE
2-11 Amniotic fluid analysis protocol used to determine fetal lung maturity.

E. Meconium aspiration syndrome

1. Aspiration of meconium (i.e., fetal stool passed into amniotic sac) predelivery, causing obstruction of airways and pneumonia
2. **H/P = meconium-stained amniotic fluid** seen during delivery; cyanosis, intercostal retractions, distended chest, tachypnea
3. **Labs** = consider blood culture to rule out sepsis
4. **Radiology** = CXR shows atelectasis, areas of hyperinflation, or pneumothorax
5. **Treatment** = suction nose, mouth, and upper airway at birth; supplemental O$_2$; intubate for worsening respiratory distress; surfactant therapy may be useful for improving respiratory function; consider empiric antibiotic therapy if concerned for development of pneumonia
6. **Complications** = pulmonary hypertension can develop if not promptly treated; increased risk of developing asthma during childhood

F. Cystic fibrosis (CF)

1. Autosomal recessive disorder caused by defect in chloride-pumping channel in exocrine glands; ducts of exocrine glands (e.g., lungs, pancreas, reproductive glands) become clogged with thick secretions
2. Presents in childhood and is universally fatal, but proper treatment may allow survival into 30s and 40s
3. Affects both pulmonary (recurrent infections, chronic sinusitis) and gastrointestinal systems (pancreatic enzyme deficiencies, malabsorption)
4. **Risk factors** = whites at higher risk than other races
5. **H/P = recurrent pulmonary infections** (e.g., *Pseudomonas, Staphylococcus aureus*), dyspnea, hemoptysis, chronic sinusitis, cough, meconium ileus at birth, steatorrhea, failure to thrive; cyanosis, digital clubbing, esophageal varices, rectal prolapse
6. **Labs** = decreased serum Na; **sweat test** shows increased Na and increased Cl (>60 mEq/L in children, >80 in adults); genetic testing can locate mutation in CF transmembrane conductance regulator (CFTR) gene in suspected cases or in carriers of the gene considering pregnancy
7. **Treatment** = deoxyribonuclease (DNase) aids in decreasing the viscosity of secretions; chest physical therapy helps to clear secretions; bronchodilators, nonsteroidal anti-inflammatory drugs (NSAIDs), antibiotics for any suspected pulmonary exacerbation or infection; supplemental pancreatic enzymes and vitamins A, D, E, and K given for malabsorption

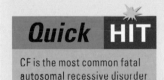

Quick HIT

CF is the most common fatal autosomal recessive disorder in the United States.

3

GASTROINTESTINAL DISORDERS

 ## I. Gastrointestinal (GI) Infections

A. Viral gastroenteritis

1. Self-limited viral infection of GI tract
2. Common agents include **Norwalk virus**, Coxsackie virus Al, echovirus, and adenovirus; **rotavirus** is common in children.
3. **History and physical (H/P)** = nausea, vomiting, diarrhea, abdominal pain, myalgias; low-grade fever
4. **Labs** = no fecal white blood cells; viral culture indicates pathogen (usually unnecessary)
5. **Treatment** = self-limited (48 to 72 hours); maintain hydration status

B. Bacterial gastroenteritis *(see Table 3-1)*

C. Parasitic and protozoan GI infections *(see Table 3-2, Figure 3-1)*

D. Hepatitis

1. Inflammatory disease of the liver is most commonly caused by **viral infection**; it can also result from alcohol or toxins.
2. Acute hepatitis is initial disease; chronic form is disease lasting >6 months
3. **Risk factors** = intravenous drug abuse (IVDA), alcoholism, travel to developing nations, poor sanitation
4. Patterns of transmission vary with virus type (see Table 3-3).
5. **H/P** = possibly asymptomatic; malaise, arthralgias, fatigue, nausea, vomiting, right upper quadrant pain; jaundice, scleral icterus, tender hepatomegaly, splenomegaly, lymphadenopathy
6. **Labs** = bilirubinuria, **increased aspartate aminotransferase (AST), increased alanine aminotransferase (ALT)**, increased bilirubin (total), increased alkaline phosphatase
   a. Hepatitis A virus (HAV): anti-HAV IgM antibodies present during illness; anti-HAV IgG antibodies present after resolution
   b. Hepatitis B virus (HBV): antigens and antibodies detected vary with disease state (see Figure 3-2, Table 3-4)
   c. Hepatitis C virus (HCV): anti-HCV antibodies and positive HCV polymerase chain reaction indicate infection (see Figure 3-3)
7. **Treatment** = rest, frequently self-limited (**except HCV**); interferon-α (IFN-α) or antivirals for HBV; IFN-α ± ribavirin for HCV; hospitalization for hepatic failure; immunoglobulin given to close contacts of patients with HAV; HAV vaccine given to travelers to developing nations; HBV vaccine routinely given to children and health care workers

TABLE 3-1 Common Pathogens in Bacterial Gastroenteritis

Pathogen	Source	Signs and Symptoms	Treatment
Bacillus cereus	Fried rice	**Vomiting** within several hours of eating, diarrhea later	Self-limited; hydration
Campylobacter jejuni	Poultry (second most common foodborne bacterial GI infection)	**Bloody** diarrhea, abdominal pain, fever; rare Guillain-Barré syndrome	Hydration, erythromycin; generally self-limited
Clostridium botulinum	Honey, home-canned foods	Nausea, vomiting, diarrhea, **flaccid paralysis**	Botulism antitoxin (not given to infants); self-limited
Clostridium difficile	**Antibiotic-induced suppression** of normal colonic flora	**Watery or bloody** diarrhea; gray pseudomembranes seen on colonic mucosa	Metronidazole, vancomycin
Escherichia coli (enterotoxigenic)	Food/water (**travelers'** diarrhea)	**Watery** diarrhea, vomiting, fever	Hydration; self-limited (often treated with FQ)
E. coli type **O157:H7** (enterohemorrhagic)	Ground beef, indirect fecal contamination	**Bloody** diarrhea, vomiting, fever, abdominal pain (risk of HUS)	Hydration; self-limited; antibiotics may actually worsen symptoms because of toxin release
Staphylococcus aureus	Room-temperature food (caused by preformed toxin)	**Vomiting** within several hours of eating; diarrhea later	Self-limited; hydration
Salmonella species	Eggs, poultry, milk, fresh produce (**most common foodborne bacterial GI infection**)	Nausea, abdominal pain, **bloody** diarrhea, fever, vomiting	Hydration; self-limited; treat immunocompromised patients with FQ
Shigella species	Food/water; associated with overcrowding	Fever, nausea, vomiting, **severe bloody** diarrhea, abdominal pain (risk of HUS)	Hydration; self-limited; ciprofloxacin, TMP-SMX in severe cases
Vibrio cholerae	Water, seafood	**Copious watery** diarrhea, signs of dehydration	**Hydration;** tetracycline or doxycycline decreases disease length
Vibrio parahaemolyticus	Seafood (oysters)	Abdominal pain, **watery** diarrhea within 24 hr of eating	Hydration; self-limited
Yersinia enterocolitica	Pork, fresh produce	Abdominal pain, **bloody** diarrhea, right lower quadrant pain, fever	Hydration; self-limited

FQ, fluoroquinolone; GI, gastrointestinal; HUS, hemolytic uremic syndrome; TMP-SMX, trimethoprim-sulfamethoxazole.

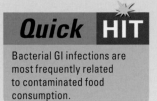

Quick HIT

Bacterial GI infections are most frequently related to contaminated food consumption.

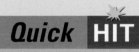

Quick HIT

Hemolytic uremic syndrome (HUS) is a complication of *E. coli* O157:H7 infection and is characterized by thrombocytopenia, hemolytic anemia, and acute renal failure; it is usually self-limited.

Gastrointestinal Disorders

TABLE **3-2**	**Common Pathogens in Parasitic and Protozoan Gastrointestinal Infections**		
Pathogen	**Source**	**Signs and Symptoms**	**Treatment**
Giardia lamblia (Figure 3-1)	Surface water (usually limited to wilderness or other countries)	**Greasy**, foul-smelling diarrhea; abdominal pain, malaise; cysts and trophozoites seen in stool sample	Metronidazole; hydration
Entamoeba histolytica	Water, areas of poor sanitation	Mild to severe **bloody** diarrhea, abdominal pain; cysts and trophozoites seen in stool sample	Metronidazole, paromomycin
Cryptosporidium parvum	Food/water; immunocompromised patients	**Watery** diarrhea, abdominal pain, malaise; acid-fast stain of stool shows parasites	Control immune suppression; nitazoxanide
Trichinella spiralis	Undercooked pork	Fever, **myalgias**, periorbital edema; eosinophilia	Albendazole, mebendazole if CNS or cardiac symptoms
Taenia solium (intestinal taeniasis)	Ingestion of cysts in undercooked pork	Nausea, abdominal pain	Praziquantel
Taenia solium (cysticercosis)	Fecal/oral transmission of eggs from feces of human with intestinal taeniasis	Cysts in muscles, subcutaneous tissues, eyes and extraocular muscles, brain (**neurocysticercosis**); may cause seizures	Albendazole plus corticosteroids for neurocysticercosis

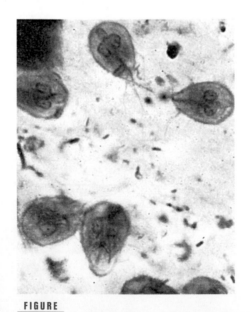

FIGURE
3-1 Giardiasis; several trophozoites are seen with characteristic pear-shaped and paired nuclei resembling owls' eyes.

(From Diallo, A.O., Chandrasekha V. [2005]. *Microbiology Recall.* Philadelphia: Lippincott Williams & Wilkins; with permission.)

TABLE **3-3**	Characteristics of Viral Hepatitis				
Hepatitis Virus	**Virus Type**	**Spread**	**Treatment**	**Prevention**	**Complications**
A (HAV)	Picornavirus (single-stranded RNA)	Food (**shellfish**), fecal–oral	Self-limited; supportive care	Vaccine before travel	Can occur in epidemics
B (HBV)	Hepadnavirus (double-stranded DNA)	Blood, other body fluids (including **sexual contact**)	HBV immediately after exposure in unvaccinated patients; IFN-α or antivirals (lamivudine, adefovir, entecavir)	**Vaccine**	5% of adults (90% of children) develop chronic hepatitis, cirrhosis, 3%–5% develop **hepatocellular carcinoma**, persistent carrier state, 1% develop fulminant hepatic failure
C (HCV)	Flavivirus (single-stranded RNA)	**Blood,** possibly-sexual contact	IFN-α; consider ribavirin	No vaccine	80% of patients develop **chronic hepatitis,** 50% with chronic HCV develop cirrhosis, slightly increased risk of hepatocellular carcinoma, persistent carrier state
D	Delta agent (incomplete single-stranded RNA)	Blood; **requires coexistent hepatitis B infection**	IFN-α	Hepatitis B vaccine	Severe hepatitis, cirrhosis, persistent carrier state
E	Calicivirus (single-stranded RNA)	Water, fecal–oral	Self limited; supportive care	No vaccine	High maternal mortality when occurring in **pregnant** women

HAV, hepatitis A virus; HBV, hepatitis B virus; HCV, hepatitis C virus; IFN, interferon.

Gastrointestinal Disorders

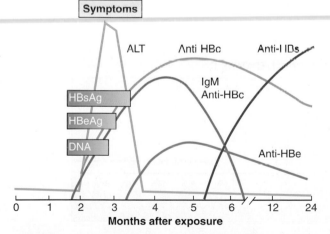

FIGURE
3-2 **Trends in serology and symptoms seen in various courses in acute hepatitis B virus (HBV) infection with resolution of disease.**

ALT, alanine aminotransferase. HBV surface antigen (HBsAg) and HBV e antigen (HBeAg) are detectable from approximately 1 to 4 months and coincide with appearance of symptoms. Antibodies are indicative of previous infection or vaccination.

(From Nettina, S. M. [2015]. *The Lippincott Manual of Nursing Practice* [10th ed., p. 715]. Philadelphia: Wolters Kluwer; with permission.)

TABLE 3-4	Serologies Seen in Various Disease States of HBV Infection			
Course of Disease	**HBV Surface Antigen(HBsAg)**	**HBV e Antigen (HBeAg)**	**HBV Surface Antibody (Anti-HBs)**	**HBV Core Antibody (Anti-HBc)**
Acute infection (4–12 wk postexposure)	Positive	Positive	Negative	Positive (IgM)
Acute infection window period (12–20 wk postexposure)	Negative	Negative	Negative	Positive (IgM)
Chronic infection, active viral replication	Positive	Positive	Negative	Positive (IgG)
Chronic infection, lesser viral replication (good prognosis)	Positive	Negative	Negative	Positive (IgG)
Past infection (recovered)	Negative	Negative	Positive	Positive (IgG)
Vaccination	Negative	Negative	Positive	Negative

HBV, hepatitis B virus.

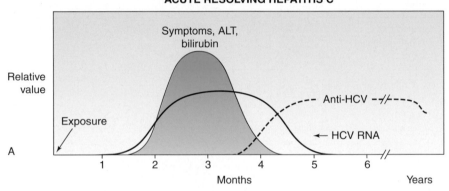

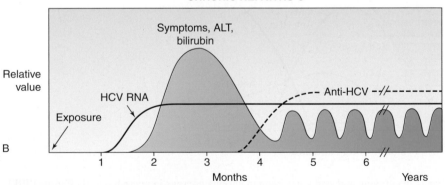

FIGURE 3-3 **Trends in serology and symptoms seen in hepatitis C virus (HCV) infection.**

ALT, alanine aminotransferase. (**A**) Acute resolving infection. (**B**) Chronic HCV infection with intermittent exacerbations of symptoms.

(From Rubin R., & Strayer D. S. [2012]. *Rubin's Pathology Image Collection* [6th ed., p. 702]. Philadelphia: Wolters Kluwer/Lippincott Williams & Wilkins; with permission.)

II. Oral and Esophageal Conditions

A. Salivary gland disorders

1. Dysfunction in sublingual, submandibular, or parotid glands resulting from ductal obstruction or inflammation
2. May be caused by sialolithiasis (ductal stone) in any salivary gland; parotid disease can also be caused by sarcoidosis, infection, or neoplasm
3. **H/P** = enlarged and painful glands; pain worsens during eating; parotid glands may have painless swelling
4. **Treatment** = warm compresses, massage, or lemon drops may help remove ductal stones; antibiotics and hydration for infection; surgery may be required for relief in refractory cases

B. Dysphagia

1. Difficulty swallowing because of oropharyngeal or esophageal transport dysfunction or pain with swallowing (i.e., odynophagia)
2. May be caused by neuromuscular disorders (e.g., achalasia, motility disorders, scleroderma) or obstruction (e.g., peptic strictures, esophageal webs or rings, cancer, radiation fibrosis)
3. **Obstructive** pathology tends to limit swallowing of **solids**; **neuromuscular** pathology tends to limit swallowing of **solids and liquids**.
4. **H/P** = feeling of **"food stuck in throat"** when swallowing, cough, solids (mechanical pathology) or solids and liquids (dysmotility) may be difficult to swallow
5. **Labs** = manometry measures esophageal pressure and may detect neuromuscular abnormality
6. **Radiology** = barium swallow and esophagogastroduodenoscopy (EGD) may be helpful for diagnosis
7. **Treatment** = varies with etiology

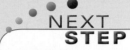

NEXT STEP

If a patient presents with dysphagia, perform a **barium swallow** before an EGD because of the lower associated risks of the former.

C. Achalasia

1. Neuromuscular disorder of esophagus with **impaired peristalsis and decreased lower esophageal sphincter (LES) relaxation** because of intramural neuron dysfunction
2. Idiopathic; most commonly affects persons 25 to 60 years of age
3. **H/P** = gradually progressive dysphagia of **solids and liquids**, regurgitation, cough, aspiration, heartburn, weight loss from poor intake
4. **Labs** = manometry shows increased LES pressure, incomplete LES relaxation, and decreased peristalsis
5. **Radiology** = barium swallow shows **"bird's beak"** sign with tapering at the LES (see Figure 3-4); EGD needed to rule out malignancy
6. **Treatment** = nitrates and calcium channel blockers relax LES but are rarely used because of simultaneous cardiac effects; pneumatic dilation, botulinum injections, or myotomy relieve obstruction
7. **Complications** = myotomy can cause gastroesophageal reflux disease (GERD)

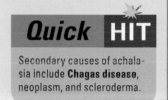

Quick HIT

Secondary causes of achalasia include **Chagas disease**, neoplasm, and scleroderma.

D. Diffuse esophageal spasm

1. Neuromuscular disorder in which nonperistaltic contractions of the esophagus occur
2. **H/P** = chest pain, dysphagia
3. **Labs** = manometry shows nonperistaltic, uncoordinated esophageal contractions
4. **Radiology** = barium swallow shows **"corkscrew"** pattern (see Figure 3-5)
5. **Treatment** = calcium channel blockers, nitrates, or tricyclic antidepressants help reduce chest pain and dysphagia

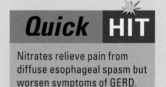

Quick HIT

Nitrates relieve pain from diffuse esophageal spasm but worsen symptoms of GERD.

E. Zenker diverticulum

1. Outpouching in upper posterior esophagus caused by smooth muscle weakness
2. **H/P** = bad breath, difficulty initiating swallowing, **regurgitation of food several days after eating**, occasional dysphagia, feeling of aspiration, neck mass that increases in size while drinking liquids

Gastrointestinal Disorders

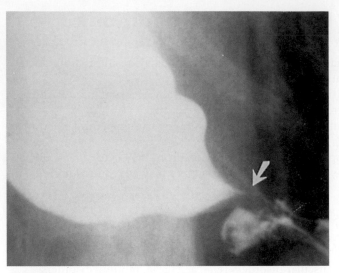

FIGURE 3-4 **Achalasia**

Barium swallow in a patient with achalasia; note the distended proximal esophagus with distal tapering and "bird's beak" sign (*white arrow*).

(From Eisenberg, R. L. [2003]. *An Atlas of Differential Diagnosis*. [4th ed., p. 397]. Philadelphia: Lippincott Williams & Wilkins; with permission.)

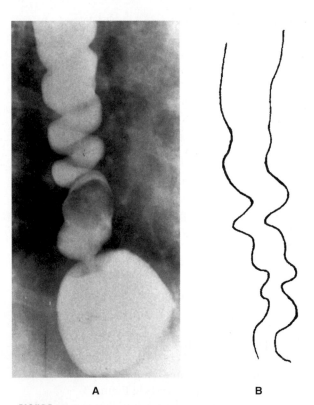

A   B

FIGURE 3-5 **Diffuse esophageal spasm**

(**A**) Barium swallow in a patient with diffuse esophageal spasm; notice the "corkscrew" pattern throughout the visible esophagus. (**B**) Illustration of diffuse esophageal spasm demonstrating twisting "corkscrew" pattern.

(From Eisenberg, R. L. [2010]. *Clinical Imaging: An Atlas of Differential Diagnosis* [5th ed.]. Philadelphia: Wolters Kluwer/Lippincott Williams & Wilkins; with permission.)

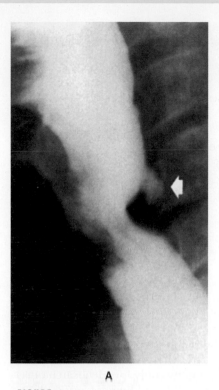 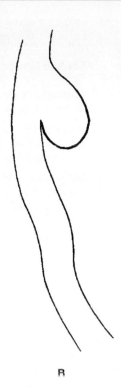

A   B

FIGURE
3-6   Zenker diverticulum

(**A**) Barium swallow in a patient with a small Zenker diverticulum (*white arrow*). (**B**) Illustration of Zenker diverticulum demonstrating outpouching of esophagus.

(From Eisenberg, R. L. [2010]. *Clinical Imaging: An Atlas of Differential Diagnosis* [5th ed.]. Philadelphia: Wolters Kluwer/Lippincott Williams & Wilkins; with permission.)

3. **Radiology** = barium swallow shows outpouching (see Figure 3-6)
4. **Treatment** = cricopharyngeal myotomy or diverticulectomy
5. **Complications** = EGD can perforate weakness in esophageal wall; vocal cord paralysis, mediastinitis possible with surgery

F. Gastroesophageal reflux disease (GERD)

1. Low pressure in LES leads to abnormal reflux of gastric contents into esophagus.
2. **Risk factors** = obesity, hiatal hernia, pregnancy, scleroderma
3. Symptoms can worsen with consumption of alcohol and fatty foods or with tobacco use.
4. **H/P** = **burning chest pain** ("heartburn") 30 to 90 min after eating, sour taste in mouth, regurgitation, dysphagia, odynophagia, nausea, cough; pain may worsen when lying down and lessen with standing
5. **Labs** = esophageal pH monitoring can detect increased acidity from reflux
6. **Radiology** = usually unneeded for diagnosis; EGD, chest radiograph, or barium swallow can help rule out neoplasm, Barrett esophagus, and hiatal hernia
7. **Treatment**
   a. Elevation of head of bed, weight loss, dietary modification
   b. Initial medications are antacids followed by H_2 antagonists or proton pump inhibitors (PPI) (see Table 3-5).
   c. Refractory disease may be treated with Nissen fundoplication or hiatal hernia repair.
8. **Complications** = esophageal ulceration, esophageal stricture, Barrett esophagus, adenocarcinoma

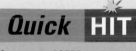

Quick HIT

Symptoms of GERD can resemble those of asthma or myocardial infarction.

Gastrointestinal Disorders

TABLE 3-5	Medications Used in Treatment of GERD		
Medication	**Mechanism**	**Adverse Effects**	**Prescription Strategy**
Antacids (calcium carbonate, aluminum hydroxide, etc.)	Neutralize gastric acid	Constipation (aluminum), nausea, diarrhea (magnesium)	Initial therapy, as needed
H_2 antagonists (cimetidine, ranitidine, etc.)	Reversibly block histamine H_2 receptors to inhibit gastric acid secretion	Headache, diarrhea, rare thrombocytopenia; cimetidine may cause gynecomastia and impotence	Patients not responding to antacids
PPIs (omeprazole, lansoprazole, etc.)	Irreversibly inhibit parietal cell proton pump (H^+/K^+ ATPase) to block gastric acid secretion	Well tolerated; may increase effects of warfarin, benzodiazepines, or phenytoin in some patients	Patients not responding to antacids

GERD, gastroesophageal reflux disease; H^+, hydrogen ion; K^+, potassium ion; LES, lower esophageal sphincter; PPIs, proton pump inhibitors.

G. Esophageal cancer
1. **Squamous cell carcinoma** (more common worldwide) or adenocarcinoma (more common in the United States) of esophagus
2. **Barrett esophagus** (intestinal metaplasia of distal esophagus secondary to chronic GERD) commonly precedes adenocarcinoma.
3. **Risk factors** = alcohol, tobacco, chronic GERD, obesity (only for adenocarcinoma)
4. **H/P** = progressive dysphagia (initially solids, later solids and liquids), weight loss, odynophagia, reflux, GI bleeding, vomiting, weakness, cough, hoarseness
5. **Labs** = biopsy used to make diagnosis
6. **Radiology** = barium swallow shows narrowing of esophagus and abnormal mass (see Figure 3-7); magnetic resonance imaging (MRI), computed tomography (CT) with contrast, or positron emission tomography (PET) scan can determine extension and metastases; EGD used to identify mass and perform biopsy

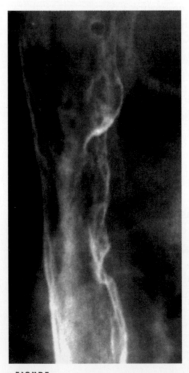

FIGURE 3-7 Barium swallow in a patient with squamous cell carcinoma of the esophagus; note the irregularity of the left esophageal wall due to neoplastic mass.

(From Eisenberg, R. L. [1996]. *Gastrointestinal Radiology: A Pattern Approach* [3rd ed.]. Philadelphia: Lippincott-Raven; with permission.)

Gastrointestinal Disorders

7. **Treatment** = surgical resection (including total esophagectomy) for early stage disease; radiation and chemotherapy used in nonoperative (advanced) cases or as neoadjuvant therapy to surgery
8. **Complications** = poor prognosis; local extension and metastases are frequently present by time of diagnosis

 ## III. Gastric Conditions

A. Hiatal hernia

1. Herniation of part of stomach above diaphragm
2. Types
   a. **Sliding:** gastroesophageal junction and stomach displaced through diaphragm (95% of cases)
   b. **Paraesophageal:** stomach protrudes through diaphragm, but gastroesophageal junction remains in normal location
3. **H/P** = possibly asymptomatic; symptoms associated with GERD
4. **Radiology** = barium swallow shows portion of stomach above diaphragm; chest radiograph may detect hernia without barium swallow if air in stomach is visible above diaphragm
5. **Treatment** = sliding hernias can be treated with reflux control; paraesophageal hernias may need surgical repair (e.g., gastropexy, Nissen fundoplication)
6. **Complications** = incarceration of stomach in herniation (seen in paraesophageal type)

B. Gastritis

1. Inflammation of gastric mucosa
2. Can be **acute (erosive)** or **chronic (nonerosive)**
3. Acute gastritis is characterized by rapidly developing, superficial lesions secondary to nonsteroidal anti-inflammatory drug (**NSAID**) use, alcohol, ingestion of corrosive materials, or **stress from severe illness**; it can involve any region of the stomach.
4. Chronic gastritis can occur in either the antrum or fundus of the stomach (see Table 3-6).
5. **H/P** = possibly asymptomatic; epigastric pain, indigestion, nausea, **vomiting**, hematemesis, melena; symptoms more common for acute form
6. **Labs** = positive urea breath test (detects increase in pH from ammonia-producing bacteria) and positive IgG antibody to *Helicobacter pylori* with existing infection; ratio of pepsinogen isoenzymes useful to detect autoimmune cause; **antral biopsy** can detect *H. pylori* infection
7. **Radiology** = EGD allows visualization of gastric mucosa to detect lesions and perform biopsy.

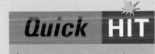

In pernicious anemia, autoantibodies destroy parietal cells, leading to low levels of intrinsic factor, vitamin B_{12} malabsorption, and megaloblastic anemia.

TABLE **3-6**	Characteristics of Type A and B Chronic Gastritis	
Characteristic	**Type A**	**Type B**
Frequency	10% of cases	90% of cases
Site	Fundus	Antrum
Pathology	Autoantibodies for parietal cells	Associated with *Helicobacter pylori* infection
Labs	Decreased gastric acid level, decreased gastrin	Increased gastric acid level
Associated conditions	Pernicious anemia, achlorhydria, thyroiditis	Peptic ulcer disease, gastric cancer

Gastrointestinal Disorders

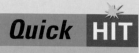

Quick HIT

Ulcers can also develop secondary to stress from severe burns (**Curling ulcers**) or intracranial injuries (**Cushing ulcers**).

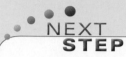

NEXT STEP

In refractory cases of PUD, gastrin level should be determined to detect Zollinger-Ellison syndrome (increased gastrin).

Quick HIT

Barium swallow radiographic findings that suggest the presence of a malignant lesion associated with an ulcer include **abnormal-appearing mucosal folds** in the region of the ulcer, presence of a **mass** near the ulcer, and irregular **filling defects** in the base of the ulcer.

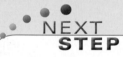

NEXT STEP

Workup for patients <40 years of age in whom concern exists for PUD can frequently be done with **noninvasive** testing; older patients or those with a previous ulcer should have an **EGD** performed.

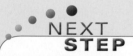

NEXT STEP

Give cyclooxygenase-2 (COX-2) selective NSAID to patients with PUD who require NSAID therapy.

Quick HIT

PPI must be stopped before gastrin level testing to collect an accurate measurement.

8. Treatment
   a. Treat acute form as peptic ulcer disease (PUD) and stop alcohol and offending medications; give H_2 antagonists or PPI to patients with severe illnesses.
   b. Type A chronic gastritis requires vitamin B_{12} replacement.
   c. Type B chronic gastritis requires eradication of *H. pylori* through multidrug treatment (typically, PPI, clarithromycin, and either amoxicillin or metronidazole for 7 to 14 days).

C. Peptic ulcer disease (PUD)

1. Erosion of gastric and duodenal mucosa secondary to impaired endothelial defenses and increased gastric acidity (see Table 3-7)
2. *H. pylori* is involved in pathology in **most gastric ulcers** and **almost all duodenal ulcers**.
3. **Risk factors** = *H. pylori* **infection**, NSAID use, tobacco, alcohol, corticosteroids; males > females
4. **H/P** = periodic **burning epigastric pain** that can change (better or worse) with eating, nausea, hematemesis, melena, hematochezia; epigastric tenderness; abdominal rigidity, rebound tenderness, and rigidity seen following acute perforation of ulcer
5. **Labs** = positive urea breath test, IgG antibodies, or biopsy detect *H. pylori*; complete blood count (CBC) can assess degree of GI bleeding
6. **Radiology** = abdominal X-ray (AXR) to detect perforation (free air under diaphragm seen following perforation); barium swallow AXR can demonstrate collections of barium in ulcerations; EGD used to perform biopsy and detect active bleeding
7. Treatment
   a. **Active bleeding** must be ruled out with CBC and EGD in patients with concerning symptoms; symptoms lasting >2 months need EGD to rule out gastric adenocarcinoma.
   b. Decrease gastric acid levels with **PPI** and **H_2 antagonist**; protect mucosa with sucralfate, bismuth subsalicylate, or misoprostol; **eliminate *H. pylori* infection** (as described previously for treatment of gastritis).
   c. Surgery is required to repair acute perforations; persistent, non-neoplastic refractory cases may require parietal cell vagotomy or antrectomy.
8. **Complications** = hemorrhage (posterior ulcers may erode into **gastroduodenal artery**), perforation (most commonly anterior ulcers), lymphoproliferative disease

D. Zollinger-Ellison syndrome

1. Syndrome secondary to gastrin-producing tumor most frequently located in duodenum (70% cases) or pancreas
2. Associated with malabsorption disorders

TABLE 3-7	Distinguishing between Gastric and Duodenal Ulcers	
Characteristic	**Gastric Ulcer**	**Duodenal Ulcer**
Patients	Age >50 yr old, *Helicobacter pylori* infection, NSAID users	Younger, *H. pylori* infection
Frequency	25% of cases	75% of cases
Timing of pain	**Soon after** eating	**2–4 hr after** eating
Gastric acid level	Normal/low	High
Gastrin level	High	Normal
Effect of eating	May **worsen** symptoms and cause nausea and vomiting	**Initial improvement** in symptoms, with later **worsening**

NSAID, nonsteroidal anti-inflammatory drug.

3. **H/P = refractory PUD**, abdominal pain, nausea, vomiting, indigestion, diarrhea, steatorrhea, possible history of other endocrine abnormalities
4. **Labs = increased fasting gastrin**; positive secretin-stimulation test (i.e., administration of secretin causes higher than expected serum gastrin levels); specific gastrin sampling in several pancreatic or abdominal veins can help localize tumor
5. **Radiology** = somatostatin receptor imaging using single-photon emission computed tomography (SPECT) can localize tumors; angiography may detect tumor if hypervascular
6. **Treatment** = surgical resection can be performed for nonmetastatic disease in which a tumor can be localized (best chance in extrapancreatic tumors); PPI and H_2 antagonists may ease symptoms; octreotide may help reduce symptoms in metastatic disease
7. **Complications** = occasionally associated with other endocrine tumors (e.g., multiple endocrine neoplasia I [MEN I]); 60% of lesions are malignant

E. Gastric cancer

1. **Adenocarcinoma** (common) or squamous cell carcinoma (rare; caused by invasion from esophagus) affecting stomach
2. Types
    a. **Ulcerating**: resembles ulcers seen in PUD
    b. **Polypoid**: large, intraluminal neoplasms
    c. **Superficial spreading**: mucosal and submucosal involvement only; best prognosis
    d. **Linitis plastica**: all layers of stomach involved; decreased stomach elasticity; poor prognosis
3. **Risk factors** = *H. pylori*, **family history**, Japanese person living in Japan, tobacco, alcohol, vitamin C deficiency, high consumption of preserved foods; males > females
4. **H/P** = weight loss, anorexia, early satiety, vomiting, dysphagia, epigastric pain; enlarged left supraclavicular lymph node (i.e., **Virchow node**) or periumbilical node (i.e., **Sister Mary Joseph node**)
5. **Labs** = increased carcinoembryonic antigen (CEA), increased 2-glucuronidase in gastric secretions, anemia if active bleeding; biopsy used for diagnosis
6. **Radiology** = barium swallow may show mass or thickened "leather bottle" stomach (linitis plastica); **EGD** used to perform biopsy and visualize ulcers
7. **Treatment** = subtotal gastrectomy for lesions in distal third of stomach, total gastrectomy for lesions in middle or upper stomach or invasive lesions; adjuvant chemotherapy and radiation therapy
8. **Complications** = early detection has high cure rate (>70%) but poor prognosis in later detection (<15% 5-year survival)

IV. Intestinal Conditions

A. Malabsorption disorders (*see Figure 3-8, Figure 3-9*)

1. Celiac disease
    a. Genetic disorder characterized by gluten intolerance (e.g., wheat, barley, rye)
    b. Immune-mediated process with IgA anti-tissue transglutaminase (TTG) and antiendomysial antibodies that cause jejunal mucosal damage
    c. **H/P** = failure to thrive, bloating, and abnormal stools in infants; diarrhea, steatorrhea, weight loss, and bloating in adults; some patients will exhibit depression, anxiety, or arthralgias; associated with Down syndrome; associated with dermatitis herpetiformis
    d. **Labs** = positive antiendomysial and antigliadin antibodies in serum; biopsy shows blunting of duodenal and jejunal villi
    e. **Treatment** = removal of gluten from diet (can still eat corn, rice); refractory disease may require corticosteroids
2. Tropical sprue
    a. Malabsorption syndrome similar to celiac sprue, with possible infectious or toxic etiology
    b. Acquired disorder in patients living in **tropical areas**; can present years after leaving tropics

---

Quick HIT

The general presentation of malabsorption includes weight loss, **bloating, diarrhea**, possible **steatorrhea**, glossitis, dermatitis, and edema.

Quick HIT

Celiac and tropical sprue exhibit the same symptoms, but only celiac sprue responds to removal of gluten from the diet, and tropical sprue occurs in patients who have spent time in the tropics.

Gastrointestinal Disorders

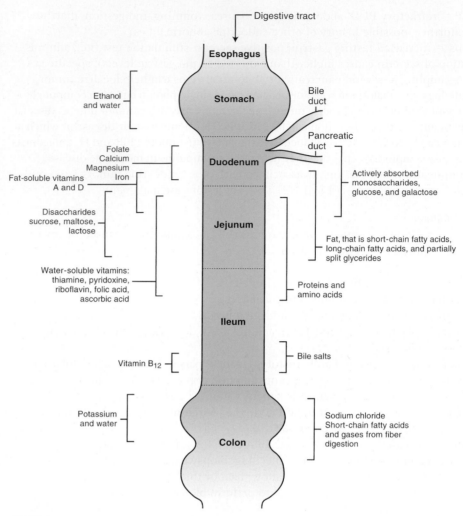

3-8 **Location of absorption of vitamins, minerals, and nutrients throughout the gastrointestinal (GI) tract.**

(Modified from Ryan, J. P. [1997]. *Physiology*. New York: McGraw Hill; Mehta, S., Milder, E. A., Mirachi, A. J., et al. [2007]. *Step-Up: A High-Yield, Systems-Based Review for the USMLE Step 1* [3rd ed.]. Philadelphia: Lippincott Williams & Wilkins.)

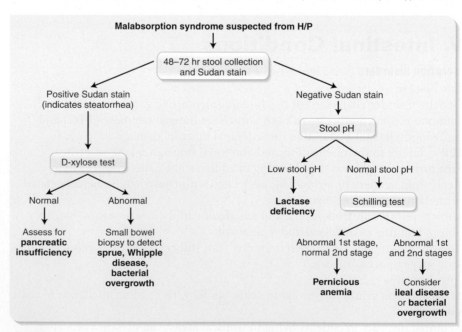

FIGURE
3-9 **Diagnostic pathway for suspected malabsorption syndrome.**

    c. **H/P** = similar presentation to celiac sprue

    d. **Labs** = no antiendomysial and anti-TTG antibodies; acute GI infection, celiac sprue, and autoimmune diseases should be ruled out with cultures and appropriate serology

    e. **Treatment** = folic acid replacement, tetracycline; removal of gluten from diet has no effect

3. **Lactose intolerance**

    a. Malabsorption syndrome resulting from deficiency of lactase; can also be secondary to Crohn's disease or bacterial overgrowth

    b. Lactose not metabolized in jejunum, leading to osmotic diarrhea

    c. **H/P** = diarrhea, abdominal pain, flatulence, and bloating after dairy consumption

    d. **Labs** = positive lactose tolerance test (i.e., minimal increase in serum glucose following ingestion of lactose), positive lactose breath hydrogen test after lactose meal

    e. **Treatment** = lactose-restricted or lactose-free diet; adequate dietary protein, fat, calcium, and vitamins; lactase replacement may benefit some patients

4. **Whipple disease**

    a. Malabsorption disorder secondary to *Tropheryma whippelii* infection and likely immune deficiency (unknown if innate to host or caused by infection); multiple organs involved

    b. **Risk factors** = white males with European ancestry

    c. **H/P** = weight loss, joint pain, abdominal pain, diarrhea, dementia, cough, bloating, steatorrhea; fever, vision abnormalities, lymphadenopathy, new heart murmur; severe wasting late in disease course

    d. **Labs** = jejunal biopsy shows foamy macrophages on periodic acid-Schiff (PAS) stain and villous atrophy

    e. **Treatment** = trimethoprim sulfamethoxazole (TMP-SMX) or ceftriaxone for 12 months

    f. **Complications** = high mortality if untreated

B. Diarrhea

1. Increased frequency of bowel movements and increased stool liquidity; **>200 g/day stool production**

2. **Risk factors** = infection, recent travel

3. Acute diarrhea (<2-week duration) is usually caused by infection (see Figure 3-10).

4. Chronic diarrhea has longer duration of symptoms and may result from malabsorption or motility disorders (see Figure 3-11).

    a. **Secretory** diarrheas are usually **hormone mediated** or caused by enterotoxic bacteria.

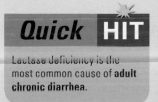

Lactase deficiency is the most common cause of **adult chronic diarrhea**.

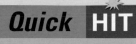

Rotavirus is the most common cause of acute diarrhea in children.

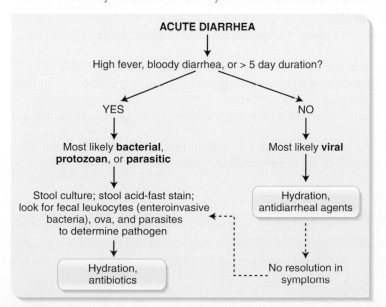

FIGURE

3-10 **Diagnostic and treatment pathways for acute diarrhea.**

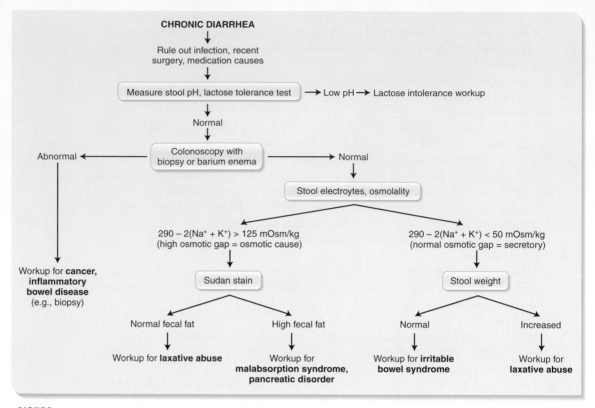

FIGURE
3-11 Diagnostic pathway for chronic diarrhea.

b. **Osmotic** diarrheas are caused by **solute collecting in bowel lumen**, leading to increased water in bowel; occur after eating, lessen with fasting
c. **Inflammatory** diarrhea results from an autoimmune inflammatory process or chronic infection.
5. Pediatric diarrhea is most commonly caused by infection, antibiotic use, or related to immunosuppression.
6. **Treatment** = hydration, treat underlying cause

C. Irritable bowel syndrome (IBS)

1. Idiopathic disorder with chronic abdominal pain and irregular **bowel habits** (see Table 3-8)
2. Most commonly begins during **teens** or **young adulthood**; females > males (2:1)
3. **H/P** = abdominal pain, diarrhea, constipation, bloating, nausea, possible vomiting; mild abdominal tenderness
4. **Labs** = rule out other GI diseases with complete blood count (CBC), electrolytes, stool culture
5. **Radiology** = consider AXR, abdominal CT, or barium studies to rule out other GI causes; colonoscopy may be performed in older patients to rule out neoplasm

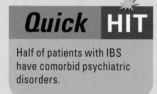

Half of patients with IBS have comorbid psychiatric disorders.

TABLE 3-8	Rome III Criteria for Diagnosis of Irritable Bowel Disease

Recurrent abdominal pain or discomfort at least 3 days per month in the last 3 months, associated with two or more of the following:
Improvement of pain with defecation
Change in frequency of stool
Change in form/appearance of stool

6. **Treatment** = assurance from physician, high-fiber diet, possible psychosocial therapy; antispasmodic, antidepressants, serotonin receptor antagonists have shown use in lessening symptoms

D. Inflammatory bowel disease (IBD) (*see Table 3-9*)

1. Disease of small and large bowel, with a constellation of symptoms associated with inflammatory bowel processes, autoimmune reactions, extraintestinal manifestations, and multiple complications
2. Types = Crohn's disease, ulcerative colitis
3. **Risk factors** = Ashkenazi Jews; whites > blacks; presents in teens or early 20s

E. Bowel obstruction (*see Figure 3-12, Figure 3-13, Table 3-10*)

1. Mechanical obstruction of small or large bowel that can lead to vascular compromise
2. The most common causes of obstruction are **adhesions**, **hernias**, and **neoplasms**.

F. Ischemic colitis

1. Ischemia and necrosis of bowel secondary to vascular compromise
2. Caused by embolus, bowel obstruction, inadequate systemic perfusion, medication, or surgery-induced vascular compromise
3. **Risk factors** = diabetes mellitus (DM), atherosclerosis, congestive heart failure (CHF), peripheral vascular disease, lupus

TABLE 3-9	**Comparison of Crohn's Disease and Ulcerative Colitis**	
	Crohn's Disease	**Ulcerative Colitis**
Site of involvement	**Entire GI tract may be involved** with multiple **"skipped"** areas; distal ileum most commonly involved; **entire bowel wall affected**	**Continuous disease beginning at rectum** and **extending possibly as far as distal ileum**; only mucosa and submucosa affected
Symptoms	Abdominal pain, weight loss, **watery** diarrhea	Abdominal pain, urgency, **bloody** diarrhea, tenesmus, nausea, vomiting, weight loss
Physical examination	Fever, right lower quadrant **abdominal mass**, abdominal tenderness, **perianal fissures and fistulas**, oral ulcers	Fever, abdominal tenderness, orthostatic hypotension, tachycardia, gross blood on rectal examination
Extraintestinal manifestations	Arthritis, ankylosing spondylitis, uveitis, nephrolithiasis	Arthritis, uveitis, ankylosing spondylitis, primary sclerosing cholangitis, erythema nodosum, pyoderma gangrenosum
Labs	ASCA frequently positive, pANCA rarely positive; hemoccult positive stool; biopsy diagnostic	ASCA rarely positive, pANCA frequently positive; biopsy diagnostic
Radiology	Colonoscopy shows colonic ulcers, strictures, **"cobblestoning,"** fissures, and **"skipped"** areas of bowel; barium enema shows fissures, ulcers, and bowel edema	Colonoscopy shows **continuous involvement**, pseudopolyps, friable mucosa; barium enema shows **"lead pipe"** colon without haustra and colon shortening
Treatment	Mesalamine, broad-spectrum antibiotics, corticosteroids, immunosuppressives; surgical resections of severely affected areas, fistulas, or strictures	Mesalamine, supplemental iron, corticosteroids, immunosuppressives; total **colectomy is curative**
Complications	Abscess formation, fistulas, fissures, malabsorption	**Significantly increased risk of colon cancer**, hemorrhage, toxic megacolon, bowel obstruction

ASCA, antiyeast *Saccharomyces cerevisiae* antibodies; GI, gastrointestinal; pANCA, perinuclear antineutrophil cytoplasmic antibodies.

Gastrointestinal Disorders

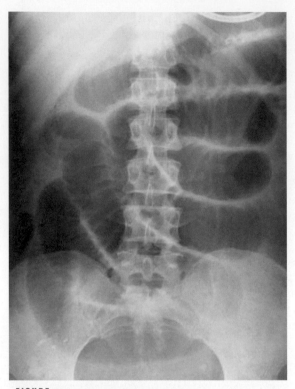

FIGURE
3-12 **Abdominal radiograph in patient with small bowel obstruction.**

Note the multiple loops of dilated bowel with a ladderlike appearance.

(From Yamada, T., Alpers D. H., Laine L., Kaplowitz N., Owyang, C., Powel, D. W. [2003]. *Textbook of Gastroenterology* [4th ed.]. Philadelphia: Lippincott Williams & Wilkins; with permission.)

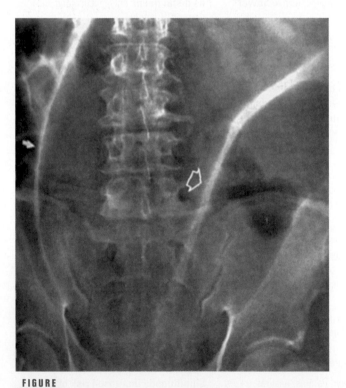

FIGURE
3-13 **Abdominal radiograph in patient with large bowel obstruction due to sigmoid volvulus; note significantly dilated bowel lumen.**

Of note are the dense line markings where the walls of two dilated loops of bowel are pressed against each other (*open arrow*) and the dense markings where a dilated loop of bowel is compressed against the cecum (*solid arrow*)

(From Eisenberg, R. L. [2003]. *Gastrointestinal Radiology: A Pattern Approach* [4th ed.]. Philadelphia: Lippincott-Raven; with permission.)

TABLE 3-10	Comparison of Small and Large Bowel Obstruction	
	Small Bowel Obstruction	**Large Bowel Obstruction**
Causes	**Adhesions, incarcerated hernias**, neoplasm, intussusception, volvulus, Crohn's disease, congenital stricture	**Neoplasm**, diverticulitis, volvulus, congenital stricture
Symptoms	Abdominal pain, **vomiting**, distention, obstipation	Abdominal pain, obstipation, distention, nausea, **late feculent vomiting**
Physical examination	Abdominal tenderness, visible peristaltic waves, high-pitched bowel sounds, absence of bowel sounds, fever	Abdominal tenderness, palpable mass, high-pitched bowel sounds, absence of bowel sounds
Radiology	AXR shows **ladderlike dilated loops of bowel**, air–fluid levels	AXR shows **bowel distention proximal to obstruction**; barium enema may detect obstruction near rectum
Treatment	Make patient NPO, maintain hydration; nasogastric decompression may relieve obstruction, but if unsuccessful, surgery is required	Make patient NPO, maintain hydration; colonoscopy may relieve obstruction, but if unsuccessful, surgery is required

AXR, abdominal X-ray; NPO, nothing by mouth.

4. **H/P** = acute abdominal pain, bloody diarrhea, vomiting; mild abdominal tenderness
5. **Labs** = increased white blood cell count (WBC), increased serum lactate
6. **Radiology** = barium enema shows diffuse submucosal changes from localized bleeding (i.e., "thumb printing"); sigmoidoscopy may show bloody and edematous mucosa; CT may show air within bowel wall and bowel wall thickening
7. **Treatment** = intravenous (IV) fluids, bowel rest, antibiotics for GI bacteria; surgical resection of necrotic bowel
8. **Complications** = high mortality in cases of irreversible damage

G. Appendicitis

1. Inflammation of appendix with possible infection or perforation
2. Caused by lymphoid hyperplasia (children), fibroid bands (adults), or fecaliths (adults)
3. **H/P** = dull periumbilical pain followed by nausea, vomiting, and anorexia; pain gradually moves to right lower quadrant and increases; **tenderness at McBurney point** (1/3 distance from right anterior superior iliac spine to umbilicus), rebound tenderness, **psoas sign** (psoas pain on passive hip extension), fever, **Rovsing sign** (right lower quadrant pain with left lower quadrant palpation); perforation produces severe pain and distention with rebound tenderness, rigidity, and guarding
4. **Labs** = increased WBC with left shift
5. **Radiology** = AXR or chest X-ray may show fecalith or free air under the diaphragm (due to perforation); **CT most sensitive test** and may show bowel wall thickening, appendicolith, abscess, phlegmon, free fluid, or right lower quadrant fat stranding
6. **Treatment** = **appendectomy**; antibiotics added (covering gram-negatives and anaerobes) for ruptured appendix
7. **Complications** = abscess formation, perforation

H. Ileus

1. **Paralytic obstruction** of bowel secondary to decreased peristalsis
2. Caused by infection, ischemia, **recent surgery**, DM, opioid use
3. **H/P** = vague abdominal pain, nausea, vomiting, bloating, no bowel movements, inability to tolerate meals; decreased bowel sounds, no rebound tenderness

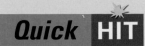
Small bowel obstruction most commonly results from **adhesion** formation, whereas **large** bowel obstruction is most commonly caused by **neoplasm**.

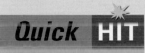
The left side of the colon is most commonly involved in ischemic colitis; the rectum is frequently spared because of collateral circulation.

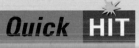
Abdominal pain for ischemic colitis is less severe than **small bowel ischemic**, which is significant and **out of proportion to examination**.

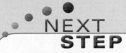
Always get a β-human chorionic gonadotropin (β-hCG) test in a woman of childbearing age with abdominal pain to **rule out pregnancy**.

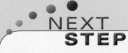
With a high clinical suspicion of appendicitis, go right to surgery and do not wait for radiologic examinations.

Gastrointestinal Disorders

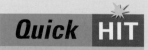

Quick HIT

Postoperative ileus typically lasts <**5 days**. Small bowel recovers in 24 hr, stomach in 48–72 hr, and large bowel in 3–5 days.

Quick HIT

Diverticular disease most frequently occurs in the sigmoid colon and is the most common cause of **acute lower GI bleeding** in patients **over 40 years of age.**

4. **Radiology** = AXR shows distention of affected bowel, air–fluid levels; barium enema can help rule out obstruction
5. **Treatment** = stop opioids, make patient NPO (i.e., nothing by mouth); colonoscopic decompression if no resolution

I. Volvulus

1. **Rotation of bowel** creates obstruction and possible ischemia; most commonly occurs at cecum and sigmoid colon
2. Tends to occur in **elderly** and **infants**
3. **H/P** = distention, abdominal pain, vomiting, obstipation; possible palpable abdominal mass
4. **Radiology** = AXR may show "**double bubble**" proximal and distal to volvulus; barium enema shows "**bird's beak**" for distal volvulus
5. **Treatment** = possibly self-limited; colonoscopic decompression of sigmoid volvulus; surgical repair or resection may be required in cecal volvulus or failed colonoscopic detorsion

J. Diverticulosis

1. Outpouchings of colonic **mucosa** and **submucosa** that herniate through muscular layer (i.e., **diverticulosis**); may erode into colonic blood vessel to cause bleeding
2. **Risk factors** = low-fiber diet, high-fat diet, >60 years of age
3. **H/P** = frequently **asymptomatic** during uncomplicated diverticulosis; occasional cramping, bloating, flatulence, irregular defecation, vague left lower quadrant abdominal pain relieved with defecation; possible painless rectal bleeding if erosion into vessel occurs
4. **Labs** = positive stool guaiac test during bleeding
5. **Radiology** = **diverticula seen on barium enema** and colonoscopy (see Figure 3-14)
6. **Treatment** = high-fiber diet may help prevent development of additional diverticula or diverticular bleeding; no evidence to support avoidance of seeds, nuts, corn, etc.
7. **Complications** = **diverticulitis**, diverticular colitis (i.e., inflammation of section of colon)

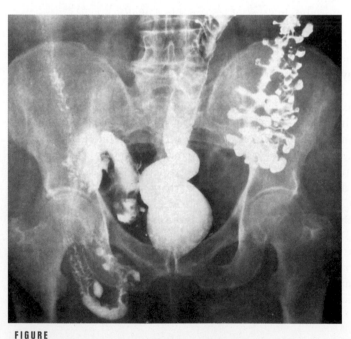

FIGURE 3-14 Barium enema in a patient with diverticular disease; numerous diverticula can be seen in the left colon.

(Modified from Daffner, R. H. & Hartman, M. [2013]. *Clinical Radiology: The Essentials* [4th ed., p. 273]. Philadelphia: Wolters Kluwer/Lippincott Williams & Wilkins; with permission.)

K. Diverticulitis

1. Obstruction of a diverticulum leading to significant inflammation, focal bowel wall necrosis, and **perforation**; poor containment of colonic rupture leads to peritonitis
2. **H/P = left lower quadrant pain**, nausea, vomiting, melena, hematochezia; abdominal tenderness, possible palpable abdominal mass, fever, abdominal distention
3. **Labs** = increased WBC
4. **Radiology** = CXR or AXR may demonstrate free air under the diaphragm; CT shows increased soft tissue density caused by inflammation, colonic diverticula, bowel wall thickening, and possible abscess formation
5. Treatment
   a. Mild early cases without perforation can be treated by bowel rest (liquids only for at least 3 days) and PO antibiotics (e.g., fluoroquinolone and metronidazole, TMP-SMX and metronidazole, or amoxicillin-clavulanate).
   b. **Surgery** required in most severe cases to resect involved segment of colon and remove any obstruction or fistula; diverting colostomy performed in cases of peritonitis (reanastomosis in 3 months)
   c. Broad-spectrum antibiotics required for any case of bowel rupture
6. **Complications** = colonic abscess, fistula formation, sepsis

L. Rectal conditions

1. Hemorrhoids
   a. Internal and external engorged rectal veins causing bleeding (**bright red blood**)
   b. **Internal** hemorrhoids arise from superior rectal veins above the pectinate line (columnar rectal epithelium); characteristically **painless**
   c. **External** hemorrhoids arise from **inferior** rectal veins below the pectinate line (squamous rectal epithelium); frequently **painful** (especially if thrombosed)
   d. **Radiology** = sigmoidoscopy used to rule out other causes of bleeding
   e. **Treatment** = warm baths, increase fiber in diet, avoid prolonged straining; sclerotherapy, ligation, or excision can be performed for worsening symptoms
2. Anal fissures
   a. Painful, bleeding tears in posterior wall of anus secondary to trauma during defecation or anal intercourse
   b. **Treatment** = stool softeners, sitz baths, topical nitroglycerin (second line); partial sphincterotomy may be performed for recurrent fissures
3. Anorectal abscesses
   a. Infection of anal crypts, internal hemorrhoids, or hair follicle leading to abscess formation
   b. **H/P** = throbbing rectal pain; fever, tenderness on digital examination
   c. **Treatment** = antibiotics, surgical incision and drainage
4. Rectal fistula
   a. Formation of tract between rectum and adjacent structures from unknown cause or secondary to **IBD** or abscess formation
   b. **H/P** = mild pain during defecation; possible visible site draining pus
   c. **Treatment** = fistulotomy; treat patients with Crohn's disease with antibiotics and immunosuppressants unless refractory disease
5. Pilonidal disease
   a. Presence of one or more cutaneous sinus tracts in the superior midline gluteal cleft
   b. Obstruction of sinus tract by hair or debris can lead to cyst and abscess formation
   c. **H/P** = usually asymptomatic; obstruction of sinus leads to mildly painful cyst with drainage (possibly purulent); small cysts can progress to larger abscesses
   d. **Treatment** = incision and drainage of abscesses; surgical closure of sinus tracts may prevent recurrence

M. Carcinoid tumor

1. Tumors arising from neuroectodermal cells that function as amine precursor uptake and decarboxylation (APUD) cells

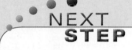

NEXT STEP

If a patient has significant rectal pain and the only finding on colonoscopy is internal hemorrhoids, a workup must be performed to locate another cause of symptoms (e.g., abscess or fissure).

2. Most commonly in bronchopulmonary tree, ileum, rectum, appendix
3. **H/P** = possibly asymptomatic; abdominal pain; possible **carcinoid syndrome** (i.e., flushing, diarrhea, bronchoconstriction, tricuspid/pulmonary valvular disease) caused by serotonin secretion by tumor (only seen with liver metastases or extra-gastrointestinal involvement)
4. **Labs** = increased 5-hydroxyindolacetic acid (5-HIAA) in urine, increased serum serotonin level
5. **Radiology** = CT or indium-labeled octreotide scintigraphy can localize tumor
6. **Treatment** = tumors <2 cm have very low incidence of metastases and should be resected; tumors >2 cm have high risk of metastases and require extensive resection; metastatic disease treated with IFN-α, octreotide, and embolization

N. Colorectal cancer

1. Neoplasm of large bowel or rectum; most commonly adenocarcinoma
2. **Risk factors** = family history, ulcerative colitis, **colonic polyps**, hereditary polyposis syndromes, low-fiber/high-fat diet, previous colon cancer, alcohol, smoking, DM
3. Spreads to regional lymph nodes; **metastasizes** most commonly to **lung** and **liver**
4. **H/P** = change in bowel habits (more common in left-sided disease), weakness, right-sided abdominal pain (in right-sided disease), constipation, hematochezia, melena, anemia due to blood loss, malaise, weight loss; abdominal or rectal mass may be palpated
5. **Labs** = **positive stool guaiac test**, decreased hemoglobin, decreased hematocrit; biopsy is diagnostic; CEA, which is increased in 70% of patients, is useful for monitoring treatment success and cancer recurrence
6. **Radiology** = barium enema may detect lesion; colonoscopy may detect lesion and obtain biopsy specimens; CT or PET used to determine local extent of disease and spread of metastases
7. **Treatment**
   a. **Surgical resection** plus regional lymph node dissection; adjuvant chemotherapy in cases of positive lymph nodes; palliative resections are helpful in metastatic disease to reduce symptoms and remove obstruction
   b. Preventative colectomy may be indicated for hereditary syndromes (see Table 3-11).
   c. Duke classification can be used for prognosis (see Table 3-12); CEA and serial colonoscopy may be followed after treatment to monitor for recurrence.

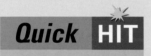

Quick HIT

Iron-deficiency anemia in elderly men and postmenopausal women is considered colon cancer until proven otherwise.

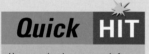

Quick HIT

Hematochezia can result from a heavy upper GI bleed.

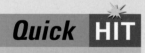

Quick HIT

Familial adenomatous polyposis (FAP), Gardner syndrome, and Turcot syndrome are caused by a mutation in the adenomatous polyposis coli (**APC**) gene.

Gastrointestinal Disorders

TABLE 3-11	Familial Colon Tumor Syndromes
Hereditary Disease	**Characteristics**
Familial adenomatous polyposis (FAP)	Hundreds of polyps in colon; near-certain development of malignant neoplasm; prophylactic subtotal colectomy recommended
Gardner syndrome	Similar to FAP with addition of common bone and soft tissue tumors
Turcot syndrome	Many colonic adenomas with high malignant potential; comorbid malignant CNS tumors
Juvenile polyposis	Hamartomatous polyps of colon, small bowel, and stomach that frequently are source of GI bleeding; slightly increased risk of malignancy later in life
Peutz-Jeghers syndrome	Polyps are hamartomas with low risk of malignancy; mucocutaneous pigmentation of mouth, hands, and genitals
Hereditary nonpolyposis colorectal cancer (HNPCC)	Multiple genetic mutations; cancer arises from normal-appearing mucosa; neoplasms tend to form in proximal colon

CNS, central nervous system; GI, gastrointestinal.

TABLE 3-12 Duke Classification System for Staging and Corresponding Prognosis of Colorectal Cancer

Class	Equivalent TNM Stage	Description	Cure Rate
A	I	Tumor confined to bowel wall	90%
B	II	Penetration of tumor into colonic serosa or perirectal fat	80%
C	III	Lymph node involvement	<60%
D	IV	Distant metastases	<5%

TNM, tumor, node, metastasis.

8. **Prevention**
   a. Regular screening for colon cancer recommended in patients >50 years of age
   b. Annual fecal occult blood test (FOBT)
   c. Flexible sigmoidoscopy every 5 years (in addition to FOBT)
   d. **Colonoscopy** is more sensitive than sigmoidoscopy but carries a 0.1% risk of perforation; it is now considered preferable over sigmoidoscopy by several expert groups and is recommended to be performed every 10 years; it should definitely be chosen over sigmoidoscopy for patients with a hereditary high risk of colon cancer.

O. GI bleeding
   1. Caused by either upper (i.e., proximal to ligament of Treitz) or lower (i.e., distal to ligament of Treitz) sources
   2. Bright red blood (e.g., hematochezia) suggests a rapid or heavy bleed; dark blood (e.g., melena, coffee-grounds emesis) suggests either blood that has passed through much of the GI tract or has been sitting in the stomach for some time (see Figure 3-15).

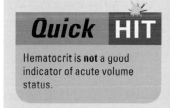

Quick **HIT**

Hematocrit is **not** a good indicator of acute volume status.

Gastrointestinal Disorders

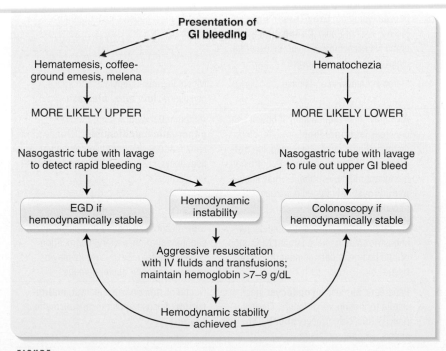

FIGURE 3-15 Diagnostic pathway for gastrointestinal (GI) bleeding.

EGD, esophagogastroduodenoscopy; IV, intravenous.

3. Common causes of upper GI bleeds are **PUD**, Mallory-Weiss tears (longitudinal esophageal tears secondary to violent retching), esophagitis, **esophageal varices**, and gastritis.
4. Common causes of lower GI bleeds are **diverticulosis**, **neoplasm**, ulcerative colitis, mesenteric ischemia, arteriovenous malformations (AVMs), hemorrhoids, and Meckel diverticulum.
5. **Diagnostics** = EGD or colonoscopy shows most sources of bleeding; barium studies may detect defects; capsule endoscopy may show sources of bleeding in the small intestine; technetium-tagged red blood cell scan may help localize intermittent bleeding; angiography can help locate AVMs
6. **Treatment** = **fluid replacement** is vital; transfusion for increased blood loss; some small bleeds stop automatically; **treat underlying cause**; PPI for upper GI bleeds until gastric cause ruled out; prophylactic antibiotics and β-blockers in patients with a known history of cirrhosis; sclerotherapy may help stop bleeding from varices; vasopressin may stop bleeding from AVMs and diverticula; surgical resection of tumors and diverticula may be needed

V. Pancreatic Disorders

A. Pancreatitis (see Table 3-13, Table 3-14)

1. **Acute** or **chronic** inflammation of pancreas associated with anatomic defects, chronic **alcohol use**, acute ductal obstruction, drugs, **gallstones**
2. Initially, results from leak of pancreatic enzymes into pancreatic and surrounding tissues; later caused by pancreatic tissue necrosis; prognosis determined by Ranson criteria

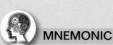

MNEMONIC

Remember the causes of acute pancreatitis by the mnemonic **PANCREATITIS**:
hyper**P**arathyroid (hypercalcemia)
Alcohol
Neoplasm
Cholelithiasis
Rx (drugs)
ERCP
Abdominal surgery
hyper**T**riglyceridemia
Infection (mumps)
Trauma
Idiopathic
Scorpion bite

TABLE **3-13**	Comparison of Acute and Chronic Pancreatitis	
	Acute Pancreatitis	**Chronic Pancreatitis**
Onset	**Sudden**, severe	**Recurrent**
Risk factors	**Gallstones**, **chronic alcohol abuse**, trauma, hypercalcemia, hyperlipidemia, drugs	**Chronic alcohol abuse**, congenital defect
History/physical	Acute epigastric pain radiating to back, nausea, vomiting, **Grey Turner sign** (ecchymosis of flank), **Cullen sign** (periumbilical ecchymosis), fever, tachycardia; hypotension, shock if severe	Recurrent epigastric pain, steatorrhea, weight loss, nausea, constipation
Labs	Increased amylase and lipase	Mildly increased amylase and lipase, glycosuria; **low fecal elastase**
Radiology	AXR may show dilated loop of bowel near pancreas (**sentinel loop**) or right colon distended until near pancreas (colon **cut-off sign**); CXR may show pleural effusion, hemidiaphragm elevation; CT may show **pseudocyst** or enlarged pancreas; US may detect gallstones	Abdominal radiograph may show **pancreatic calcifications**; CT may show calcifications, pancreatic enlargement, or pseudocyst; MRCP or ERCP may be helpful for diagnosis
Treatment	Hydration, pain control with opioids, nasogastric suction, make patient NPO, stop offending agent; debridement of necrotic tissue	Stop alcohol use, opioid analgesia, enzyme supplementation, dietary modification (small, low-fat meals); surgery may be required to repair ductal damage
Complications	Pancreatic abscess, **pseudocyst**, necrosis, fistula formation, renal failure, chronic pancreatitis, hemorrhage, **shock**, DIC, sepsis, respiratory failure	Ductal obstruction, pseudocyst, **malnutrition**, glucose intolerance, pancreatic cancer

CT, computed tomography; CXR, chest X-ray; DIC, disseminated intravascular coagulation; ERCP, endoscopic retrograde cholangiopancreatography; MRCP, magnetic resonance cholangiopancreatography; US, ultrasound.

TABLE 3-14	Ranson Criteria for Determining Prognosis during Acute Pancreatitis	
Increased Mortality Associated with Three or More of the Following:		
On Admission	**During Initial 48 hr After Admission**	
Serum glucose >200 mg/dL	Serum calcium <8 mg/dL	
Serum AST >250 IU/L	Hematocrit decreases >10%	
Serum LDH >350 IU/L	Pao₂ <60 mm Hg	
>55 yr of age	BUN increases >5 mg/dL	
WBC >16,000/mL	Base deficit >4 mEq/L	
	Fluid sequestration >6 L	

BUN, blood urea nitrogen; LDH, lactate dehydrogenase; Pao₂, partial pressure of arterial oxygen; WBC, white blood cell count.

MNEMONIC

Remember Ranson criteria for increased mortality from acute pancreatitis on **admission** by the mnemonic **GA LAW:**
Glucose >200 mg/dL
AST >250 IU/L
LDH >350 IU/L
Age >55 years
WBC >16,000/mL

MNEMONIC

Ranson criteria for increased mortality from acute pancreatitis **during initial 48 hrs after admission** may be remembered by the mnemonic **Calvin & HOBBeS:**
Calcium <8 mg/dL
Hct decrease >10%
O₂ (PaO₂) <60 mm Hg
BUN increase >5 mg/dL
Base deficit >4 mEq/L
Sequestration of fluid >6 L

B. Pancreatic pseudocyst
1. Fluid collection arising from pancreas consisting of enzyme-rich fluids contained in sac of inflamed membranous tissue
2. **H/P** = usually asymptomatic; recent acute pancreatitis, epigastric pain; fever
3. **Labs** = increased WBC, increased amylase; aspiration of pseudocyst demonstrates very high amylase content
4. **Radiology** = pseudocyst visible on ultrasound (US) or CT
5. **Treatment** = possibly self-resolving, drainage (surgical, endoscopic, or percutaneous) indicated if lasting >6 weeks, painful, or rapidly growing; debride necrotic pancreatic tissue
6. **Complications** = rupture, hemorrhage, abscess or pseudoaneurysm formation

C. Exocrine pancreatic cancer
1. Adenocarcinoma of pancreas most commonly in head of pancreas
2. **Risk factors** = chronic pancreatitis, DM, family history, tobacco, high-fat diet; male > female, obesity, sedentary lifestyle
3. **H/P** = **abdominal pain radiating to back**, anorexia, nausea, vomiting, weight loss, fatigue, steatorrhea; jaundice if bile duct obstructed (painless jaundice is possible); palpable, nontender gallbladder (i.e., **Courvoisier sign**); splenomegaly (if in tail), palpable deep abdominal mass, ascites
4. **Labs** = possible hyperglycemia; increased **CEA** and **CA 19–9** tumor markers; increased bilirubin (total and direct) and increased alkaline phosphatase with bile duct obstruction; biopsy used to make diagnosis
5. **Radiology** = CT shows mass, dilated pancreas, local spread, and dilated bile ducts; US also useful for imaging mass, but not as sensitive as CT; endoscopic retrograde cholangiopancreatography (ERCP) locates tumors not seen with CT; endoscopic US often helpful for staging and to guide fine-needle aspiration biopsy
6. **Treatment**
   a. Nonmetastatic disease limited to head of pancreas may be resected with **Whipple procedure** (i.e., removal of pancreatic head, distal stomach, duodenum, proximal jejunum, common bile duct, and gallbladder).
   b. Lesions in body or tail rarely amenable to surgery but can be resected via subtotal pancreatectomy if found early
   c. Adjuvant chemotherapy may be beneficial in resectable disease.
   d. Enzyme deficiency treated with replacement therapy
   e. Stenting of pancreatic ducts, biliary ducts, or duodenum can be performed as palliative therapy in advanced disease.

Gastrointestinal Disorders

7. **Complications** = usually not detected until progressed; **5-year survival <2%**; 20% to 30% 5-year survival following successful Whipple procedure; migratory thrombophlebitis (i.e., **Trousseau syndrome**)

D. Endocrine pancreatic cancers
1. Neoplasms involving glandular pancreatic tissue
2. Frequently difficult to locate; may be seen with CT or MRI
3. **Zollinger-Ellison syndrome** (see earlier discussion under "Gastric Conditions" section)
4. **Insulinoma**
   a. Insulin-secreting β-islet cell tumor causing **hypoglycemia**
   b. **H/P** = headache, visual changes, confusion, weakness, mood instability, palpitations, diaphoresis
   c. **Labs** = **increased fasting insulin**, spontaneous hypoglycemia, high C-peptide
   d. **Radiology** = CT, US, or indium-labeled octreotide scintigraphy may be useful for localizing tumor
   e. **Treatment** = surgical resection; diazoxide or octreotide may relieve symptoms in nonresectable disease
5. **Glucagonoma**
   a. Glucagon-secreting α-cell tumor causing hyperglycemia
   b. May present as refractory DM
   c. **H/P** = abdominal pain, diarrhea, weight loss, mental status changes; exfoliating rash (**necrolytic migratory erythema**); **symptoms of DM**
   d. **Labs** = hyperglycemia, **increased glucagon**; biopsy confirms diagnosis
   e. **Radiology** = CT or endoscopic US may localize tumor
   f. **Treatment** = surgical resection if localized lesion; octreotide, IFN-α, chemotherapy, and embolization may be used in metastatic disease
   g. **Complications** = frequently malignant; poor prognosis
6. **VIPoma**
   a. Vasoactive intestinal peptide (VIP)-producing tumor of non–β-islet cells
   b. **H/P** = **watery diarrhea**, weakness, nausea, vomiting, abdominal pain
   c. **Labs** = increased serum VIP, stool osmolality suggests secretory cause
   d. **Radiology** = CT may detect tumor
   e. **Treatment** = surgical resection for localized tumors; corticosteroids, chemotherapy, octreotide, and embolization used in metastatic disease

⬡ VI. Biliary Disorders

A. Cholelithiasis
1. Gallstone formation in the gallbladder that can cause cystic duct obstruction
2. **Risk factors** = age >40 years, obesity, female, multiparity, oral contraceptive use, total parenteral nutrition (TPN), recent rapid weight loss, family history, DM,
3. Most stones are composed of **cholesterol**; others are calcium bilirubinate (i.e., **pigmented stones**) secondary to chronic hemolysis
4. **H/P** = possibly asymptomatic; postprandial abdominal pain (**worst in right upper quadrant [RUQ]**), nausea, vomiting, indigestion, flatulence; RUQ tenderness, palpable gallbladder
5. **Radiology** = US may show gallstones (see Figure 3-16); AXR will only show some pigmented stones (because of calcium content and high iron content from bilirubin)
6. **Treatment** = dietary modification (decrease fatty food intake), bile salts (dissolve stones), shock wave lithotripsy (uses sound waves to break up stones); **cholecystectomy** is typically performed in symptomatic patients
7. **Complications** = recurrent stones, **acute cholecystitis, pancreatitis**

B. Acute cholecystitis
1. Inflammation of gallbladder commonly caused by **gallstone obstruction of cystic duct**; acalculous cholecystitis can occur in patients on TPN or in those who are critically ill

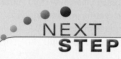

NEXT **STEP**

If Whipple's triad is seen **(symptoms of hypoglycemia while fasting, hypoglycemia, and improvement in symptoms with carbohydrate load),** perform a workup for insulinoma.

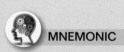

Quick HIT

Insulinomas are almost always **solitary**; multiple insulinomas may be seen in **MEN 1.**

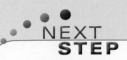

MNEMONIC

Remember the **5 Fs** for patients susceptible to gallstone formation: **F**emale, **F**ertile, **F**at, **F**orty (years of age), and **F**amily history.

NEXT **STEP**

If a positive Murphy sign **(palpation of RUQ during inspiration stops inspiration secondary to pain)** is detected, suspect acute cholecystitis and perform an US.

Gastrointestinal Disorders

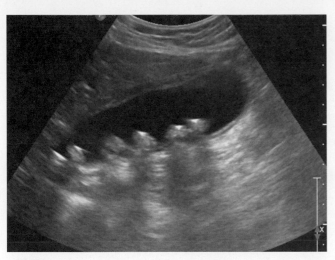

FIGURE 3-16 Ultrasound demonstrating multiple gallstones in the gallbladder.

Note the shadow caused by gallstones, which may be more apparent than the gallstones themselves in several cases.

(From Kawamura, D. M. and Lunsford, B. M. [2012]. *Diagnostic Medical Sonography, Abdomen and Superficial Structures* [3rd ed., p. 180]. Philadelphia: Lippincott Williams & Wilkins; with permission.)

2. **H/P** = RUQ pain radiating to back, nausea, vomiting, anorexia; fever, palpable gallbladder, RUQ tenderness; symptoms more severe and longer in duration than typical cholelithiasis
3. **Labs** = increased WBC; increased bilirubin (total and direct) and increased alkaline phosphatase seen when condition is related to impacted stone or cholangitis
4. **Radiology** = US may show gallstones, sludge, thickened gallbladder wall, or sonographic Murphy sign; hepatic iminodiacetic acid (**HIDA**) scan will detect cystic duct obstruction (gallbladder fails to fill normally during scan)
5. **Treatment** = hydration, antibiotics, cholecystectomy (frequently delayed after 24 to 48 hours of supportive care); patients with more mild symptoms can be treated with lithotripsy and bile salts; patients who are not stable for surgery can be treated with ERCP delivery of stone solvents
6. **Complications** = perforation, gallstone ileus, abscess formation

C. Cholangitis

1. Infection of bile ducts secondary to ductal obstruction
2. **Risk factors** = cholelithiasis, anatomic duct defect, biliary cancer
3. **H/P** = RUQ pain, chills; **jaundice, fever, RUQ tenderness**; change in mental status or signs of shock seen in severe cases (see Figure 3-17)
4. **Labs** = increased WBC, increased bilirubin (total and direct), increased alkaline phosphatase, increased AST and ALT, increased amylase with associated pancreatic inflammation, **positive blood cultures**
5. **Radiology** = US may detect obstruction; HIDA scan is more sensitive
6. **Treatment** = hydration, IV antibiotics, endoscopic biliary drainage followed by delayed cholecystectomy; severe symptoms demand **emergency bile duct decompression** and relief of obstruction

D. Gallbladder cancer

1. Adenocarcinoma of gallbladder associated with cholelithiasis, chronic infection, and biliary tract disease; generally poor prognosis
2. **H/P** = similar symptoms to acute cholecystitis; anorexia, weight loss, abdominal pain radiating to back; palpable gallbladder, jaundice
3. **Labs** = increased bilirubin (total and direct), increased alkaline phosphatase, increased cholesterol; biopsy provides diagnosis

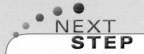

NEXT STEP

If Charcot triad (**RUQ pain, jaundice, and fever**) is seen, suspect cholangitis and perform an US or HIDA scan.

Gastrointestinal Disorders

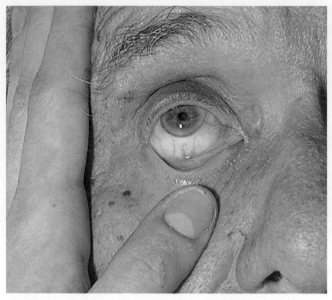

FIGURE 3-17 **Jaundice in a patient with hyperbilirubinemia.**

Note the yellow sclera and skin compared with the normal hue of the examiner's hand.

(From Bickley, L. S., & Szilagyi, P. [2012]. *Bates' Guide to Physical Examination and History Taking* [11th ed., p. 184]. Philadelphia: Lippincott Williams & Wilkins; with permission.)

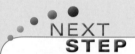

NEXT STEP

A **calcified gallbladder** is highly suggestive of chronic cholecystitis but may represent cancer in 10%–30%, and cholecystectomy should be performed promptly to confirm diagnosis.

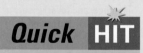

***Quick* HIT**

Gender, presence or absence of antimitochondrial antibodies, and ERCP distinguish PBC from PSC.

4. **Radiology** = abdominal radiograph may show **calcified gallbladder** (i.e., porcelain gallbladder); US or endoscopic US may detect invasive mass; ERCP can localize lesion and perform biopsy
5. **Treatment** = cholecystectomy, lymph node dissection, partial removal of adjacent hepatic tissue; adjuvant radiation therapy and chemotherapy may reduce recurrence rates and are used as primary therapies in unresectable disease

E. Primary biliary cirrhosis (PBC)

1. Autoimmune disease with intrahepatic bile duct destruction leading to accumulation of cholesterol, bile acids, and bilirubin
2. **Risk factors** = rheumatoid arthritis, Sjögren syndrome, scleroderma; **female > male**
3. **H/P** = possibly asymptomatic; fatigue, pruritus, arthralgias; jaundice, xanthomas, skin hyperpigmentation, hepatosplenomegaly
4. **Labs** = increased alkaline phosphatase, increased GGT, normal AST and ALT, increased cholesterol, increased bilirubin (total and direct) later in disease course; positive antinuclear antibody (ANA), **positive antimitochondrial antibodies**; workup may indicate comorbid autoimmune diseases; biopsy shows inflammation and necrosis in bile ducts
5. **Treatment** = ursodeoxycholic acid improves liver function and reduces symptoms; colchicines or methotrexate can be added in more severe cases; liver transplant needed in progressive disease

F. Primary sclerosing cholangitis (PSC)

1. Progressive destruction of intrahepatic and extrahepatic bile ducts leading to fibrosis and cirrhosis
2. **Risk factors** = ulcerative colitis; **male > female**
3. **H/P** = possibly asymptomatic; fatigue, pruritus, RUQ pain; fever, night sweats, jaundice, xanthomas
4. **Labs** = increased alkaline phosphatase, increased GGT, normal AST and ALT, increased cholesterol, increased bilirubin (total and direct), possible positive perinuclear antineutrophil cytoplasmic antibodies (pANCA); biopsy appears similar to that for PBC

5. **Radiology** = ERCP shows stricturing and irregularity of extrahepatic and intrahepatic bile ducts (i.e., "**beads on string**")
6. **Treatment** = endoscopic stenting of strictures; surgical resection of affected ducts and liver transplant may be required in progressive cases

G. Disorders of hepatic bilirubin transport

1. **Normal bilirubin transport**
   a. Unconjugated bilirubin from red blood cell count (RBC) hemolysis exists in venous circulation.
   b. Unconjugated bilirubin enters hepatocytes and is conjugated by glucuronosyltransferase.
   c. Conjugated bilirubin reenters venous circulation.
   d. Abnormal levels of unconjugated bilirubin versus conjugated bilirubin versus both types can help indicate location of pathology and narrow differential diagnosis (see Table 3-15).
2. **Gilbert disease**
   a. Autosomal recessive or dominant disease with **mild deficiency** of glucuronosyltransferase
   b. **H/P** = mild jaundice following fasting, exercise, or stress
   c. **Labs** = increased indirect bilirubin <5 mg/dL
   d. **Treatment** = none necessary
3. **Crigler-Najjar syndrome type I**
   a. Autosomal recessive disease with **severe deficiency** in glucuronosyltransferase
   b. **H/P** = persistent jaundice and central nervous system (CNS) symptoms (due to kernicterus) in infants
   c. **Labs** = increased indirect bilirubin >5 mg/dL
   d. **Treatment** = phototherapy, plasmapheresis, calcium phosphate combined with orlistat; liver transplantation is an option
   e. **Complications** = early kernicterus can cause permanent CNS damage

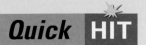

Prehepatic conditions cause an increase in **indirect bilirubin; posthepatic** conditions cause an increase in **direct bilirubin; intrahepatic** conditions can cause an increase of **either** or **both** types of bilirubin.

Gastrointestinal Disorders

TABLE 3-15 **Causes of Conjugated and Unconjugated Bilirubinemia**

Increased Total Bilirubin		
Hyperbilirubinemia	**Cause**	**Examples**
Unconjugated (indirect)	Excess bilirubin production	Hemolytic anemia Disorders of erythropoiesis Internal hemorrhage resorption
	Impaired conjugation	Physiologic jaundice of newborn Deficiency of glucuronosyltransferase (Gilbert disease, Crigler-Najjar syndrome) Hepatocellular disease (cirrhosis, hepatitis)
Conjugated (direct)	Decreased hepatic bilirubin excretion	Impaired bilirubin transport (Dubin-Johnson syndrome, Rotor syndrome) Hepatocellular disease (cirrhosis, hepatitis) Drug impairment
	Extrahepatic biliary obstruction	Intrahepatic bile duct disease (PBC, PSC) Gallstone obstruction of bile ducts (choledocholithiasis) Pancreatic or biliary cancer Biliary atresia

PBC, primary biliary cirrhosis; PSC, primary sclerosing cholangitis.

4. **Crigler-Najjar syndrome type II**
   a. Mild deficiency of glucuronosyltransferase; phenotypically similar to Gilbert syndrome
   b. Can be treated with phenobarbital, which induces hepatic synthesis of glucuronyltransferase, and reduces jaundice

VII. Hepatic Disorders

A. Alcohol-related liver disease

1. Progressive liver damage secondary to **chronic alcohol abuse**
2. Initially characterized by fatty deposits in liver; reversible with alcohol cessation
3. Continued alcoholism causes hepatic inflammation and early necrosis
4. Progressive damage results in cirrhosis
5. H/P = asymptomatic for many years of alcoholism; anorexia, nausea, vomiting late in disease course; abdominal tenderness, ascites, splenomegaly, hepatomegaly, fever, jaundice, testicular atrophy, gynecomastia, digital clubbing
6. **Labs** = increased ALT, increased AST, increased γ-glutamyl transferase (GGT), increased alkaline phosphatase, increased bilirubin (total and direct), prolonged prothrombin time (PT), decreased lipids, increased WBC; biopsy provides diagnosis (**fatty liver**, many polymorphonuclear leukocytes (PMNs), areas of necrosis)
7. **Treatment** = **cessation of alcohol use**, thiamine, folate, high caloric intake (2,500 to 3,000 kcal/day); liver transplant is a consideration in patients who are able to maintain abstinence from alcohol
8. **Complications** = cirrhosis, hepatic encephalopathy, coagulation disorders

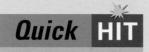

Quick HIT

In viral hepatitis, AST and ALT are equally high; in alcohol-related liver disease, AST > ALT by >2:1 ratio

B. Cirrhosis

1. **Persistent liver damage** leading to **necrosis** and **fibrosis** of hepatic parenchyma
2. Caused by **alcoholism**, chronic **HBV** or **HCV** infection, chronic bile duct obstruction and chronic cholestasis (PBC/PSC), and hepatic parenchymal diseases (hemochromatosis, Wilson disease, α_1-antitrypsin deficiency, NASH, autoimmune hepatitis)
3. **H/P** = general signs and symptoms may include weakness, weight loss, digital clubbing, Dupuytren contractures in hands; **portal hypertension** leads to esophageal varices and possibly variceal bleeding, abdominal wall varicosities (**caput medusae**), hepatosplenomegaly, **ascites**; **liver failure** leads to jaundice, coagulopathy, peripheral edema, mental status changes (from encephalopathy), asterixis (asynchronous flapping of hands), testicular atrophy and gynecomastia (in men), spider telangiectasias, palmar erythema
4. **Labs** = increased ALT, increased AST, increased GGT, increased alkaline phosphatase, decreased albumin, anemia, decreased platelets, prolonged PT; paracentesis of ascites shows fluid with <2.5 g/dL protein, WBC <300/μL, normal glucose level, and decreased amylase; biopsy shows fibrosis and hepatic necrosis
5. **Radiology** = US detects small, nodular liver
6. **Treatment** = **nonreversible**, but progression may be halted; stop offending agent (e.g., alcohol); treat varices with β-blockers or sclerotherapy to reduce bleeding risk; lactulose and rifaximin may improve encephalopathy; liver transplant may be needed in progressive cases
7. **Complications** = **portal hypertension**, varices (caused by venous hypertension), ascites, **hepatic encephalopathy** (because of poor filtering of blood), renal failure, spontaneous bacterial peritonitis

C. Portal hypertension

1. Increase in portal vein pressure giving it a **higher pressure than the inferior vena cava**; may result from prehepatic, intrahepatic, or posthepatic causes
2. Prehepatic causes include portal vein thrombosis.
3. Intrahepatic causes include **cirrhosis**, schistosomiasis, parenchymal disease, and granulomatous disease.
4. Posthepatic causes include **right-sided heart failure**, hepatic vein thrombosis, and Budd-Chiari syndrome (i.e., hepatic vein thrombosis secondary to hypercoagulability)
5. Shunting of blood into systemic veins causes varices in several locations (see Figure 3-18)

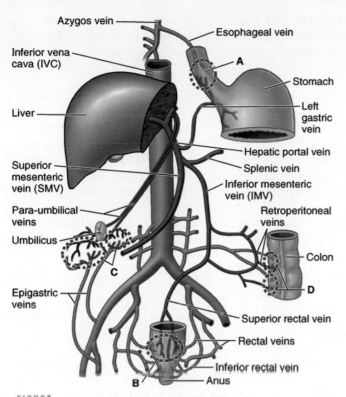

FIGURE
3-18 **Portal-systemic anastomoses and common sites of varices in portal hypertension.**

These anastomoses provide collateral circulation in cases of obstruction in the liver or hepatic portal vein. Darker blue, portal tributaries; lighter blue, systemic tributaries; A, anastomoses between esophageal veins; B, anastomoses between rectal veins; C, anastomoses between paraumbilical veins (portal) and small epigastric veins of the anterior abdominal wall; D, anastomoses between the twigs of colic veins (portal) and the retroperitoneal veins.

(From Moore, K. L., Agur, A. M. R., and Dalley, A. F. [2013]. *Clinically Oriented Anatomy* [5th ed., p. 167]. Philadelphia: Lippincott Williams & Wilkins; with permission.)

6. **H/P** = **ascites**, abdominal pain, change in mental status (from hepatic encephalopathy), hematemesis (caused by esophageal varices), symptoms of cirrhosis; hepatomegaly, splenomegaly, fever, abdominal wall varices, testicular atrophy, gynecomastia
7. **Labs** = paracentesis shows ascites with serum-ascites albumin gradient (SAAG) ≥1.1
8. **Radiology** = CT may show ascites and obstructing mass; EGD may show esophageal varices
9. **Treatment**
   a. Salt restriction and diuretics (furosemide and spironolactone) for ascites
   b. IV antibiotics for bacterial peritonitis (or with variceal hemorrhage)
   c. Dialysis for renal failure
   d. Vasopressin or sclerotherapy for bleeding varices
   e. **Hepatic shunting** via laparotomy or transjugular intrahepatic portosystemic shunting (TIPS) is short-term solution for severe disease; **liver transplant** often required as eventual treatment in progressive cases

D. Hemochromatosis

1. Autosomal recessive disease of iron absorption
2. **Excess iron absorption** causes iron deposition in liver, pancreas, heart, and pituitary, leading to eventual fibrosis.
3. Rarely is result of chronic blood transfusions or alcoholism
4. **H/P** = abdominal pain, polydipsia, polyuria, arthralgias, impotence, lethargy; **pigmented rash** (bronze hue), hepatomegaly, testicular atrophy; may see symptoms and signs that resemble DM and CHF
5. **Labs** = increased iron, increased ferritin, increased transferrin saturation, slightly increased AST and ALT; biopsy shows increased iron content in liver, but diagnosis is usually made by genetic testing

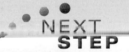

NEXT STEP

If paracentesis detects very high albumin and LDH equal to 60% serum LDH, worry about a neoplastic etiology and do a full workup for cancer.

Quick HIT

Spontaneous bacterial peritonitis can result from systemic infection and comorbid portal hypertension; paracentesis will show >250 PMN/μL total protein >1 g/dL, glucose <50 mg/dL, and lactate dehydrogenase (LDH) > normal serum LDH.

Gastrointestinal Disorders

6. **Treatment = weekly or biweekly phlebotomy** until normal iron, then monthly phlebotomy; avoid excess alcohol consumption; deferoxamine for iron chelation
7. **Complications** = cirrhosis, hepatoma, CHF, DM, hypopituitarism

E. Wilson disease

1. Autosomal recessive disorder of impaired copper secretion, primarily in young adults
2. **Excess copper deposits** in liver, brain, cornea
3. **H/P** = psychiatric disturbances (e.g., depression, neuroses, **personality changes**), **loss of coordination**, dysphagia; jaundice, tremor, possible green-brown rings in cornea (i.e., **Kayser-Fleischer rings**), hepatomegaly; signs may precede symptoms
4. **Labs** = decreased serum ceruloplasmin, increased urinary copper, slightly increased AST and ALT; biopsy shows increased copper deposits in liver
5. **Treatment = trientine** or penicillamine for copper chelation; lifelong zinc for maintenance therapy; dietary copper restriction (no organ meats, shellfish, chocolate, nuts, or mushrooms), supplementary vitamin B_6; liver transplantation may be needed in cases of liver failure
6. **Complications** = fulminant hepatic failure, cirrhosis

F. α₁-Antitrypsin deficiency

1. Codominant disorder with decreased α_1-antitrypsin production leading to cirrhosis and panlobular **emphysema**
2. Most symptoms arise from emphysemic component of disease.
3. **Labs** = increased AST, increased ALT; **pulmonary function tests (PFTs) demonstrate obstructive disease**
4. **Treatment** = liver transplant or lung transplant may be needed in severe cases; enzyme replacement may be helpful in stopping disease progression

G. Hepatic neoplasms

1. **Benign tumors** (e.g., hepatic adenoma, focal nodular hyperplasia, hemangiomas, hepatic cysts)
   a. Benign hepatic tumors found more commonly in **women with history of oral contraceptive use**
   b. **H/P** = frequently asymptomatic; possible RUQ fullness
   c. **Radiology** = CT, MRI, or angiography detects hypervascular liver mass
   d. **Treatment** = frequently untreated; larger tumors may be resected or embolized to prevent rupture
2. **Hepatocellular carcinoma** (hepatoma)
   a. Malignant tumor of hepatic parenchyma
   b. **Risk factors = HBV or HCV infection**, cirrhosis, hemochromatosis, excessive consumption of aflatoxin from *Aspergillus*-infected food, schistosomiasis
   c. **H/P** = RUQ pain, weight loss, malaise, anorexia, diarrhea, dyspnea; jaundice, hepatomegaly, bruit over liver, ascites
   d. **Labs** = slightly increased AST and ALT, increased alkaline phosphatase, increased bilirubin (total and direct), **increased α-fetoprotein**; biopsy provides diagnosis but risks causing substantial hemorrhage
   e. **Radiology** = CT, MRI, or US shows liver mass; angiography may show increased vascularity; PET can be used to determine extent of spread
   f. **Treatment** = surgical resection of small tumors (lobectomy or partial hepatectomy) and chemotherapy; transplant may be an option for limited disease; radiofrequency ablation and chemoembolization are options for unresectable tumors
   g. **Complications** = poor prognosis; portal vein obstruction, Budd-Chiari syndrome, liver failure

VIII. Pediatric GI Disorders

A. Tracheoesophageal fistula

1. Malformation of trachea and esophagus resulting in tract formation between structures (see Figure 3-19)

Gastrointestinal Disorders

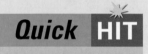

Quick HIT

Liver metastases from breast, lung, or colon cancers are much more common than primary liver cancers.

Quick HIT

Biopsy of hepatic masses is usually contraindicated because of hypervascularity and risk of hemorrhage.

Quick HIT

Paraneoplastic syndromes associated with hepatoma include hypoglycemia, excessive RBC production, refractory watery diarrhea, hypercalcemia, and variable skin lesions.

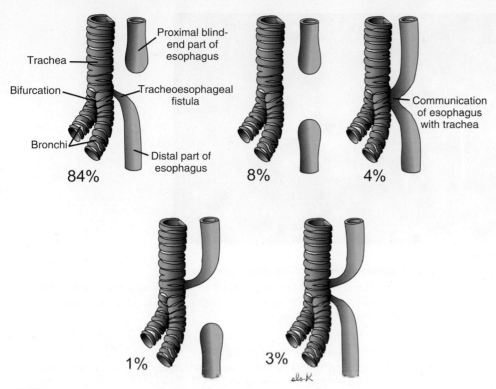

Trachea

Bifurcation

Bronchi

Proximal blind-
end part of
esophagus

Tracheoesophageal
fistula

Distal part of
esophagus

84%

8%

4%

Communication
of esophagus
with trachea

1%

3%

**FIGURE
3-19** **Variations of tracheoesophageal fistulas.**

(Modified from Sadler, T. W. (2012). *Langman's Medical Embryology* (12th ed., p. 212). Baltimore: Wolters Kluwer Health; with permission.)

2. Frequently associated with esophageal atresia
3. **H/P** = coughing and cyanosis during feeding, food may fill blind pouch, abdominal distention, possible history of aspiration pneumonia
4. **Radiology** = chest radiograph following nasogastric tube insertion demonstrates malformation (tube in lung or blind pouch)
5. **Treatment** = surgical repair

B. Pyloric stenosis

1. Hypertrophy of pyloric sphincter causing obstruction of gastric outlet
2. **H/P** = symptoms begin a few weeks after birth; nonbilious emesis, **projectile emesis; palpable epigastric olive-sized mass**
3. **Labs** = hypochloremic, hypokalemic metabolic alkalosis
4. **Radiology** = barium swallow shows thin pyloric channel (i.e., **string sign**); US shows increased pyloric muscle thickness (see Figure 3-20)
5. **Treatment** = pyloromyotomy

C. Necrotizing enterocolitis

1. Idiopathic mucosal necrosis and epithelial cell sloughing
2. **Risk factors** = preterm birth, low birth weight
3. **H/P** = bilious vomiting, lethargy, poor feeding, diarrhea, **hematochezia**; abdominal distention, abdominal tenderness; signs of shock in severe cases
4. **Labs** = metabolic acidosis, decreased Na^+
5. **Radiology** = abdominal radiograph shows bowel distention, **air in bowel wall**, portal vein gas, or free air under the diaphragm
6. **Treatment** = TPN, IV antibiotics, broad-spectrum antibiotics, nasogastric suction, surgical resection of affected bowel

D. Hirschsprung disease

1. Absence of bowel autonomic innervation causing bowel spasm and obstruction
2. **H/P** = vomiting, **obstipation**, failure to pass stool; abdominal distention

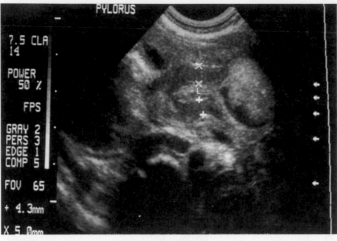

FIGURE 3-20 Abdominal ultrasound demonstrating pyloric stenosis.

Note the thin pyloric lumen (L) and the thickened pyloric musculature (defined by region between ×'s and +'s).

(From Daffner, R. H. & Hartman, M. [2013]. *Clinical Radiology: The Essentials* [4th ed. p. 298]. Philadelphia: Wolters Kluwer/Lippincott Williams & Wilkins; with permission.)

3. **Labs** = bowel biopsy shows **absence of ganglia**
4. **Radiology** = AXR demonstrates dilated bowel; barium enema shows proximal dilation (megacolon) with distal narrowing
5. **Treatment** = colostomy and resection of affected area

E. Intussusception

1. **Telescoping of bowel into adjacent segment** of bowel, leading to obstruction; most frequently proximal to ileocecal valve
2. **Risk factors** = Meckel diverticulum, Henoch-Schönlein purpura, adenovirus infection, cystic fibrosis
3. **H/P** = sudden abdominal pain that lasts <1 min and is episodic; pallor, sweating, vomiting, bloody mucus in stool (i.e., **currant jelly stool**); abdominal tenderness; **palpable, sausage-like abdominal mass**
4. **Labs** = increased WBC
5. **Radiology** = barium enema will show obstruction; US or CT may detect abnormal bowel
6. **Treatment** = barium enema may reduce defect; surgery required for refractory cases
7. **Complications** = bowel ischemia (appendix particularly susceptible)

F. Meckel diverticulum

1. Common **remnant of vitelline** duct that exists as **outpouching of ileum** and may contain **ectopic tissue**
2. **H/P** = asymptomatic; occasionally presents with painless rectal bleeding, **intussusception**, diverticulitis, or abscess formation
3. **Radiology** = gastric mucosa may be detected by technetium radionucleotide scan (i.e., **Meckel scan**)
4. **Treatment** = surgical resection if symptomatic

G. Neonatal jaundice

1. Hyperbilirubinemia in the newborn may be due to **physiologic, hepatic, or hematologic** causes
   a. Physiologic (**common**): **physiologic undersecretion**, breastfeeding failure
   b. Increased hemolysis: maternal–fetal ABO incompatibility, hereditary RBC abnormalities, glucose-6-phosphate dehydrogenase (G6PD) deficiency
   c. Bilirubin overproduction without hemolysis: hemorrhage, maternal–fetal transfusion
   d. Hepatic abnormalities: Gilbert syndrome, Crigler-Najjar syndrome, biliary atresia
2. Physiologic causes frequently resolve within 2 weeks.

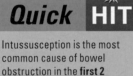

Quick HIT

Intussusception is the most common cause of bowel obstruction in the **first 2 years of life.**

Quick HIT

Intussusception in an adult is considered cancer until proven otherwise and usually will require surgical reduction.

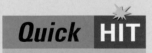

Quick HIT

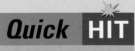

Meckel diverticulum rule of 2s—males **2 times** more common than females, occurs within **2 ft** of ileocecal valve, **2 types** of ectopic tissue (gastric, pancreatic), found in **2%** of the population, most complications occur before **2** years of age.

3. **Kernicterus** is deposition of bilirubin in the basal ganglia and hippocampus and may cause permanent damage; results from extremely high serum bilirubin and is typically only seen with hepatic abnormalities

4. **H/P** = jaundice, scleral icterus; lethargy, high-pitched cry, seizures, and apnea seen with kernicterus

5. **Labs** = frequently indirect hyperbilirubinemia (due to hemolysis); jaundice developing with initial 24 hrs after birth, total bilirubin >15 mg/dL, or direct bilirubin >2 mg/dL suggests nonphysiologic cause

6. **Treatment** = phototherapy used for physiologic jaundice lasting several days; suspected nonphysiologic causes should be worked up and may require exchange transfusion; intravenous immunoglobulin may reduce need for exchange transfusion in cases of maternal–fetal blood type incompatibility

H. Failure to thrive

1. Children below third percentile weight for age or failure to gain weight appropriate for age

2. May be due to underlying illness or neglect

3. **H/P** = look for leads to organic causes; screen for abuse

4. **Labs** = urinalysis, CBC, blood culture, urine culture, serum electrolytes, cystic fibrosis testing, and caloric intake records may be helpful in making diagnosis

5. **Treatment** = high-calorie diet, treat underlying disorder; educate parents in proper nutrition and feeding; contact social support services in cases of neglect or abuse

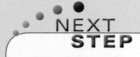

NEXT STEP

Always look for signs of abuse and neglect in a child with failure to thrive.

4 GENITOURINARY DISORDERS

I. Normal Renal Function

A. Physiology (*see Figure 4-1*)

1. Kidneys function to filter serum plasma, regulate fluid volume and electrolyte levels, maintain body fluid homeostasis, and secrete several hormones important in systemic hemodynamics.

2. **Proximal convoluted tubule** (cortex)

   a. Almost all glucose, bicarbonate (HCO_3^-), amino acids, and metabolites are reabsorbed.

   b. Two-thirds of sodium (Na^+) is reabsorbed; chloride (Cl^+) and water (H_2O) are reabsorbed passively along osmotic gradient.

   c. Organic acids (e.g., uric acid, etc.) and bases are secreted into tubules.

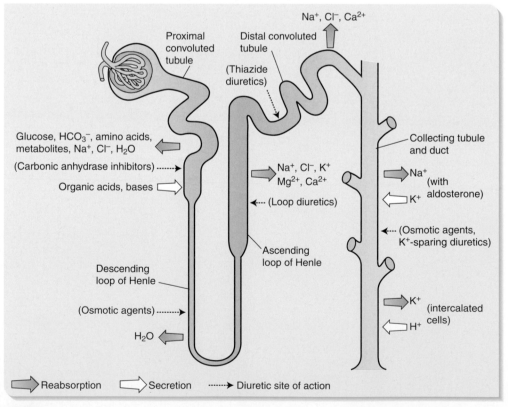

FIGURE 4-1 Anatomy of the nephron and major sites of ion, water, and molecule exchange.

3. **Descending loop of Henle** (medulla)
   a. Increasing interstitial osmotic gradient causes water reabsorption and concentration of tubule fluid.
   b. Descending limb is the only segment of the loop that is permeable to H_2O.
4. **Ascending loop of Henle** (medulla)
   a. Active reabsorption of Na^+, Cl^-, and potassium (K^+) by $Na^+/K^+/Cl^-$ cotransporter
   b. Reabsorption of magnesium (Mg^{2+}), calcium (Ca^{2+}), and K^+ through paracellular diffusion
5. **Distal convoluted tubule** (cortex)
   a. Cells impermeable to water
   b. Na^+ and Cl^- reabsorbed by Na^+/Cl^- transporter
   c. Ca^{2+} reabsorbed via parathyroid hormone activity
6. **Collecting tubule** (cortex) **and duct** (medulla)
   a. Principal cells drive Na^+ reabsorption and K^+ secretion when stimulated by aldosterone.
   b. Intercalated cells secrete H^+ and reabsorb K^+.
   c. Antidiuretic hormone (ADH) drives H_2O reabsorption.

B. Diuretics (*see Table 4-1*)
1. Affect electrolyte and fluid resorption at distinct locations along the renal tubular system
2. Renal activity of diuretics affects body fluid composition and volume.

TABLE 4-1	Common Diuretics and Effects within the Nephron			
Diuretic	**Site of Action**	**Mechanism of Action**	**Indications**	**Adverse Effects**
Carbonic anhydrase inhibitors (acetazolamide)	Proximal convoluted tubule	Inhibition of carbonic anhydrase causes mild diuresis and prevents HCO_3 reabsorption	Glaucoma, epilepsy, altitude sickness, metabolic alkalosis, idiopathic intracranial hypertension	Mild metabolic acidosis, hypokalemia, nephrolithiasis
Osmotic agents (mannitol, urea)	Proximal convoluted tubule, loop of Henle, collecting tubule	Increased tubular osmotic gradient increases H_2O excretion	Increased intracranial pressure, acute kidney injury (from shock or drug toxicity), acute glaucoma	No effect on Na^+ excretion, hyponatremia initially, followed by relative hypernatremia
Loop diuretics (furosemide, bumetanide, torsemide, ethacrynic acid)	Ascending loop of Henle	Inhibits $Na^+/Cl^-/K^+$ cotransporter to decrease reabsorption and indirectly inhibits Ca^{2+} reabsorption	CHF, pulmonary edema, hypercalcemia; rapid onset useful in emergent situations	Ototoxicity, hyperuricemia, hypokalemia, hypocalcemia
Thiazides (hydrochlorothiazide, chlorthalidone, metolazone)	Distal convoluted tubule	Inhibits Na^+/Cl^- cotransporter to decrease reabsorption and indirectly increases K^+ excretion and increases Ca^{2+} reabsorption	HTN, CHF, hypercalciuria, nephrogenic diabetes insipidus	Hypokalemia, hyponatremia, hyperuricemia, hypercalcemia
K^+-sparing aldosterone antagonists (spironolactone, eplerenone)	Collecting tubules	Aldosterone receptor antagonists, inhibits Na^+-K^+ exchange	Hyperaldosteronism, CHF, post-MI, cirrhosis; acne, PCOS (spironolactone only)	Hyperkalemia; gynecomastia, menstrual irregularity (spironolactone only)
Other K^+-sparing (triamterene, amiloride)	Collecting tubules	Blocks Na^+-K^+ exchanger in cortical collecting tubules	HTN, K^+-preserving diuresis	Hyperkalemia

CHF, congestive heart failure; HTN, hypertension; MI, myocardial infarction.

II. Disorders of the Kidney

A. Pyelonephritis

1. Infection of renal parenchyma most commonly caused by *Escherichia coli*; *Staphylococcus saprophyticus*, *Klebsiella*, and *Proteus* are less common pathogens; *Candida* is a potential cause in immunocompromised patients
2. Most commonly occurs as **sequelae of ascending urinary tract infection (UTI)**
3. **Risk factors** = urinary obstruction, immunocompromise, history of previous pyelonephritis, diabetes mellitus (DM), sexual intercourse >3 times/week, new sexual partner, spermicide use
4. **History and Physical (H/P)** = **flank pain**, chills, nausea, vomiting, urinary frequency, dysuria, urgency; fever (>101.5°F/38°C), **costovertebral tenderness**
5. **Labs** = increased white blood cell count (WBC), erythrocyte sedimentation rate (ESR), and C-reactive protein (CRP); **white blood cell casts in urine**; positive urine cultures with >10^5 bacteria/mL urine (possibly negative when due to hematogenous spread)
6. **Treatment** = intravenous (IV) fluoroquinolones, aminoglycosides, or cephalosporins (third generation) for 1 to 2 days, followed by outpatient oral antibiotics; severe or complicated cases may require 14 to 21 days of IV antibiotics; early mild cases in reliable patients may be amenable to oral antibiotics alone
7. **Complications** = increased risk of preterm labor and low birth weight in **pregnant** women

B. Nephrolithiasis *(see Table 4-2)*

1. Formation of "kidney" stones; stone formation can also occur elsewhere in the urinary tract; symptoms arise when stones become stuck in the urinary tract and cause **obstruction**.
2. **Risk factors** = family history, prior nephrolithiasis, low fluid intake, frequent UTIs, hypertension (HTN), DM, gout, renal tubular acidosis, **hypercalcemia**, **hyperparathyroidism**, certain drugs (e.g., acetazolamide, loop diuretics); males > females
3. **H/P** = **acute severe colicky flank pain** that may extend to inner thigh or genitals, nausea, vomiting, dysuria; possible gross hematuria
4. **Labs** = urinalysis shows hematuria (see Table 4-3)
5. **Radiology** = abdominal X-ray shows stones in most cases (except uric acid stones); computed tomography (CT) or ultrasound (US) may locate stones; intravenous pyelogram (IVP) shows filling defect but is used infrequently

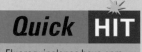

Quick HIT

Fluoroquinolones have comparable bioavailability for the oral and IV formulations.

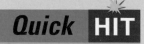

Quick HIT

The **uretero–vesical junction** is the most common site of renal stone impaction.

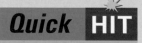

Quick HIT

Patients with **impacted stones** will be in pain and will **shift position frequently** in unsuccessful attempts to find a comfortable position; patients with **peritonitis** will remain **rigid**.

Quick HIT

In an IVP, water-soluble contrast dyes are injected IV and excreted by the kidneys; an appropriately timed X-ray will demonstrate excretion of the dye through the urinary tract and may show urinary defects and obstructions.

Genitourinary Disorders

TABLE 4-2	Types of Nephrolithiasis (Renal Stones)			
Type	**Frequency**	**Cause**	**Radiology**	**Notes**
Calcium oxalate	72%	**Idiopathic hypercalciuria**, small bowel diseases	Radiopaque	Most patients have no identifiable cause
Struvite (Mg-NH$_4$-PO$_4$)	12%	**Urinary tract infection** (with urease-positive bacteria: *Proteus*, *Klebsiella*)	Radiopaque	More common in **women**; may form staghorn calculi
Calcium phosphate	8%	**Hyperparathyroidism**, renal tubular acidosis	Radiopaque	
Uric acid	7%	Chronic acidic/concentrated urine, chemotherapeutic drugs, gout	**Radiolucent**	Treat by alkalinizing urine
Cystine	1%	Cystinuria, amino acid transport defects	Radiopaque	May form staghorn calculi

TABLE 4-3	Common Causes of Hematuria	
Age	**Temporary Hematuria**	**Persistent Hematuria**
<20 yr	Idiopathic UTI Exercise Trauma Endometriosis (women)	Glomerular disease
20–50 yr	Idiopathic UTI Nephrolithiasis Exercise Trauma Endometriosis (women)	Adult polycystic kidney disease Neoplasm (bladder, kidney, prostate) Glomerular disease
>50 yr	Idiopathic UTI Nephrolithiasis Trauma	Adult polycystic kidney disease BPH (men) Neoplasm (bladder, kidney, prostate) Glomerular disease

BPH, benign prostatic hyperplasia; UTI, urinary tract infection.

6. **Treatment** = hydration and pain control (possibly narcotics and/or ketorolac); shockwave lithotripsy can break up stones <3 cm diameter so that they pass through the ureters; surgery may be required for larger stones
7. **Complications** = hydronephrosis, recurrent stones

C. Hydronephrosis

1. **Dilation of renal calyces** as a result of increased pressure in the distal urinary tract
2. Caused by increased intrarenal pressure from urinary tract obstruction (e.g., stones, anatomic defects, extraurinary/intraurinary mass)
3. Can lead to permanent damage of renal parenchyma
4. **H/P** = possibly asymptomatic; dull or intermittent flank pain with history of UTI; anuria suggests significant bilateral ureteral obstruction
5. **Radiology** = US or IVP detects dilation (see Figure 4-2)

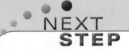

NEXT STEP

Rule out bladder or urethral obstruction in an anuric patient by attempting bladder catheterization.

Genitourinary Disorders

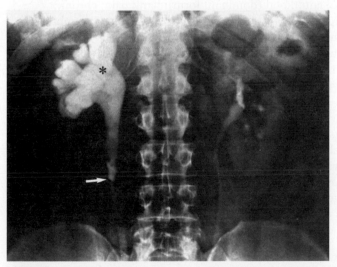

FIGURE 4-2 Intravenous pyelogram demonstrating hydronephrosis in the right kidney (*asterisk*); renal pelvis dilation is evident as is a radiopaque stone in the right ureter (*arrow*); the left kidney appears normal.

(From Daffner, R. H., & Hartman M. [2013]. *Clinical Radiology: The Essentials* [4th ed., p. 315]. Philadelphia, PA: Wolters Kluwer/Lippincott Williams & Wilkins.)

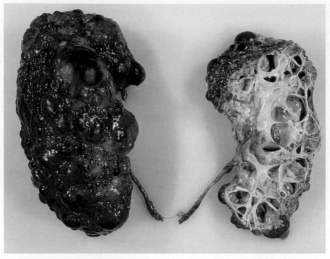

Autosomal dominant polycystic kidney disease.

Note enlargement of the kidney with many cysts of various sizes.

(From Rubin R., & Strayer, D. S. [2012]. *Rubin's Pathology* [6th ed., p. 759]. Philadelphia, PA: Wolters Kluwer/Lippincott Williams & Wilkins; with permission.)

6. **Treatment** = drainage via nephrostomy tube; treat underlying obstruction (balloon dilation of ureter and placement of double-J stent in ureter may allow urine flow)
7. **Complications** = renal failure

D. Polycystic kidney disease

1. Hereditary syndrome characterized by the formation of cysts in one or both kidneys leading to eventual kidney functional impairment and failure (see Figure 4-3)
2. Types
   a. **Autosomal dominant: most common form**; affects **adults**; large multicystic kidneys that function poorly
   b. **Autosomal recessive**: rare form; presents in **children**; fatal in initial years of life (without transplant)
3. **H/P** = asymptomatic until adulthood (dominant form); flank pain, chronic UTI, gross hematuria; large, palpable kidneys; possible hypertension; symptoms exacerbated by cyst rupture
4. **Labs** = increased blood urea nitrogen (BUN), increased creatinine (Cr), anemia; urinalysis shows hematuria and proteinuria
5. **Radiology** = US or CT will show **large multicystic kidneys**; stones may be a comorbid finding
6. **Treatment** = vasopressin receptor antagonists and amiloride can help prevent collection of fluid in cysts; preserve kidney function by treating UTI and HTN; drainage of large cysts helps with pain control; dialysis or transplant may be required if function deteriorates into renal failure
7. **Complications** = end-stage renal disease, hepatic cysts, intracranial aneurysms, subarachnoid hemorrhage, mitral valve prolapse; more severe symptoms and quicker deterioration occur in the recessive form

E. Renal cell carcinoma

1. Most common primary malignant neoplasm of renal parenchyma
2. **Risk factor** = **tobacco smoking**, exposure to cadmium and asbestos
3. **H/P** = flank pain, weight loss; abdominal mass, HTN, fever, hematuria

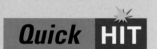

Quick **HIT**

15% of patients with polycystic kidney disease develop a **subarachnoid hemorrhage**.

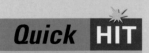

Quick **HIT**

Malignancies that cause increased erythropoietin: renal cell carcinoma, hepatocellular carcinoma, pheochromocytoma, and hemangioblastoma

4. **Labs** = polycythemia (secondary to increased erythropoietin activity); urinalysis shows hematuria; biopsy can be performed but is usually foregone in favor of immediate surgical resection
5. **Radiology** = US, magnetic resonance imaging (MRI), or CT with contrast may show renal mass
6. **Treatment** = nephrectomy or renal-sparing resection with lymph node dissection (typically performed without biopsy for solid mass with adequate radiographic imaging); immunotherapy, radiation therapy, and chemotherapy used for metastatic or unresectable disease but infrequently improve survival
7. **Complications** = poor prognosis if not caught in early stages; early recognition significantly improves prognosis

F. Interstitial nephropathy (acute interstitial nephritis)

1. Damage of renal tubules or parenchyma caused by **drugs, toxins**, infection, or autoimmune processes
2. Medication causes include β-lactam antibiotics, sulfonamides, **aminoglycosides**, nonsteroidal anti-inflammatory drugs (NSAIDs), allopurinol, proton pump inhibitors (PPIs), and diuretics (in addition to several other drugs).
3. Toxic causes include **cadmium, lead**, copper, mercury, and some poisonous mushrooms.
4. Other causes include infection, sarcoidosis, amyloidosis, myoglobinuria (from muscle injury or excessive exercise), and high uric acid levels.
5. **H/P** = symptoms of acute kidney injury, nausea, vomiting, malaise, rash; fever
6. **Labs** = increased Cr, eosinophilia; urinalysis may show granular or epithelial casts; toxin screens may detect offending agents; renal biopsy shows infiltration of inflammatory cells and renal tubular necrosis
7. **Treatment** = stop offending agent; supportive care until renal recovery; corticosteroids may be beneficial in refractory cases
8. **Complications** = acute tubular necrosis (ATN) (i.e., progressive damage of renal tubules), acute or chronic renal failure, renal papillary necrosis (ischemic necrosis of renal parenchyma), end-stage renal disease

III. Glomerular Diseases

A. Nephritic syndromes (*see Table 4-4*)

1. Acute **hematuria** and proteinuria that result secondary to **glomerular inflammation**
2. **H/P** = varies with pathology; oliguria and gross hematuria (evidenced by brown urine) are common
3. **Labs** = vary with pathology; generally increased BUN, increased Cr; hematuria and proteinuria seen on urinalysis; 24-hr urine collection measures protein as <3.5 g/day
4. **Treatment** = varies with pathology; dialysis or renal transplantation may be required in cases of renal failure

B. Nephrotic syndromes (*see Table 4-5*)

1. Significant proteinuria (**>3.5 g/day**) associated with hypoalbuminemia and hyperlipidemia
2. Frequently subsequent to glomerulonephritis
3. **H/P** = varies with pathology; generally **edema**, foamy urine, dyspnea, hypertension, ascites
4. **Labs** = vary with pathology; generally decreased albumin and hyperlipidemia; proteinuria >3.5 g/day seen on 24-hr urine collection
5. **Treatment** = varies with pathology; frequently includes diuretics and dietary salt and protein restriction

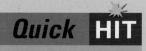

Quick HIT

Both nephritic and nephrotic syndromes involve diseases of the glomeruli; they are differentiated by the absence (nephritic) or presence (nephrotic) of proteinuria >3.5 g/day.

Genitourinary Disorders

TABLE 4-4 Nephritic Syndromes

Type	Pathology	H/P	Labs	Treatment
Postinfectious glomerulonephritis	Sequelae of systemic infection (most commonly **group A streptococcus**)	Recent infection, oliguria, edema, brown urine, hypertension; more common in **children**	Hematuria and proteinuria in urinalysis, high antistreptolysin O titer, **subepithelial "humps"** of IgG and C3 on renal basement membrane on electron microscopy	Self-limited, supportive treatment (decrease edema and hypertension)
IgA nephropathy (Berger disease)	Uncertain but may be related to infection; deposition of IgA immune complexes in mesangial cells	Hematuria, flank pain, low-grade fever	**Increased serum IgA**, mesangial cell proliferation on electron microscopy	Occasionally self-limited; give ACE-I and statins for persistent proteinuria; give corticosteroids if nephrotic syndrome develops
Goodpasture syndrome	Deposition of antiglomerular and antialveolar basement membrane antibodies (renal disease is a subtype of RPGN)	Dyspnea, hemoptysis, myalgias, hematuria	**Serum IgG antiglomerular basement membrane antibodies**, anemia, pulmonary infiltrates on CXR, **linear pattern of IgG antibody deposition** on fluorescence microscopy of glomeruli	Plasmapheresis, corticosteroids, immunosuppressive agents; can progress to renal failure
Alport syndrome	Hereditary defect in collagen IV in basement membrane	Hematuria, symptoms of renal failure, **high-frequency hearing loss, eye disease** (cataracts, lenticonus)	Red cell casts, hematuria, proteinuria, and pyuria on urinalysis; **"split basement membrane"** on electron microscopy	Variable prognosis with no therapy identified to halt cases of renal failure; ACE-I may reduce proteinuria; renal transplant may be complicated by Alport-related development of Goodpasture syndrome
Rapidly progressive (crescentic) glomerulonephritis (RPGN)	**Rapidly progressive renal failure** from idiopathic causes or associated with other glomerular diseases or systemic infection	Sudden renal failure, weakness, nausea, weight loss, dyspnea, hemoptysis, myalgias, fever, oliguria	Deposition of inflammatory cells and eventually fibrous material in Bowman capsule, and crescent formation (basement membrane wrinkling) on electron microscopy; pauci-immune RPGN is ANCA+	Poor prognosis with rapid progression to renal failure; corticosteroids, plasmapheresis, and immunosuppressive agents may be helpful; renal transplant frequently required
Lupus nephritis (mesangial, membranous, focal proliferative, and diffuse proliferative types)	Complication of systemic lupus erythematosus involving proliferation of endothelial and mesangial cells	Possibly asymptomatic, possible hypertension or renal failure; may develop nephrotic syndrome	**ANA, anti-DNA antibodies**; hematuria and possible proteinuria on urinalysis	Corticosteroids or immunosuppressive agents can delay renal failure; ACE-I and statins help reduce proteinuria
Granulomatosis with polyangiitis (Wegener)—also see Pulmonary chapter	Similar to crescentic disease with addition of **pulmonary involvement** granulomatous inflammation of airways and renal vasculature	Weight loss, respiratory symptoms, hematuria, fever	**c-ANCA**; deposition of immune complexes in renal vessels seen on electron microscopy; pulmonary biopsy helpful in diagnosis	Corticosteroids, cytotoxic agents (cyclophosphamide); variable prognosis

ACE-I, angiotensin-converting enzyme inhibitor; ANA, antinuclear antibody; ANCA, antineutrophil cytoplasmic antibody; c-ANCA, cytoplasmic antineutrophil cytoplasmic antibody; CXR, chest X-ray; H/P, history and physical.

Genitourinary Disorders

TABLE 4-5	Nephrotic Syndromes			
Type	**Pathology**	**H/P**	**Labs**	**Treatment**
Minimal change disease	Idiopathic; may involve effacement (flattening) of foot processes on basement membrane	Possible hypertension, increased frequency of infections; most common cause of nephrotic syndrome in **children**	Hyperlipidemia, hypoalbuminemia; proteinuria on urinalysis; flattening of basement membrane foot processes seen on electron microscopy	Corticosteroids, cytotoxic agents
Focal segmental glomerular sclerosis	Frequently idiopathic or associated with drug use or **HIV**; segmental sclerosis of glomeruli	Possible hypertension; most common cause of nephrotic syndrome in **adults** in the United States (especially in blacks and Latinos)	Hyperlipidemia, hypoalbuminemia; hematuria and high proteinuria on urinalysis; sclerotic changes seen in some glomeruli on electron microscopy	Corticosteroids, cytotoxic agents, ACE-I, statins; progressive cases that require renal transplant (uncommon) frequently have recurrence
Membranous nephropathy	Idiopathic or associated with infection, systemic lupus erythematosus, neoplasm, or drugs; thickening of basement membrane	Edema, dyspnea; history of infection or medication use may lead to diagnosis; associated with hepatitis B and C	Hyperlipidemia, hypoalbuminemia; proteinuria on urinalysis; **"spike and dome" basement membrane thickening** on electron microscopy	Corticosteroids, cytotoxic agents, ACE-I, statins; variable rates of renal failure and renal vein thrombosis (requires anticoagulation)
Membranoproliferative glomerulonephritis	Idiopathic or associated with infection or autoimmune disease; thickening of basement membrane; associated hepatitis B and C, SLE, and subacute bacterial endocarditis	Edema, HTN; history of systemic infection or autoimmune condition; gradual progression to renal failure	Hyperlipidemia, hypoalbuminemia, possible hypocomplementemia; proteinuria and possible hematuria on urinalysis; IgG deposits may be seen on basement membrane on fluorescence microscopy; **basement membrane thickening with double-layer "train track" appearance** on electron microscopy	Corticosteroids combined with either aspirin or dipyridamole may delay progression to renal failure
Diabetic nephropathy (diffuse, nodular)	Basement membrane and mesangial thickening related to diabetic vascular changes	History of DM, hypertension, progressive renal failure	Hyperlipidemia, hypoalbuminemia, proteinuria on urinalysis; basement membrane thickening on electron microscopy seen in both types, round nodules (**Kimmelstiel-Wilson nodules**) seen within glomeruli in nodular type	Treat underlying DM, dietary protein restriction; ACE-I; tight blood pressure control
Amyloidosis	Deposition of amyloid protein fibrils in glomeruli and/or renal vasculature; may also involve many other tissues (heart, GI tract nerve tissue, etc.)	Edema, may progress to renal failure; other findings depend on extrarenal tissues involved	Hyperlipidemia, hypoalbuminemia, may have elevated creatinine; proteinuria on urinalysis; Congo red stain of biopsy shows **apple-green birefringence** on polarized light	Melphalan, hematopoietic stem cell transplant, renal transplant

ACE-I, angiotensin-converting enzyme inhibitor; DM, diabetes mellitus; GI, gastrointestinal; H/P, history and physical; HTN, hypertension.

Genitourinary Disorders

IV. Renal Failure

A. Acute kidney injury (AKI)

1. Sudden decrease in renal function (e.g., glomerular filtering, urine production, or chemical excretion abnormalities with BUN and Cr retention) resulting from prerenal, intrarenal, or postrenal causes
   a. Prerenal causes include **hypovolemia**, sepsis, renal artery stenosis, and drug toxicity.
   b. Intrarenal causes include **ATN** (drugs, toxins), glomerular disease, and renal vascular disease.

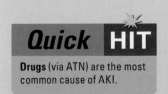

Quick **HIT**

Drugs (via ATN) are the most common cause of AKI.

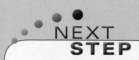

c. Postrenal disease is caused by **obstruction** of renal calyces, ureters, or the bladder (e.g., stones, tumor, adhesions).

2. **H/P** = may initially be asymptomatic; possible fatigue, anorexia, nausea, oliguria, gross hematuria, flank pain, or mental status changes; possible pericardial friction rub, hypertension, fever, diffuse rash, edema

3. **Labs**
   a. **Increased BUN, increased Cr** (azotemia)
   b. Urinalysis may show hematuria and red cell casts (glomerular or vasculitic disease), epithelial casts (ATN), pyuria with waxy casts (interstitial disease or obstruction), or pyuria alone (infection).
   c. Fractional excretion of Na^+ (FENa) <1% suggests a prerenal cause, >2% suggests ATN.

$$FENa = \frac{[(urine\ Na)/(serum\ Na)]}{[(urine\ Cr)/(serum\ Cr)]}$$

   d. Findings consistent with nephritic or nephrotic syndromes should prompt renal biopsy.

4. **Radiology** = US, CT, IVP, or renal angiography may be useful to detect masses, hydronephrosis, abnormal blood flow, obstruction, or vasculitis

5. **Treatment** = prevent fluid overload, stop drugs causing ATN; dietary protein restriction, corticosteroids, dialysis

B. Chronic kidney disease (CKD)

1. Progressive damage of renal parenchyma that can take several years to develop
2. HTN and DM are the most common causes.
3. **H/P** = gradual development of uremic syndrome (i.e., changes in mental status, decreased consciousness, HTN, pericarditis, anorexia, nausea, vomiting, gastrointestinal (GI) bleeding, peripheral neuropathy, brownish coloration of skin)
4. **Labs** = increased K^+, decreased Na^+, increased phosphate, decreased Ca^{2+}, anemia, metabolic acidosis, increased BUN, increased Cr; urine osmolality is similar to serum osmolality
5. **Radiology** = US may show hydronephrosis or shrunken kidneys
6. **Treatment** = restrict dietary salt and protein, correct electrolyte abnormalities, treat underlying condition; dialysis or renal transplant may be needed in progressive cases
7. **Complications** = end-stage renal disease (i.e., chronic kidney disease with severe symptoms and electrolyte abnormalities requiring dialysis for survival), renal osteodystrophy (i.e., bone degeneration secondary to low serum Ca^{2+}), encephalopathy, severe anemia (caused by decreased erythropoietin)

C. Dialysis

1. Induced filtering of blood required when kidney function is inadequate or serum composition increases risk of mortality.
2. Types
   a. **Hemodialysis**: machine filters blood and returns filtered plasma to vasculature; synthetic grafts or surgical arteriovenous fistulas in the forearm are utilized for access
   b. **Peritoneal dialysis**
      (1) Dialysate fluid temporarily pumped into peritoneum via a permanent catheter
      (2) Substances in the blood diffuse across the peritoneum from the surrounding vasculature to the dialysate fluid according to osmotic drive (peritoneum serves as a filter)
      (3) Dialysate fluid containing solutes is pumped out of peritoneal cavity.
3. **Indications** = severe hyperkalemia, severe metabolic acidosis, fluid overload, uremic syndrome, CKD with Cr >12 mg/dL and BUN >100 mg/dL
4. **Complications** = infection at access sites, fluid overload with dyspnea, hypotension (hemodialysis)
5. Frequently precedes renal transplant

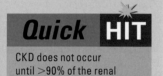

Genitourinary Disorders

V. Acid-base Disorders

A. Renal tubular acidosis (*see Table 4-6*)

1. Abnormalities in renal tubular H^+ secretion or HCO_3^- reabsorption
2. Leads to nonanion gap metabolic acidosis

TABLE 4-6	Characteristics of Types of Renal Tubular Acidosis		
	Distal (Type 1)	**Proximal (Type 2)**	**Low Renin/ Aldosterone (Type 4)**
Defect	Impaired H^+ secretion leading to secondary hyperaldosteronism	HCO_3^- reabsorption	Primary or secondary hypoaldosteronism
Cause	Idiopathic, autoimmune diseases, drugs, chronic infection, nephrocalcinosis, cirrhosis, SLE, obstructive nephropathy	Idiopathic, multiple myeloma, Fanconi syndrome, Wilson disease, amyloidosis, vitamin D deficiency, autoimmune diseases	Primary renin or aldosterone deficiency, **DM**, Addison disease, sickle cell disease, interstitial disease
Urine pH	**>5.3**	<5.3	<5.3
Serum electrolytes	Low K^+, variable HCO_3^-	Low K^+, low HCO_3^-	**High K^+**, high Cl^-
Radiology	Possible **stones**	**Bone lesions**	
Treatment	Oral HCO_3^-, K^+, thiazide diuretic	Oral HCO_3^-, K^+; thiazide or loop diuretic	Fludrocortisone, K^+ restriction

DM, diabetes mellitus; SLE, systemic lupus erythematosus.

B. Acid-base physiology

1. In a healthy person, serum pH is regulated by HCO_3^- reabsorption (proximal tubule of kidneys) and blood Pco_2 (respiratory activity).
2. In a healthy person:
   a. pH = 7.40
   b. Pco_2 = 40 mm Hg
   c. Po_2 = 100 mm Hg
   d. HCO_3^- = 24 mEq/L
3. Pco_2 and pH can be measured with arterial blood gas; HCO_3^- is calculated by the Henderson-Hasselbach equation:

$$pH = pKa + \log\left(\frac{[HCO_3^-]}{0.03 \times Pco_2}\right)$$

4. pH >7.42 → alkalosis; pH <7.3 → acidosis
5. Disturbances because of HCO_3^- abnormalities are metabolic; disturbances caused by Pco_2 levels are **respiratory**.
6. For any disturbance, the body tries to compensate and normalize serum pH.

C. Acid-base disturbances (*see Figure 4-4, Table 4-7*)

1. Anion gap
   a. Difference between serum Na^+ and Cl^- and HCO_3^- ion concentrations
   b. **Anion gap = $[Na^+] - [Cl^-] - [HCO_3^-]$** (normal = 8 to 12)
   c. Normal anion gap acidosis suggests HCO_3^- loss
   d. Increased anion gap acidosis suggests H^+ excess

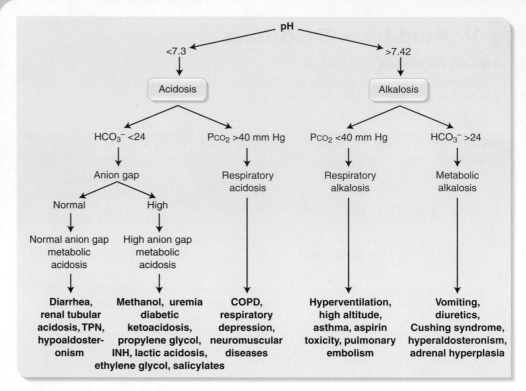

MNEMONIC

Remember the causes of high anion gap metabolic acidosis by the mnemonic **MUD PILES**:
Methanol
Uremia
Diabetic ketoacidosis
Propylene glycol
Isoniazid/**I**ron
Lactic acidosis
Ethylene glycol
Salicylates

FIGURE
4-4   **Differentiation of acid-base disturbances and related causes.**

Note: Compensatory mechanisms should be checked to differentiate solitary from mixed disturbances.

COPD, chronic obstructive pulmonary disease; TPN, total parenteral nutrition.

2. **Mixed disorder**
   a. Combination of multiple acid-base disturbances
   b. Detected when corrected, HCO_3^- is different from measured value.
   c. Corrected HCO_3^- = measured anion gap − normal anion gap + measured HCO_3^- (for which 12 = value of normal anion gap)
   d. If corrected, HCO_3^- is
      (1) Normal, disturbance is solitary high anion gap acidosis
      (2) Increased, disturbance is metabolic alkalosis with high anion gap acidosis
      (3) Decreased, disturbance is nonanion gap acidosis with high anion gap acidosis

TABLE **4-7**	Acid-Base Disturbances and Compensatory Mechanisms					
Disorder	**pH**	**(H⁺)**	**(HCO₃⁻)**	**Pco₂**	**Compensation**	**Common Causes**
Metabolic acidosis	↓	↑	↓↓	↓	Hyperventilation	Diarrhea, diabetic ketoacidosis, lactic acidosis, renal tubular acidosis
Metabolic alkalosis	↑	↓	↑↑	↑	Hypoventilation	Vomiting, diuretics, Cushing syndrome, hyperaldosteronism, adrenal hyperplasia
Respiratory acidosis	↓	↑	↑	↑↑	Increased HCO₃⁻ reabsorption	COPD, respiratory depression, neuromuscular diseases
Respiratory alkalosis	↑	↓	↓	↓↓	Decreased HCO₃⁻ reabsorption	Hyperventilation, high altitude, asthma, aspirin toxicity, pulmonary embolism

COPD, chronic obstructive pulmonary disease; ↑, high; ↓, low; ↑↑, very high; ↓↓, very low.

VI. Electrolyte Disorders

A. Hypernatremia

1. Serum Na^+ >155 mEq/L
2. Caused by **dehydration**, loss of fluid from skin (e.g., burns, sweating), loss of fluid from GI tract (e.g., vomiting, diarrhea), diabetes insipidus, iatrogenic (see Figure 4-5)
3. **H/P** = oliguria, thirst, weakness, lethargy, decreased consciousness, mental status changes, seizures
4. **Treatment**
   a. Gradual hydration with normal saline for inadequate fluid intake or excess fluid loss (maximal Na^+ reduction = 12 mEq/day)
   b. Approximate required correction in a patient with purely fluid losses as a cause of hypernatremia can be determined through calculation of the **water deficit**:

$$\text{Water Deficit} = \text{Total body water} \times \left(\frac{[Na]}{140} - 1 \right)$$

$$\text{Water Deficit} = (0.60 \times [\text{mass in kg}]) \times \left(\frac{[Na]}{140} - 1 \right)$$

   c. Half of deficit is given in 24 hr in addition to maintenance fluids, remainder is given over following 24 to 48 hr; close monitoring of Na^+ is required to avoid excessive correction.
   d. Because total body water will be slightly greater than patient's body water content at time of hypernatremia (because of fluid loss), calculated water deficit may be artificially high.
5. Complications = seizures, CNS damage; too rapid hydration can cause **cerebral edema**

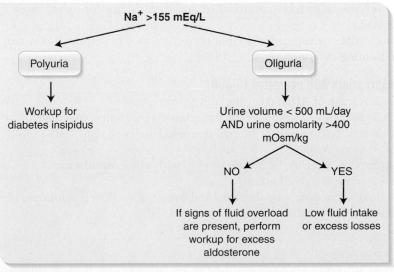

FIGURE 4-5 Evaluation of hypernatremia.

Na$^+$ >155 mEq/L

Polyuria → Workup for diabetes insipidus

Oliguria → Urine volume < 500 mL/day AND urine osmolarity >400 mOsm/kg

NO → If signs of fluid overload are present, perform workup for excess aldosterone

YES → Low fluid intake or excess losses

Genitourinary Disorders

B. Diabetes insipidus (DI)

1. Disorders of ADH-directed water reabsorption leading to dehydration and hypernatremia
2. Types
   a. **Central**: failure of posterior pituitary to secrete ADH; can result from idiopathic causes, cerebral trauma, pituitary tumors, hypoxic encephalopathy, or anorexia nervosa
   b. **Nephrogenic**: kidneys do not respond to ADH; can result from hereditary renal disease, **lithium toxicity**, hypercalcemia, or hypokalemia
3. **H/P** = polydipsia, polyuria, signs of dehydration
4. **Labs**
   a. Hypernatremia
   b. Low urine osmolality with large urine volume
   c. Water deprivation test
      (1) 2 to 3–hr water deprivation followed by ADH administration
      (2) Failure of urine osmolality to rise after water deprivation suggests DI.
      (3) A rise in urine osmolality following ADH administration suggests central DI.
      (4) Failure of urine osmolality to rise after ADH administration suggests nephrogenic DI.
5. **Radiology** = CT with contrast or MRI may show pituitary tumor
6. **Treatment**
   a. Treat underlying condition
   b. Central DI: desmopressin (DDAVP) given as ADH analogues
   c. Nephrogenic DI: salt restriction, increased H_2O intake; thiazide diuretics may reduce fluid loss (cause mild hypovolemia through activity at distal convoluted tubule to induce increased water absorption at proximal tubule); treat underlying condition (stop medications, treat tumor or renal disease)

C. Hyponatremia

1. Serum Na^+ <135 mEq/L
2. Caused by renal H_2O retention (e.g., congestive heart failure, syndrome of inappropriate ADH secretion [SIADH]), thiazide diuretics (i.e., salt wasting), **hyperglycemia** (i.e., osmotic hyponatremia), or high fluid intake (see Figure 4-6)
3. **H/P** = confusion, nausea, weakness, decreased consciousness
4. **Treatment** = treat underlying condition (stop offending agent, correct hyperglycemia or hyperlipidemia, etc.); salt administration and H_2O restriction unless hypovolemic and serum osmolality <280 mOsm/kg (rehydrate with saline no faster than 12 mEq/day); give loop diuretics or hypertonic saline for severe cases (Na^+ <120 mEq/L)
5. **Complications** = CNS damage; overly rapid correction with hypertonic saline can cause **central pontine myelinolysis**

D. Syndrome of inappropriate ADH secretion (SIADH)

1. **Nonphysiologic release of ADH**, resulting in hyponatremia
2. Caused by CNS pathology, sarcoidosis, **paraneoplastic syndromes**, psychiatric drugs, major surgery, pneumonia, or human immunodeficiency virus (HIV)
3. **H/P** = chronic hyponatremia
4. **Labs** = serum hypo-osmolarity (<280 mOsm/kg) with urine osmolarity >100 mOsm/kg; urine Na^+ >20 mEq/L
5. **Treatment** = fluid restriction; loop diuretics and hypertonic saline if symptomatic; demeclocycline may help maintain normal Na^+ levels

E. Hyperkalemia

1. Serum K^+ >5.0 mEq/L
2. Caused by metabolic acidosis, aldosterone deficiency, tissue breakdown, insulin deficiency, adrenal insufficiency, renal failure, K^+-sparing diuretics
3. **H/P** = weakness, nausea, vomiting; **arrhythmias**; paralysis or paresthesia in severe cases

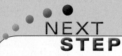

Quick HIT

Pseudohyponatremia is an artifact of hyperlipidemia in which serum Na^+ falsely appears to be low.

NEXT STEP

To calculate (Na^+) that will result from correction of hyperglycemia, add 1.6 mEq/L Na^+ for every 100 mg/dL glucose >100 mg/dL.

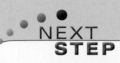

NEXT STEP

Pseudohyperkalemia occurs from red blood cell hemolysis following blood collection, so K^+ should be measured **immediately** in drawn blood and increased serum K^+ should be confirmed with a **repeat blood sample** using a large-gauge needle.

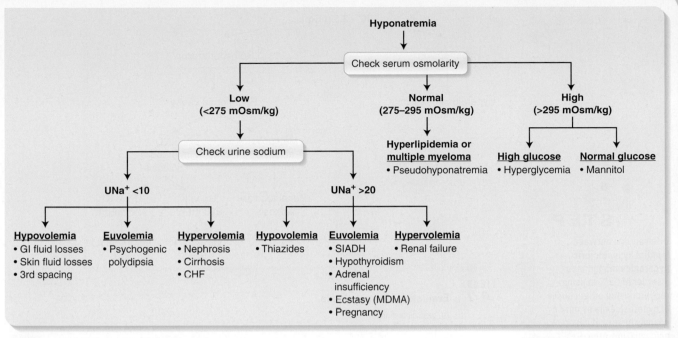

FIGURE 4-6 Evaluation of hyponatremia.

ACE-I, angiotensin-converting enzyme inhibitor; CHF, congestive heart failure; FENa, fractional excretion of Na = (Urine [Na⁺] × serum Cr) / (serum [Na⁺] × Urine Cr); SIADH, syndrome of inappropriate ADH secretion

4. Electrocardiogram (ECG) = tall, peaked T waves
5. Treatment = calcium gluconate (treats cardiac effects but does not change K⁺ level), $NaHCO_3$, or glucose with insulin to encourage K^+ uptake by cells; sodium polystyrene sulfonate binds K^+ and removes it through the GI tract; **dialysis** may be required in severe cases

F. Hypokalemia

1. Serum K^+ <3.5 mEq/L
2. Due to poor dietary intake, metabolic/respiratory alkalosis, hypothermia, vomiting, diarrhea, hyperaldosteronism, insulin excess (e.g., treatment of diabetic ketoacidosis), K^+-wasting diuretics (loop, thiazide), or renal tubular acidosis types I and II (see Figure 4-7)
3. H/P = Fatigue, weakness, paresthesias and/or paralysis; hyporeflexia, arrhythmias
4. ECG = T-wave flattening, ST depression, U waves
5. Treatment = treat underlying disorder; give oral or IV KCl (10 to 20 mEq/hr)
6. Complications = overly rapid replacement can lead to **arrhythmias**

G. Hypercalcemia

1. Serum Ca^{2+} >10.5 mg/dL
2. Caused by **hyperparathyroidism**, **neoplasm**, immobilization, thiazide diuretics, high ingestion of calcium carbonate and milk (milk-alkali syndrome; more often seen in children), sarcoidosis, or hypervitaminosis A or D
3. H/P = deep pain, easy fractures, possible nephrolithiasis, nausea, vomiting, constipation, weakness, mental status changes, polyuria
4. Labs = increased parathyroid hormone in hyperparathyroidism; very high Ca^{2+} and normal or low parathyroid hormone frequently seen with neoplasm; increased vitamins A or D seen in hypervitaminoses
5. EKG = shortened QT interval
6. Treatment = treat underlying disorder; hydration; calcitonin and **bisphosphonates** in cases of excess bone reabsorption; glucocorticoids decrease intestinal absorption in severe cases; surgery indicated for hyperparathyroidism and resectable neoplasms

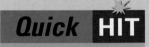

Hypercalcemia is characterized by "bones" (fractures), "stones" (nephrolithiasis), "groans" (GI symptoms), and "psychiatric overtones" (changes in mental status).

Genitourinary Disorders

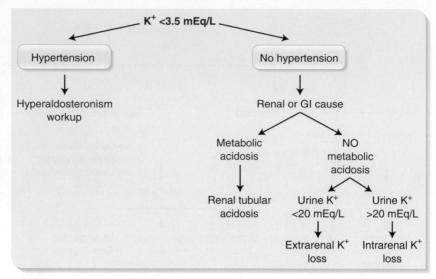

FIGURE 4-7 Evaluation of hypokalemia.

GI, gastrointestinal.

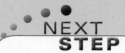

NEXT STEP

Differentiate between **familial hypocalciuric hypercalcemia** (genetic disorder of Ca^{2+}-sensing receptors) and other causes of hypercalcemia by noting a family history of hypercalcemia, low urine Ca^{2+}, and absence of osteopenia, nephrolithiasis, and mental status changes in the former.

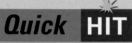

Quick HIT

Loop diuretics are "Ca^{2+}-wasting" and can **cause** hypocalcemia.

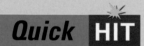

Quick HIT

Thiazide diuretics are "Ca^{2+}-sparing" and can **cause** hypercalcemia.

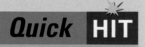

Quick HIT

Cultured urine should be from a midstream sample (**clean catch**) to avoid contamination from skin flora.

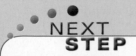

NEXT STEP

Perform a workup for sexually transmitted urethritis in any **man** with a suspected UTI because the symptoms may appear similar.

H. Hypocalcemia

1. Serum Ca^{2+} <8.5 mg/dL
2. Caused by hypoparathyroidism, hyperphosphatemia, chronic renal failure, vitamin D deficiency, **loop diuretics**, pancreatitis, or alcoholism
3. H/P = abdominal pain, dyspnea; tetany, **Chvostek sign** (i.e., tapping facial nerve causes spasm), carpopedal spasm when blood pressure cuff inflated (i.e., **Trousseau sign**)
4. **Labs** = decreased serum Ca^{2+} (total serum Ca^{2+} should be adjusted for hypoalbuminemia, lower limit of normal Ca^{2+} decreases 0.8 mg/dL for each 1 g/dL albumin <4; ionized calcium will not be affected by albumin levels); increased phosphate seen with hypoparathyroidism and renal failure
5. EKG = prolonged QT interval
6. **Treatment** = treat underlying disorder; oral Ca^{2+} or IV Ca^{2+} for severe symptoms; vitamin D supplementation, if necessary

VII. Bladder and Ureteral Disorders

A. Urinary tract infection (UTI)

1. Ascending infection of urethra, bladder, and ureters resulting from inoculation of lower urinary tract (rarely hematogenous spread)
2. Most commonly due to *E. coli, S. saprophyticus, Proteus, Klebsiella, Enterobacter, Pseudomonas,* and enterococcus
3. **Risk factors** = **obstruction**, Foley catheter, vesicoureteral reflux, pregnancy, DM, sexual intercourse, immunocompromise; female > male
4. **H/P** = **urinary frequency**, dysuria (i.e., painful urination), suprapubic pain, **urgency**
5. **Labs** = urinalysis shows increased nitrates, increased leukocyte esterase, and white blood cells in urine; urine culture will show >10^5 **pathogen colonies/mL**; blood tests usually not helpful unless due to hematogenous spread
6. **Treatment** = amoxicillin, trimethoprim-sulfamethoxazole (TMP-SMX), or fluoroquinolones for 3 days; relapsing infection should be treated for 14 days
7. **Complications** = abscess formation, pyelonephritis, renal failure, prostatitis

B. Urinary incontinence

1. Involuntary leakage of urine; more common in the elderly
2. First step in evaluation is to evaluate for causes of secondary incontinence (UTI, impaired mobility, fecal impaction, atrophic vaginitis, or delirium)

3. **Urge incontinence** (detrusor overactivity)
   a. Leakage of urine due to uninhibited bladder contractions
   b. **H/P** = diagnosis usually made by history of urgency, frequent voiding of small amounts of urine, and possibly incontinence
   c. **Treatment** = bladder training, antimuscarinics (oxybutynin, tolterodine, solifenacin, etc.)
4. **Stress incontinence**
   a. Leakage of urine during any maneuver that increases abdominal pressure due to decreased anatomic support of and function of the urinary sphincter
   b. **Risk factors** = female sex, multiparity, obesity
   c. **H/P** = incontinence accompanies coughing, sneezing, laughing, exercise, lifting heavy objects; diagnosis usually made by history and bladder diary; urodynamic testing by a urologist may be helpful but is usually not necessary
   d. **Treatment** = conservative therapy (weight loss, Kegel exercises), surgical therapy (midurethral sling)
5. **Overflow incontinence**
   a. Continuous leakage of urine due to incomplete bladder emptying
   b. More common in men
   c. **Causes** = bladder outlet obstruction (benign prostatic hyperplasia, urethral strictures), impaired detrusor contractility, neurogenic bladder
   d. **H/P** = weak urinary stream, dribbling, frequency, hesitancy, and nocturia; bladder diary is very helpful; palpable distended bladder
   e. **Testing** = automated bladder scanner or catheterized postvoid residual detects full bladder after voiding
   f. **Treatment** = decompress bladder with Foley catheter initially; treat underlying obstruction with surgery as needed; treat detrusor underactivity with sacral nerve stimulation; intermittent self-catheterization is sometimes required

C. Bladder cancer
1. **Transitional cell carcinoma** (common), squamous cell cancer (uncommon), or adenocarcinoma of the bladder (uncommon)
2. **Risk factors** = **tobacco**, schistosomiasis, cyclophosphamide, aniline dyes, petroleum byproducts, recurrent UTI; male 3× > female
3. **H/P** = **painless gross hematuria**; suprapubic pain, frequency, dysuria, and urgency occur later in disease; palpable suprapubic mass
4. **Labs** = urinalysis shows hematuria; urine cytology shows malignant cells; biopsy confirms diagnosis
5. **Radiology** = cystoscopy is important for visualization of lesions, urine specimen collection, and lesion biopsy; pelvic CT, MRI, or IVP may detect mass
6. **Treatment** = transurethral cystoscopic resection for superficial tumors; partial or total cystectomy for more invasive tumors; adjuvant intravesical chemotherapy and radiation therapy commonly utilized; regional radiation therapy and systemic chemotherapy for large tumors and metastatic disease
7. **Complications** = frequent recurrence

VIII. Male Reproduction

A. Urethritis
1. Infection of urethra caused by sexually transmitted *Neisseria gonorrhoeae* or *Chlamydia trachomatis*
2. **H/P** = dysuria, frequency, urgency, **burning urination**; **purulent urethral discharge** seen with *N. gonorrhoeae*
3. **Labs** = Gram stain shows gram-negative diplococci for *N. gonorrhoeae*; Thayer-Martin culture will detect *N. gonorrhoeae*; negative Gram stain suggests *C. trachomatis*; diagnosis of *Chlamydia* may be confirmed with nucleic acid amplification testing

4. **Treatment** = single-dose ceftriaxone with doxycycline or azithromycin used to treat both possible infections simultaneously; **treat sexual partners**; report of cases to public health office may be required
5. **Complications** = urethral strictures, frequent reinfection when sexual partners not treated

B. Prostatitis
1. Inflammation of prostate from unknown cause or as complication of UTI
2. **H/P** = perineal pain, dysuria, frequency, urgency; fever, tender prostate on digital rectal examination
3. **Labs** = may be suggestive of UTI; possible hematuria; white blood cells seen in prostatic secretions
4. **Treatment** = TMP-SMX (frequently for 4 to 6 weeks); treat for sexually transmitted diseases (STDs) in sexually active males

C. Benign prostatic hyperplasia (BPH)
1. **Benign enlargement of prostate** seen with increasing frequency as men age beyond 40 years
2. **H/P** = urinary **hesitancy**, straining, **weak or intermittent stream**, dribbling; frequency, urgency, **nocturia**, and overflow incontinence develop secondary to incomplete emptying or UTI; digital examination detects uniformly enlarged, rubbery prostate
3. **Labs** = possible mild increase in prostate-specific antigen (PSA); rule out infection (urinalysis), cancer (biopsy), and renal failure (serum electrolytes, BUN, Cr)
4. **Radiology** = transrectal US shows enlarged prostate
5. **Treatment** = α_1-receptor blockers (e.g., terazosin, etc.) and **5 α-reductase inhibitors** (e.g., finasteride, etc.) improve symptoms; surgery needed for refractory cases (i.e., transurethral resection of prostate [TURP]); transurethral needle ablation may be performed in men who are poor surgical candidates

D. Prostate cancer
1. Adenocarcinoma occurring in peripheral zone of prostate
2. **Risk factors** = increased age, family history, high-fat diet, prostatitis
3. **H/P** = frequently asymptomatic; weakened urinary stream, urinary retention, weight loss, back pain in later disease; **nodular or irregular prostate on digital examination**, lymphedema
4. **Labs** = urinalysis may show hematuria and pyuria; **increased PSA**, increased alkaline phosphatase; biopsy provides diagnosis
5. **Radiology** = transrectal US shows irregular prostate; bone scan, chest X-ray (CXR), and CT may detect metastases
6. **Treatment**
   a. Good prognosis with early treatment
   b. Radical retropubic, perineal, laparoscopic, or robotic prostatectomy; retropubic approach used for more extensive tumors
   c. Radiation therapy via external beam radiation or brachytherapy (i.e., implantation of radioactive seeds in prostate) may be used in early tumors in place of surgery.
   d. Follow up with PSA posttreatment to monitor for metastases and recurrence.
   e. Antiandrogen therapy (i.e., hormone therapy or orchiectomy) with chemotherapy can be used to improve symptoms in high-grade or metastatic disease.
   f. Older men may not be treated because tumors are frequently slow growing.
7. **Complications** = **incontinence** and **impotence** are common with radical prostatectomy

E. Epididymitis
1. Inflammation of epididymis associated with testicular inflammation
2. Caused by prostatitis, **STDs** (especially *Chlamydia*), urinary reflux
3. **H/P** = epididymal **pain relieved by supporting scrotum**, dysuria; scrotal tenderness, and induration

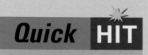
Quick HIT

Nonbacterial prostatitis is more common than bacterial prostatitis.

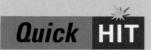
Quick HIT

BPH develops in the **central zone** of the prostate adjacent to the urethra and does not predispose patients to prostate cancer.

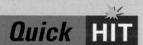
Quick HIT

Prostate cancer is the **most common nondermatologic cancer** in men; however, **lung** cancer is the greatest cause of **cancer-related death** in males, whereas **prostate** cancer is the **second** highest.

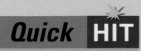
Quick HIT

Supporting the scrotum does **not** relieve pain in testicular torsion but does relieve pain in epididymitis.

4. **Labs** = urinalysis shows white blood cells; urine culture with specialized culture media may help diagnose STDs

5. **Treatment** = ceftriaxone and doxycycline or fluoroquinolone; NSAIDs and scrotal support for noninfectious causes

F. Testicular torsion

1. **Twisting of spermatic cord** leading to **vascular insufficiency** of testes
2. **H/P** = very painful and swollen testes, nausea, vomiting; fever, **testes displaced superiorly**, mass in spermatic cord may be felt, absent cremasteric reflex
3. **Radiology** = US may show torsion
4. **Treatment** = **emergent surgical reduction** of torsion within several hours of onset; manual detorsion can be attempted before surgery (may be difficult to determine correct direction to rotate); testes attached to scrotal wall (i.e., orchiopexy) to prevent recurrence
5. **Complications** = testicular ischemia or infarction without prompt treatment

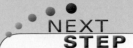

NEXT STEP

If testicular torsion is suspected and US is suggestive of the diagnosis, proceed to surgery without waiting for other tests.

G. Testicular cancer

1. Germ cell (seminomatous, nonseminomatous) or stromal cell (Leydig, Sertoli, or granulosa cell) tumors of testicles
2. **Risk factors** = prior history of testicular cancer, undescended testes, family history
3. **H/P** = **painless testicular mass**, possible gynecomastia or lower abdominal pain; GI or pulmonary symptoms can result from metastases
4. **Labs** = increased β-human chorionic gonadotropin (β-hCG) and increased α-fetoprotein in germ cell tumors; increased estrogen in stromal cell tumors
5. **Radiology** = US may detect dense testicular mass, CXR or CT can detect extent of tumor and metastases
6. **Treatment** = radical orchiectomy with/without chemotherapy and radiation therapy for early stage seminomas; radical orchiectomy with/without retroperitoneal lymph node dissection or chemotherapy for early stage nonseminomas; chemotherapy and possible postchemotherapy debulking performed for more extensive disease
7. **Complications** = **prognosis is very good**, but nonseminomas have lower cure rates and increased risk of recurrence

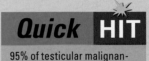

Quick HIT

95% of testicular malignancies are of a germ cell origin.

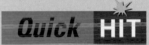

Quick HIT

Testicular cancer is the most common cancer in men between 15 and 35 years of age.

H. Infertility (male)

1. Inability of couple to achieve pregnancy following 1 year of normal sexual activity **without use of contraception**
2. **H/P** = history of testicular trauma, surgery, chemotherapy, or infection can be contributory; varicocele (collection of veins in scrotum), undescended testes, or penile defects may be seen on examination
3. **Labs** = hormone analysis, complete blood count (CBC), and urinalysis may be useful for diagnosis; semen analysis for sperm motility, morphology, volume, and concentration may be useful
4. **Treatment** = treat underlying condition; surgical correction of anatomic defects, hormone therapy, education in sexual technique, or in vitro fertilization may help in achieving pregnancy

I. Impotence

1. Inability to obtain or maintain erection during sexual activity
2. Caused by denervation, **vascular insufficiency**, endocrine abnormalities, psychological concerns, drugs, or alcoholism
3. **H/P** = history of trauma, surgery, or infection can be contributory; examination should consider vascular (decreased pulses and perfusion), hormonal (testicular atrophy or gynecomastia), and neurologic (decrease anal wink reflex and paresthesias) etiologies
4. **Labs** = possible decreased testosterone, decreased luteinizing hormone (LH), or increased prolactin
5. **Treatment** = treat underlying condition; stop offending agents; psychological counseling and sexual education; papaverine injection or oral phosphodiesterase-5 inhibitors may help maintain penile vascular engorgement

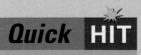

Quick HIT

Frequent infections in the presence of infertility may necessitate a workup for **cystic fibrosis**.

Genitourinary Disorders

IX. Pediatric Genitourinary Concerns

A. Wilms tumor

1. Malignant tumor of renal origin presenting in **children <4 years of age**
2. **Risk factors** = family history, neurofibromatosis, other genitourinary abnormalities
3. **H/P** = weight loss, nausea, vomiting, dysuria, polyuria; palpable abdominal or flank mass, hypertension, fever
4. **Labs** = measure BUN, Cr, and CBC to assess kidney function
5. **Radiology** = CT or US shows renal mass; CXR and CT can show metastases
6. **Treatment** = surgical resection or nephrectomy, chemotherapy, and possible radiation; good prognosis without extensive involvement

B. Urethral displacement

1. Urethral opening on top (i.e., epispadias) or underside (i.e., hypospadias) of penis associated with other penile anatomic abnormalities
2. **H/P** = defect apparent on examination and during urination
3. **Treatment** = surgical correction (ideally during infancy); do not circumcise before surgical correction
4. **Complications** = may contribute to infertility

C. Enuresis

1. Nocturnal bedwetting seen in young children
2. Seen in all children; **most cases resolve by age 4 years**; rare cases associated with disease
3. **H/P** = **almost always nonpathologic**; unusual findings in history and examination should prompt further workup
4. **Treatment** = education, enuresis alarms, dietary modifications (no fluids near bedtime); desmopressin or imipramine used in refractory cases

D. Undescended testes (cryptorchidism)

1. Testes lying in abdominal cavity and not consistently located within scrotum
2. **H/P** = empty scrotal sac, testes inconsistently found in scrotum
3. **Treatment** = exogenous hCG administration or orchiopexy before age 5 years to reduce risk of cancer and allow testicular development
4. **Complications** = testicular cancer (risk reduced but not eliminated by surgical correction), infertility

E. Posterior urethral valves

1. Abnormal folds of tissue in the distal prostatic urethra, causing bladder outlet obstruction and weak urinary stream
2. **H/P** = Often diagnosed on prenatal US; weak urinary stream, UTI; abdominal distention
3. **Imaging** = ultrasound reveals thick-walled bladder, bilateral hydronephrosis, and/or megaureter; voiding cystourethrogram (VCUG) shows elongation and dilation of the posterior urethra during voiding
4. **Treatment** = cystoscopic transurethral ablation of abnormal tissue or urinary diversion (vesicostomy)

5

ENDOCRINE DISORDERS

I. Disorders of Glucose Metabolism

A. Normal glucose metabolism
1. Regulated by pancreatic enzymes insulin and glucagon
2. **Insulin**
   a. Secreted by pancreatic β-islet cells in response to glucose intake and feeding (strongest stimuli, but also influenced by other protein and neural input)
   b. Secretion decreases with fasting and exercise (i.e., feedback relationship with nutrient supply)
   c. Induces glucose and amino acid uptake by muscle, adipose cells, and liver
   d. Drives conversion of glucose to glycogen, fatty acids, and pyruvate
   e. Induces storage of glucose metabolites in tissue (e.g., glycogen in liver, fatty acids in adipose cells, protein anabolism)
   f. Inhibits lipolysis in adipose tissue
3. **Glucagon**
   a. Secreted by α-islet cells primarily in response to decreased glucose and protein intake
   b. Promotes mobilization of glycogen and fatty acids
4. Insulin:glucagon ratio determines state of glucose metabolism.

B. Diabetes mellitus (DM) type I (juvenile onset diabetes, insulin-dependent diabetes)
1. **Loss of ability to produce insulin** most likely caused by autoimmune destruction of β-islet cells
2. Association with human leukocyte antigens HLA-DR3, HLA-DR4, and HLA-DQ genotypes
3. Age of presentation has a bimodal age distribution (first peak at 4 to 6 years, second peak at 10 to 14 years).
4. **History and Physical (H/P)** = polyuria, polydipsia, polyphagia, weight loss; more rapid onset than type II DM
5. **Labs** = hyperglycemia, glycosuria (i.e., glucose in urine), serum and urine ketones, increased hemoglobin A_{1c} (indicates hyperglycemia over prior 3 months and used to monitor adequacy of control) (see Table 5-1)
6. **Treatment** = scheduled insulin injections (see Figure 5-1, Table 5-2) or continuous insulin infusion via insulin pump; monitoring of serum glucose at home to guide insulin and dietary adjustments; close multidiscipline follow-up to monitor development of complications
7. **Complications** = **diabetic ketoacidosis** (DKA), hypoglycemia (secondary to excess insulin administration), retinopathy, neuropathy, nephropathy, atherosclerosis

C. Diabetes mellitus type II (adult onset diabetes, non–insulin-dependent diabetes)
1. Development of **tissue resistance to insulin**, leading to hyperglycemia and gradual decrease in the ability of β-islet cells to produce insulin (see Table 5-3)
2. **Risk factors** = family history, obesity, metabolic syndrome, lack of exercise, gestational diabetes

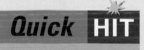

Quick **HIT**

Rubella, Coxsackie virus, and mumps have been associated with onset of β-islet cell destruction leading to DM type I.

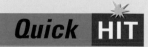

Quick **HIT**

Hemoglobin A_{1c} is a good measure for how well therapy has controlled serum glucose over a 3-month period or for how compliant a patient has been with prescribed therapy.

TABLE **5-1**	Plasma Glucose Diagnostic Criteria for Diabetes Mellitus[a]	
Plasma Glucose Test	**Level (mg/dL)**	**And . . .**
Random plasma glucose	≥200	With symptoms of DM
Fasting plasma glucose	≥126	On 2 separate occasions
Plasma glucose	≥200	2 hr after 75 g oral glucose load[b]
Hemoglobin A$_{1c}$	≥6.5%	

[a]Diagnosis is based on the occurrence of at least one of the above findings.
[b]This is a positive oral glucose tolerance test.
DM, diabetes mellitus.

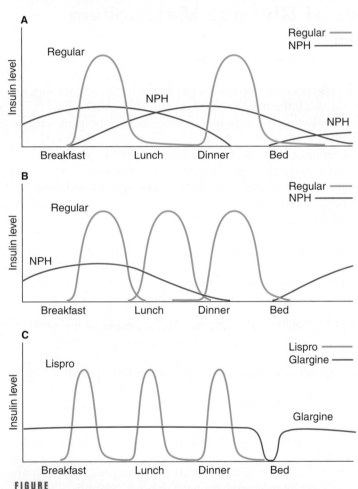

FIGURE
5-1 **Examples of insulin regimens in diabetes mellitus.**

(A) Injection of regular and NPH insulin (in 2:1 ratio) together at breakfast followed by a second regular insulin dose at dinner and a second NPH dose at bedtime. In some cases, the second dose of NPH can be given concomitantly with the second regular insulin dose at dinner. (B) Adjustment in regimen A to achieve tighter, shorter time control by adding an additional dose of regular insulin at lunch and only administering NPH at bedtime. In patients with overnight hypoglycemia, insulin detemir can be substituted for NPH. (C) Tight control regimen using very rapid acting insulin at meals and a bedtime dose of insulin glargine. NPH, neutral protamine Hagedorn insulin.

3. Historically diagnosed **after age 40 years**, but mean age of diagnosis is decreasing
4. H/P = asymptomatic in early stages with **gradual onset** of symptoms; polyuria, polydipsia, polyphagia, acanthosis nigricans; symptoms related to complications can present before actual diagnosis
5. **Labs** = similar to those for DM type I (see Table 5-1); serum insulin can be increased, normal, or decreased

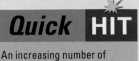

Quick HIT

An increasing number of obese patients with DM type II are being diagnosed at ages **<40 yr** because of the increasing prevalence of **obesity**.

TABLE 5-2 Formulations of Injected Insulin

Type of Insulin	Time of Onset of Action	Peak Effect	Duration of Action
Very rapid acting[a] (e.g., lispro, aspart, glulisine)	10 min	1 hr	2–4 hr
Regular[a]	30 min	2–4 hr	5–8 hr
NPH	2 hr	6–10 hr	18–24 hr
Insulin glargine	2 hr	No peak	24+ hr
Insulin detemir	2 hr	No peak	6–24 hr

[a]Appropriate for use in continuous infusion pump.
NPH, neutral protamine Hagedorn insulin.

TABLE 5-3 Comparisons of Diabetes Mellitus Types I and II

	DM Type I	DM Type II
Cause	Likely autoimmune destruction of β-islet cells	Development of insulin resistance in tissues
Inheritance/genetics	HLA linked	Strong family history
Age of onset	Usually <15 yr of age	Frequently >40 yr of age
Onset of symptoms	Rapid	Gradual
Pancreatic effects	β-Islet cell depletion	Gradual decrease in β-islet cells
Serum insulin	Low	Increased or normal; low in later disease
Body type	Thin	Obese
Acute complications	DKA	HHS
Treatment	Insulin	Oral hypoglycemic agents, possibly insulin

DKA, diabetic ketoacidosis; DM, diabetes mellitus; HHS, hyperosmolar hyperglycemic state, HLA, human leukocyte antigen

6. Treatment
   a. Initial therapy focuses on nutrition (reduced calorie intake, carbohydrate control, and consistency), exercise, and weight loss.
   b. Metformin is frequently the first oral agent prescribed (see Table 5-4).
   c. If hemoglobin A_{1c} remains >7 after 2 to 3 months of monotherapy, add sulfonylurea, thiazolidinedione, or insulin.
   d. If patient begins to exhibit signs of decreased insulin production or if hemoglobin A_{1c} is consistently >8.5, add insulin regimen.
   e. Close monitoring of blood glucose levels is important to directing therapy.
7. **Complications = hyperosmolar hyperglycemic nonketotic syndrome** (HHNS), retinopathy, nephropathy, neuropathy, atherosclerosis

D. Complications of diabetes
1. **Diabetic ketoacidosis (DKA)**
   a. Extremely low insulin and glucagon excess cause degradation of triglycerides into fatty acids and eventual conversion into **ketoacids**.
   b. Occurs in patients with DM type I who do not take prescribed insulin or those who have infections, high stress, myocardial infarction (MI), or high alcohol use
   c. **H/P** = weakness, polyuria, polydipsia, abdominal pain, vomiting; dry mucous membranes, decreased skin turgor, fruity odor on breath, hyperventilation

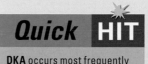

Quick HIT

DKA occurs most frequently in patients with **DM type I** and is **uncommonly seen** in **DM type II**.

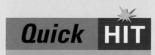

Quick HIT

HHS is seen in patients with **DM type II** and is **not seen** in patients with **DM type I** because sufficient insulin production is required to prevent DKA from occurring first.

Endocrine Disorders

TABLE 5-4 Noninsulin Drugs Used in Treatment of Diabetes Mellitus Type II

Drug	Mechanism	Role	Adverse Effects
Biguanides (metformin)	**Decrease hepatic gluconeogenesis, increase insulin sensitivity**, reduce LDL, raise HDL	Frequently first-line drug	GI disturbance, rare lactic acidosis, decreased vitamin B_{12} absorption; contraindicated in patients with hepatic or renal insufficiency
Sulfonylureas (glyburide, glimepiride, glipizide)	**Stimulate insulin release** from β-islet cells, reduce serum glucagon, increase binding of insulin to tissue receptors	Frequently used after metformin	**Hypoglycemia**; contraindicated in patients with hepatic or renal insufficiency (greater risk of hypoglycemia)
Thiazolidinediones (pioglitazone, rosiglitazone)	Decrease hepatic gluconeogenesis, **increase insulin sensitivity**	Adjunct to other drugs or monotherapy	Weight gain and fluid retention (contraindicated in CHF), increase serum LDL
DPP-IV inhibitors (sitagliptin, saxagliptin, linagliptin, alogliptin)	**Inhibit degradation of incretin** hormones → decreased glucagon, increased insulin, delay gastric emptying	Adjunct to other drugs	Diarrhea, constipation, edema
Incretin mimetics (exenatide, liraglutide)	Agonize GLP-1 receptors → decrease glucagon, increase insulin, delay gastric emptying	SC injection; adjunct to other drugs	Mild weight loss, **nausea**, hypoglycemia, slight risk of pancreatitis
SGLT-2 inhibitors (dapagliflozin, canagliflozin)	Inhibit renal reabsorption of glucose, lowering blood glucose	Adjunct therapy for patients inadequately controlled on two drugs; only useful in patients with normal renal function	Mild hypoglycemia, recurrent UTI, **genital fungal infections**
α-Glucosidase inhibitors (acarbose)	**Decrease GI absorption** of starch and disaccharides	Adjunct to other drugs; may be used in patients with DM type I	Diarrhea, flatulence, GI disturbance
Meglitinides (repaglinide, nateglinide)	**Stimulate insulin release** from β-islet cells	Used as secondary drug with metformin or rarely as initial drug	**Hypoglycemia**; significantly more expensive than sulfonylureas with no therapeutic advantage
Pramlintide	Amyline analog; delay gastric emptying, promote satiety	Injectable drug used only in conjunction with insulin (type 1 or type 2 DM)	Nausea, hypoglycemia

DM, diabetes mellitus; DPP-IV, dipeptidyl peptidase-IV; GI, gastrointestinal; GLP-1, glucagon-like peptide-1; LDL, low-density lipoprotein; MI, myocardial infarction; SGLT, sodium-glucose linked transporter; UTI, urinary tract infection.

(Kussmaul respirations = deep, labored, regular breathing); mental status changes develop with worsening dehydration

   d. **Labs = glucose 300 to 800 mg/dL** (rarely >1,000), decreased Na^+, normal or increased serum K^+ (total body K^+ is decreased), decreased phosphate, high anion gap metabolic acidosis, **serum and urine ketones**

   e. **Treatment** = intravenous (IV) fluids, insulin, KCl; treat underlying disorder (success of treatment may be confirmed by closure of anion gap)

2. **Hyperosmolar hyperglycemic state (HHS)**

   a. Extremely high glucose with profound dehydration

   b. Occurs in patients with DM type II with lengthy infections, stress, or illness; insulin production is sufficient to prevent DKA by suppressing lipolysis and ketogenesis

   c. **H/P** = polyuria, polydipsia, dehydration, mental status changes; seizures and stroke can occur in severe cases

   d. **Labs = glucose >800 mg/dL** (frequently >1,000), no acidosis

   e. **Treatment** = IV fluids, insulin, correction of electrolyte abnormalities; treat underlying disorder

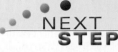

NEXT **STEP**

Differentiate DKA from HHS using serum glucose, presence of acidosis, and history of type of DM.

3. **Diabetic retinopathy**
   a. Vascular occlusion and ischemia, with or without neovascularization in retina, leading to visual changes
   b. Associated with microaneurysms, hemorrhages, infarcts, and macular edema
   c. **Background retinopathy (no neovascularization)** makes up most cases; **proliferative retinopathy (with neovascularization)** has increased risk of hemorrhages.
   d. **H/P = progressive vision loss**; retinal changes seen on funduscopic examination (e.g., arteriovenous nicking, hemorrhages, edema, infarcts)
   e. **Treatment = control diabetes**, antihypertension (HTN) therapy, annual follow-up with ophthalmology, laser photocoagulation for neovascularization, injection of intervitreal corticosteroids to reduce macular edema
   f. **Complications =** vision loss, early cataracts and glaucoma, retinal detachment
4. **Diabetic nephropathy**
   a. Intercapillary glomerulosclerosis, mesangial expansion, and basement membrane degeneration that develops after long-term DM
   b. Slightly greater risk in DM type I than in DM type II
   c. Initially presents with proteinuria; renal insufficiency later develops with nephrotic syndrome
   d. **H/P =** develops after several years with DM (20+); lab abnormalities may appear well before symptoms; symptoms and signs of renal insufficiency (e.g., HTN, uremia) develop as renal function deteriorates
   e. **Labs =** hypoalbuminemia, increased creatinine (Cr), increased blood urea nitrogen (BUN); urinalysis shows proteinuria and microalbuminuria, electron microscopy shows basement membrane thickening and Kimmelstiel-Wilson nodules in glomeruli
   f. **Treatment = control diabetes**; angiotensin-converting enzyme inhibitor (ACE-I) or angiotensin receptor blocker (ARB) to decrease blood pressure, low-protein diet, infection prevention; dialysis may eventually be required
   g. **Complications =** end-stage renal disease
5. **Diabetic neuropathy**
   a. Neural damage and conduction defects leading to sensory, motor, and autonomic nerve dysfunction
   b. **Sensory** neuropathy begins in feet and progresses in stocking-glove pattern; symptoms include paresthesias, neural pain, and decreased vibratory and pain sensation.
   c. **Motor** neuropathy may be distally or proximally distributed and may be characterized by weakness or loss of coordination.
   d. **Autonomic** neuropathy can cause postural hypotension, impotence, incontinence, and diabetic gastroparesis (i.e., delayed gastric emptying).
   e. **Treatment = control diabetes**; neural pain can be treated with tricyclic antidepressants, carbamazepine, or gabapentin; narcotics or tramadol can be considered for persistent neural pain; patients should be taught how to perform regular foot examinations
   f. **Complications = Charcot joints, diabetic foot ulcers**; amputation may be needed to treat progressive infections and deformity
6. **Atherosclerosis**
   a. Incidence greatly increased in diabetic patients secondary to macrovascular disease
   b. Increased risk of coronary artery disease and peripheral vascular disease (PVD), leading to increased risk of MI, distal ischemia, and ulcer formation secondary to poor healing and infection
   c. **Treatment =** control HTN and hyperlipidemia; daily aspirin (ASA) therapy
   d. **Complications =** MI (frequently silent), PVD, poor healing of trauma and infections

E. Hypoglycemia *(see Table 5-5)*
   1. Inadequate blood glucose that can result in an inadequate supply of glucose to tissues and brain damage

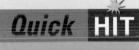

Patients with sensory neuropathy are at **increased risk** for developing **foot infections** and need to be taught to check their feet regularly to avoid ulcer formation.

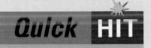

Repetitive foot trauma in cases of impaired pain sensation can lead to severe foot deformity and joint destruction (**Charcot joints**).

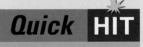

Diabetic patients are at an increased risk of **silent MI** because of impaired pain sensation.

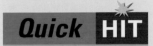

Cardiac complications are the **greatest cause of death** in diabetic patients.

Endocrine Disorders

TABLE 5-5	Causes of Hypoglycemia			
Cause	**Pathology**	**Diagnosis**	**Treatment**	
Reactive	Decrease in serum glucose **after eating** (postsurgical or idiopathic)	Hypoglycemia and symptoms improve with carbohydrate meal	Frequent small meals	
Iatrogenic (excess insulin)	**Excess insulin** administration or adverse effect of **sulfonylurea** or meglitinide use	**Increased insulin in presence of hypoglycemia**, adjustment of drug regimen reduces symptoms	Adjust insulin regimen, consider different oral hypoglycemic drug	
Insulinoma[a]	**β-Islet cell tumor** producing excess insulin	Increased insulin in presence of hypoglycemia, may be detected on CT or MRI	Surgical resection if able to locate	
Fasting	**Underproduction of glucose** because of hormone deficiencies, malnutrition, or liver disease	Lab abnormalities and history associated with particular etiology	Proper nutrition, enzyme replacement	
Alcohol induced	Glycogen depletion and **gluconeogenesis inhibition** by high concentrations of alcohol	History of alcohol use, serum ethanol >45 mg/dL	Proper nutrition, stopping high quantity alcohol use	
Pituitary/adrenal insufficiency	Decreased cortisol production leads to insufficient hepatic gluconeogenesis in response to hypoglycemia	Low serum cortisol; site of defect determined by ACTH activity tests; possible other comorbid endocrine abnormalities	Cortisol replacement	

[a]A similar presentation would be expected for tumors with paraneoplastic production of insulin or insulin-like substance.
ACTH, adrenocorticotropic hormone; CT, computed tomography; MRI, magnetic resonance imaging.

2. H/P = faintness, weakness, diaphoresis, and palpitations because of responsive excess secretion of epinephrine (attempt to mobilize glycogen); headache, confusion, mental status changes, and decreased consciousness because of inadequate supply of glucose to the brain

II. Thyroid Disorders

A. Thyroid function

1. Thyroid hormones induce central nervous system (CNS) maturation during growth, increase basal metabolic rate, increase cardiac output, and promote bone growth.
2. Thyrotropin-releasing hormone (TRH) secretion from hypothalamus is stimulated by cold and inhibited by stress (see Figure 5-2).
3. TRH induces secretion of thyroid-stimulating hormone (TSH) in the anterior pituitary.
4. TSH secretion is also controlled by feedback inhibition from thyroxine (T_4) thyroid hormone.
5. Metabolic effects are determined by free T_4 and triiodothyronine (T_3); remaining thyroid hormones bound to thyroid-binding globulin (TBG).

B. Hyperthyroidism

1. Excess production of thyroid hormones
2. Multiple causes, but **Graves disease** is most common (see Table 5-6)
3. **H/P** = weight loss, increased appetite, **heat intolerance**, **anxiety**, diaphoresis, palpitations, increased bowel frequency; staring or lid lag, tremor, tachycardia, increased pulse pressure, warm skin, hyperreflexia, possible atrial fibrillation
4. **Labs** = **decreased TSH**, increased total T_4, free T_4, total T_3, and T_3 resin uptake
5. **Complications** = thyroid storm

C. Thyroid storm

1. Severe hyperthyroidism induced by infection, surgery, or stress in patients with preexisting hyperthyroidism
2. **H/P** = existing symptoms of hyperthyroidism, severe diaphoresis, vomiting, diarrhea; tachycardia, fever, **mental status changes**

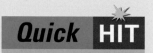

Quick HIT

T_4 is converted to T_3 in serum; T_3 is more potent than T_4 but has a shorter half-life.

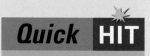

Quick HIT

If TBG levels increase (e.g., pregnancy, oral contraceptive use), total T_4 increases but free T_4 remains normal.

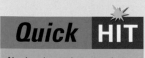

Quick HIT

Nephrotic syndrome and androgen use decrease TBG levels, leading to decreased total T_4 but normal free T_4.

Endocrine Disorders

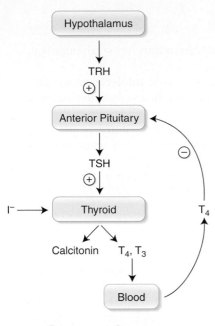

FIGURE
5-2 **Hypothalamopituitary regulation of thyroid hormone production.**

I⁻, iodine; T₃, triiodothyronine; T₄, thyroxine; TRH, thyroid-releasing hormone; TSH, thyroid-stimulating hormone.

TABLE 5-6 — Causes of Hyperthyroidism

Etiology	Pathology	Aids in Diagnosis	Treatment
Graves disease	Autoimmune **TSI antibodies** bind to TSH receptors in thyroid and stimulate thyroid hormone production	**Exophthalmos, pretibial myxedema**, painless goiter; TSI found in serum; **high uptake on thyroid scan**	Thionamides (methimazole, PTU) achieve euthyroidism in many cases; **radioablation** with radioactive iodine or **subtotal thyroidectomy** for definitive cure; atenolol can be used for symptomatic relief
Toxic adenoma (Plummer disease)/toxic multinodular goiter	**Single or multiple hyperactive nodules** produce excess thyroid hormones	Thyroid scan shows **increased uptake** at site(s) of nodule(s)	Thionamides, radioactive iodine, or surgical resection
Subacute thyroiditis (de Quervain thyroiditis)	Enlarged thyroid due to possible viral stimulus	**Painful goiter**, mild symptoms of hyperthyroidism, neck pain, **fever**; increased ESR; **decreased uptake on thyroid scan**	Self-limited; NSAIDs and β-blockers to treat symptoms; thyroid replacement may be needed if hypothyroidism occurs during gland recovery
Silent thyroiditis	Temporary thyroiditis that **may follow pregnancy**	Painless goiter; **low uptake on thyroid scan; biopsy shows inflammation**	Self-limited; β-blockers to treat symptoms
Factitious hyperthyroidism	Excess thyroid hormone ingestion	**No goiter** in cases of hyperthyroidism; **normal** thyroid scan	Stop excess ingestion

ESA, erythrocyte sedimentation rate; NSAIDs, nonsteroidal anti-inflammatory drugs; PTU, propylthiouracil; TSH, thyroid-stimulating hormone; TSI, thyroid-stimulating immunoglobulin.

3. **Labs** = increased T₄ and T₃, decreased TSH
4. **Treatment** = similar to treatment of hyperthyroidism but higher doses of medications given in greater frequency; β-blockers, thionamides, IV sodium iodine (helps block thyroid hormone release), hydrocortisone (inhibits conversion of T₄ to T₃); surgery or radioablation when patient is stable
5. **Complications** = 25% to 50% mortality

Endocrine Disorders

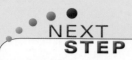

NEXT STEP

To determine if an enlarged thyroid or thyroid mass is caused by excess thyroid activity or a malignancy, perform a thyroid scan (measures uptake of radioactive iodine to indicate normal, excessive, or absent thyroid function).

Quick HIT

Hypothyroidism can result from autoimmune processes, **thyroid surgery**, thyroid radioablation, pituitary dysfunction, chronic lithium use, and chronic iodide use.

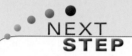

NEXT STEP

If decreased TSH and hypothyroidism are seen, suspect a pituitary or hypothalamic etiology.

Quick HIT

Two frequent complications of thyroid surgery are **hoarseness** (secondary to damage of the recurrent laryngeal nerve) and **hypocalcemia** (secondary to surgical hypoparathyroidism).

D. Hashimoto thyroiditis

1. Most common cause of hypothyroidism
2. Autoimmune condition characterized by chronic thyroiditis; most commonly in middle-aged women
3. H/P = weakness, fatigue, decreased exercise capacity, **cold intolerance, weight gain**, constipation, irregular menstruation, **depression**, hoarseness; hyporeflexia, bradycardia, dry skin, edema, **painless goiter**
4. Labs = **increased TSH**, decreased total T_4, decreased free T_4, **antithyroid peroxidase (anti-TPO)** and **antithyroglobulin antibodies**; lymphocytic infiltrates and fibrosis seen on biopsy
5. Radiology = **decreased uptake** on thyroid scan (i.e., "cold scan")
6. Treatment = lifelong levothyroxine replacement

E. Thyroid carcinoma

1. Workup of thyroid nodules
   a. Thyroid nodules are usually benign and increase in frequency with age.
   b. Nodules should be evaluated with TSH levels, thyroid function tests, ultrasound (US), and fine needle aspiration (FNA) with biopsy.
   c. "Cold" nodules exhibit decreased radioactive iodide (I^-) uptake (from decreased metabolic activity); "hot" nodules exhibit increased iodide uptake (from increased metabolic activity).
   d. Increased risk of malignancy = male, children, adults over age 60 years and under age 30 years, history of neck irradiation, poor iodide uptake on thyroid scan (cold nodule), solid nodule on US
   e. Malignant nodules can arise from a variety of thyroid cell types (see Table 5-7).
2. H/P = nontender nodule in anterior neck, dysphagia, hoarseness; possible cervical lymphadenopathy
3. Labs = biopsy provides diagnosis; thyroid hormones normal or decreased
4. Radiology = US used to determine size and local extension; thyroid scan may differentiate hot from cold nodule (malignant nodules more likely to be cold)
5. Treatment
   a. Benign small cystic nodules may be observed.
   b. Benign solid nodules are treated with surgery, radioablation, and postoperative levothyroxine to stop thyroid hormone overproduction and decrease risk of malignant conversion.
   c. Malignant tumors require surgical resection (lobectomy for nonanaplastic tumors <1 cm diameter, total thyroidectomy for larger tumors) and radioiodine ablation.
   d. Radiation therapy for tumors with local extension; chemotherapy for metastatic tumors
   e. Thyroid replacement (levothyroxine) needed after surgery

TABLE 5-7	Types of Thyroid Carcinoma			
Type	**Cells Affected**	**Frequency**	**Characteristics**	**Prognosis**
Papillary	Columnar cells of gland	**Most common form** (78% cases); most common in younger patients; follicular variant (17% cases) is most common variant	Begins as slow-growing nodule; eventually metastasizes to local cervical lymph nodes	**Good**; few recurrences; follicular type has slightly worse prognosis (50% 10-yr survival)
Medullary	Parafollicular C cells	4% of thyroid cancers	**Produces calcitonin**; may present with other endocrine tumors (MEN IIa and IIb)	Worse in older patients; metastases common at diagnosis
Anaplastic	Poorly differentiated neoplasm	1% of thyroid cancers	**Very aggressive**; local extension causes hoarseness, dysphagia	Poor

MEN IIa, multiple endocrine neoplasia type IIa.

III. Parathyroid Disorders

A. Parathyroid function

1. Plasma calcium (Ca^{2+}) regulation (see Figure 5-3)
   a. **Parathyroid hormone** (PTH): **secreted in response to low serum Ca^{2+}**; induces osteoclasts to reabsorb bone and increases plasma Ca^{2+}; induces kidneys to increase conversion of 25-(OH) vitamin D to 1,25-(OH)$_2$ vitamin D, decreases phosphate reabsorption, and increases distal tubule Ca^{2+} reabsorption for net increase in plasma Ca^{2+}
   b. **1,25-(OH)$_2$ vitamin D**: metabolite of dietary vitamin D; production in kidneys increases with PTH secretion; increases intestinal Ca^{2+} absorption; increases renal proximal tubule phosphate reabsorption (in opposition to PTH-induced phosphate wasting)
   c. **Calcitonin**: secreted by thyroid parafollicular cells; inhibits bone reabsorption

B. Primary hyperparathyroidism

1. **Excess PTH secretion**, leading to **hypercalcemia** and osteopenia
2. Most cases result from **single adenoma**; remaining cases mostly occur with hyperplasia of all four glands; parathyroid cancer is rare
3. H/P = frequently asymptomatic; symptoms of hypercalcemia may be present (e.g., bone pain, nausea and vomiting, mental status changes, renal stones, constipation, weakness, increased risk of fracture) (see Chapter 4, **Genitourinary Disorders**, for further discussion of hypercalcemia)
4. Labs = increased Ca^{2+}, decreased phosphate, increased urine Ca^{2+}, increased PTH
5. Radiology = decreased bone density on dual X-ray absorptiometry (DXA) scan
6. Treatment = surgical resection (i.e., parathyroidectomy) of single adenoma; for four-gland hyperplasia, all glands are removed, and a portion of one gland

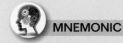

MNEMONIC

Remember the **"bones," "stones," "groans,"** and **"psychiatric overtones"** of hypercalcemia in cases of hyperparathyroidism.

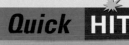

Decreased Ca^{2+} with increased PTH suggests a hyperparathyroidism secondary to **malnutrition**, malabsorption, **renal disease**, or calcium-wasting drugs.

Endocrine Disorders

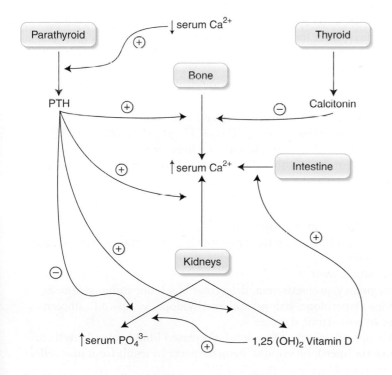

FIGURE

5-3 Serum Ca^{2+} regulation.

PTH, parathyroid hormone.

is implanted in the muscle of forearm to maintain some PTH production; treat hypercalcemia with IV fluids and bisphosphonates

C. Hypoparathyroidism

1. PTH deficiency caused by **surgical removal** of parathyroids (most common) or autoimmune degeneration of glands (uncommon), leading to hypocalcemia
2. **H/P** = tingling in lips and fingers, dry skin, weakness, abdominal pain, tetany, dyspnea; possible tachycardia, seizures, movement disorders, cataracts, dental hypoplasia, positive Trousseau (i.e., carpal spasm when blood pressure cuff inflated) and Chvostek signs (i.e., tapping of facial nerve causes spasm) (see Chapter 4, **Genitourinary Disorders**)
3. **Labs** = decreased Ca^{2+}, increased phosphate, decreased PTH
4. **Radiology** = X-rays may demonstrate osteosclerosis or increased bone density
5. **Treatment** = Ca^{2+} and vitamin D supplementation

D. Pseudohypoparathyroidism

1. Hypocalcemia resulting from tissue **nonresponsiveness to PTH**
2. Associated with developmental and skeletal abnormalities (e.g., **Albright hereditary osteodystrophy**)
3. **H/P** = symptoms of hypocalcemia, short stature, seizures, poor mental development in children
4. **Labs** = decreased Ca^{2+}, increased phosphate, **increased PTH**; administration of PTH causes no change in serum or urine Ca^{2+}
5. **Treatment** = Ca^{2+} and vitamin D supplementation

IV. Pituitary and Hypothalamic Disorders

A. Hypothalamic-pituitary function

1. Hypothalamus responds to stimuli by modulating pituitary activity (see Figure 5-4).
   a. Hormones are released into the hypophyseal portal system to regulate subsequent hormone release from the anterior pituitary.
   b. Anterior pituitary hormone secretion is regulated by feedback mechanisms in addition to the hypothalamus.
   c. Impulses sent through the hypothalamo-hypophyseal tract regulate hormone release from the posterior pituitary.
2. Anterior pituitary lacks nerve terminals and is responsible for secretion of prolactin, adrenocorticotropic hormone (ACTH), TSH, growth hormone (GH), follicle-stimulating hormone (FSH), and luteinizing hormone (LH).
3. Posterior pituitary is a neural extension of the hypothalamus and is responsible for antidiuretic hormone (ADH) and oxytocin secretion.

B. Hyperprolactinemia

1. Excess **prolactin** secretion by anterior pituitary
   a. Causes decreased LH and FSH secretion, galactorrhea (i.e., milk secretion), and amenorrhea in women
   b. Causes gynecomastia in men
2. Can result from **pregnancy, prolactinoma**, drugs that block dopamine synthesis (e.g., phenothiazines, risperidone, haloperidol, methyldopa, verapamil), dopamine-depleting drugs, or hypothalamic damage
3. **H/P** = **amenorrhea and galactorrhea (women)**; decreased libido, erectile dysfunction, and **gynecomastia (men)**; bitemporal hemianopsia can result from mass effect of tumor in sella turcica
4. **Labs** = increased prolactin; if adenoma, prolactin >300 ng/mL and TRH administration causes no additional prolactin secretion
5. **Radiology** = magnetic resonance imaging (MRI) may detect pituitary tumor
6. **Treatment** = dopamine agonists (e.g., cabergoline, bromocriptine, pergolide), stopping offending agents; transsphenoidal surgery and radiation therapy should be performed in refractory cases

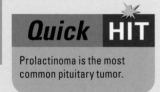

Quick HIT

Prolactinoma is the most common pituitary tumor.

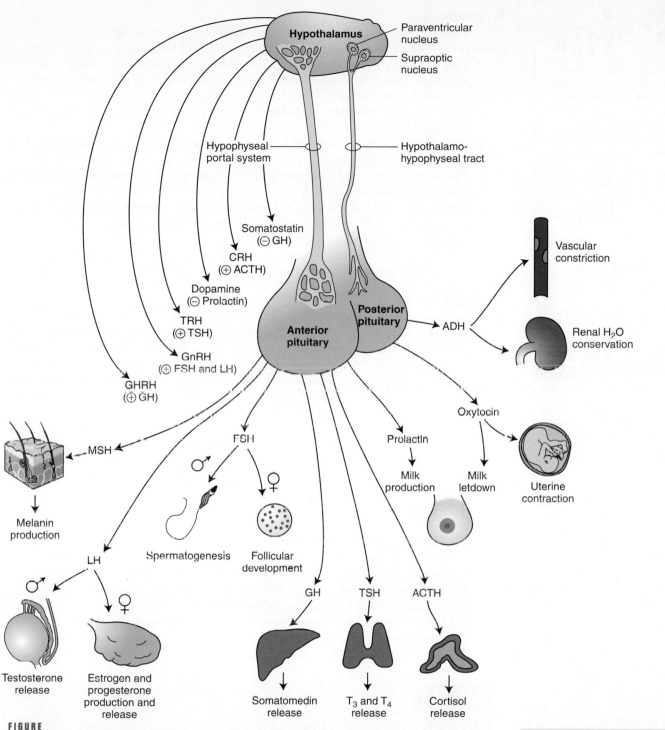

FIGURE
5-4
Hypothalamopituitary axis.

ACTH, adrenocorticotropic hormone; ADH, antidiuretic hormone; CRH, corticotrophin-releasing hormone; GH, growth hormone; GHRH, growth hormone-releasing hormone; GnRH, gonadotropin-releasing hormone; FSH follicle-stimulating hormone; LH, luteinizing hormone; PRH, prolactin-releasing hormone; T_3, triiodothyronine; T_4, thyroxine; TRH, thyrotropin-releasing hormone; TSH, thyroid-stimulating hormone. (From Mehta, S., Milder, E. A., Mirachi, A. J., & Milder, E. [2006]. *Step-Up: A High-Yield, Systems-Based Review for the USMLE Step 1* [3rd ed., p. 165]. Philadelphia, PA: Lippincott Williams & Wilkins.)

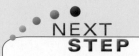

NEXT STEP

Compare current appearance of adult patients to multiple pictures at younger ages to aid in the detection of a gradual enlargement in features seen in acromegaly.

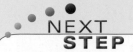

NEXT STEP

For a child with extremely **advanced growth for the given age** (gigantism), perform a workup for increased GH.

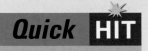

Quick HIT

Patients with acromegaly have **insulin resistance** (similar to DM type II) and develop diabetes in 10% of cases.

C. Acromegaly

1. Excess secretion of **GH** by anterior pituitary caused by adenoma
2. H/P = **enlargement** of hands and feet, coarsening of facial features (e.g., enlargement of nose, jaw, and skin folds), thickened skin, increased body hair growth, joint pain (caused by osteoarthritis), neural pain (because of nerve entrapment); changes may be gradual
3. Heart, lungs, spleen, liver, and kidneys become enlarged and can cause symptoms secondary to dysfunction.
4. **Labs** = increased GH, increased GH 1 to 2 hr following 100 g glucose load (GH decreases in normal cases)
5. **Radiology** = computed tomography (CT) or MRI may detect tumor; X-rays may demonstrate increased bone density
6. **Treatment** = surgical resection of adenoma; dopamine agonists or octreotide to lessen effects of GH; radiation therapy may be useful in cases unresponsive to surgical or medical treatment
7. **Complications** = **cardiac failure**, DM, spinal cord compression, vision loss secondary to pressure of tumor on optic nerve

D. Hypopituitarism

1. **Deficiency of all anterior pituitary hormones** caused by tumor, hemorrhagic infarction (i.e., pituitary apoplexy), surgical resection, trauma, sarcoidosis, tuberculosis, postpartum necrosis (i.e., Sheehan syndrome), or dysfunction of the hypothalamus
2. Some pituitary hormones are kept in storage, and target organs may maintain some autonomous function, so symptoms specific to deficiency of each type of hormone appear at various times (see Table 5-8).
3. Labs
   a. LH/FSH: decreased LH, FSH, estrogen (women), and testosterone (men); menstruation does not occur following administration of medroxyprogesterone
   b. GH: decreased GH; no increase in GH after administration of insulin
   c. TSH: decreased TSH, T_4, and T_3 uptake
   d. Prolactin: decreased prolactin (most noticeable postpartum)
   e. ACTH: decreased ACTH; cortisol does not increase following administration of insulin (normally should increase at least 10 μg/dL); ACTH and 11-deoxycortisol do not increase following administration of metyrapone
4. **Treatment** = treat underlying cause, if possible; treatment depends on which hormones are deficient
   a. GH: **recombinant hormone replacement therapy**
   b. LH/FSH: testosterone replacement in men; estrogen-progesterone pill for women; gonadotropin-releasing hormone (GnRH) can be used in men or women desiring fertility

TABLE 5-8	Progression of Hormone Deficiency in Hypopituitarism	
Order of Loss	**Hormone(s)**	**Symptoms**
1	GH	Growth failure and short stature in children
2	LH, FSH	Infertility, decreased libido, and decreased pubic hair; amenorrhea and genital atrophy in women; impotence and testicular atrophy in men
3	TSH	Hypothyroidism leading to fatigue and cold intolerance; no goiter
4	Prolactin	No postpartum lactation
5	ACTH, MSH	Adrenal insufficiency leading to fatigue, weight loss, decreased appetite, and poor response to stress; decreased skin pigment because of low MSH

ACTH, adrenocorticotropic hormone; FSH, follicle-stimulating hormone; GH, growth hormone; LH, luteinizing hormone; MSH, melanocyte-stimulating hormone; TSH, thyroid-stimulating hormone.

   c. TSH: levothyroxine

   d. Prolactin: no need to treat (women will be unable to lactate)

   e. ACTH: hydrocortisone, dexamethasone, or prednisone

E. Disorders of posterior pituitary

1. Syndrome of inappropriate ADH secretion (SAIDH) (see Chapter 4, **Genitourinary Disorders**)
2. Diabetes insipidus (see Chapter 4, **Genitourinary Disorders**)

V. Adrenal Disorders

A. Adrenal function *(see Table 5-9)*

TABLE 5-9	Function of Zones in Adrenal Cortex and Medulla		
Region	**Stimulation**	**Secretory Products**	**Action of Secretory Products**
Zona glomerulosa (cortex)	Renin-angiotensin system	Aldosterone	Conserve body sodium, maintains body fluid volume
Zona fasciculata (cortex)	ACTH	Cortisol	Maintains glucose production from proteins, aids in fat metabolism, aids in vascular regulation, influences immune response, aids in nervous regulation
Zona reticularis (cortex)	ACTH	Androgens	Development of secondary sexual characteristics, increased bone and muscle mass, promotes male sexual differentiation and sperm production
Medulla	Preganglionic sympathetic neurons	Epinephrine, norepinephrine	Postsynaptic neurotransmitter in sympathetic autonomic system, induces sympathetic effects (glucose mobilization, increase heart contractility and rate, etc.)

ACTH, adrenocorticotropic hormone.

B. Cushing syndrome

1. Syndrome of **excess cortisol** is caused by **excess corticosteroid administration**, **pituitary adenoma** (i.e., Cushing disease), paraneoplastic ACTH production, or adrenal tumor.
2. **H/P** = weakness, depression, menstrual irregularities, polydipsia, polyuria, increased libido, impotence; HTN, **acne**, **increased hair growth**, central obesity, "**buffalo hump**" (i.e., hunchback-like hump on back), "**moon facies**" (i.e., rounded face caused by increased fat deposition), **purple striae** on abdomen, cataracts
3. **Labs** = (in addition to those depicted in Figure 5-5) hyperglycemia, glycosuria, decreased K$^+$
4. **Treatment** = adjust corticosteroid dosing in cases of excess administration; surgical resection or pituitary irradiation for pituitary tumors; surgical resection for some nonpituitary tumors; octreotide may improve symptoms in paraneoplastic syndromes; cortisol replacement may be needed after surgery
5. **Complications** = increased risk of mortality from cardiovascular or thromboembolic complications; increased infection risk, **avascular necrosis of hip**, hypopituitarism, or adrenal insufficiency after surgery

C. Hyperaldosteronism

1. Primary hyperaldosteronism is due to an adrenal adenoma (i.e., Conn syndrome); secondary hyperaldosteronism is due to activation of the renin-angiotensin-aldosterone system secondary to perceived low blood pressure in the kidneys (e.g., renal artery stenosis, heart failure, cirrhosis, nephrotic syndrome).

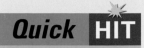

Quick HIT

ACTH and melanocyte-stimulating hormone (**MSH**) arise from the same precursors and follow the same trend in their serum concentrations.

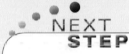

Quick HIT

Excess corticosteroid administration is the **most common** cause of Cushing syndrome.

NEXT STEP

To determine the cause of cortisol excess, screen patients with symptoms of Cushing syndrome with:

- **Low dexamethasone suppression test**: 1–2 mg dexamethasone given at night; low cortisol normally found next morning; no decrease in cortisol seen in Cushing syndrome;
- **High-dose dexamethasone suppression test**: 8 mg/day for 2 days; used to determine cause of cortisol excess.

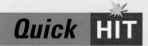

Quick HIT

Symptoms of Cushing syndrome can take up to a year to resolve following therapy.

Endocrine Disorders

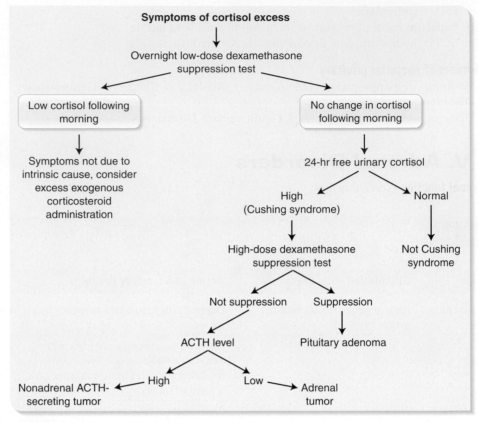

FIGURE

5-5 Example of diagnostic algorithm for a patient with suspected Cushing syndrome caused by cortisol excess.

ACTH, adrenocorticotropic hormone.

2. **H/P** = headache, weakness, paresthesias; recalcitrant **HTN**, tetany
3. **Labs** = **decreased K⁺, metabolic alkalosis,** mildly increased Na⁺, decreased renin (Conn syndrome only), **increased 24-hr urine aldosterone; high ratio of plasma aldosterone concentration (PAC) to plasma renin activity (PRA)** indicates primary hyperaldosteronism
4. **Radiology** = CT or MRI may detect adrenal mass
5. **Treatment** = surgical resection of tumor (primary hyperaldosteronism); treat underlying disorder causing renin-angiotensin system hyperactivity (in secondary hyperaldosteronism); aldosterone antagonists (e.g., spironolactone) improve hypokalemia until definitive therapy administered

D. Adrenal insufficiency

1. **Mineralocorticoid** (i.e., aldosterone) or **glucocorticoid** (i.e., cortisol) **deficiency** caused by adrenal disease or ACTH insufficiency
2. Type
   a. **Addison disease** (primary insufficiency): autoimmune destruction of adrenal cortices caused by autoimmune disease, infection, or hemorrhage; can occur with other endocrine autoimmune processes
   b. **Secondary corticoadrenal insufficiency:** due to insufficient ACTH production by pituitary
   c. **Tertiary corticoadrenal insufficiency:** because of insufficient corticotropin-releasing hormone (CRH) secretion by hypothalamus, most commonly due to chronic corticosteroid use
3. **H/P** = weakness, **fatigue,** anorexia, weight loss, nausea and vomiting (more common in primary disease), myalgias, arthralgias, decreased libido (women), memory impairment, depression, mild psychosis; **hypotension,** possible **increased skin pigmentation** (because of feedback influence of melanocyte-stimulating hormone [MSH])

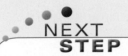

NEXT STEP

Examine patients with adrenal insufficiency for **increased skin pigmentation**; this finding is **seen in Addison disease** (secondary to increased MSH production accompanying increased ACTH production) but **not in secondary or tertiary insufficiency.**

Endocrine Disorders

4. Labs
   a. Decreased Na^+ and increased K^+ secondary to low aldosterone, eosinophilia, decreased cortisol
   b. Increased ACTH with Addison disease, decreased ACTH with secondary or tertiary insufficiency
   c. Decreased cortisol that increases following ACTH analogue (cosyntropin) administration in secondary or tertiary insufficiency but not in Addison disease
5. **Treatment** = treat underlying disease; **glucocorticoid replacement** (e.g., hydrocortisone, dexamethasone, prednisone), **mineralocorticoid replacement** (may not be needed in secondary or tertiary disease), dehydroepiandrosterone (DHEA), and hydration to achieve adequate volume status; titrate cortisol levels for periods of stress (increased need) and to avoid exacerbating secondary adrenal insufficiency
6. **Complications** = **Addisonian crisis** (i.e., severe weakness, fever, mental status changes, and vascular collapse caused by stress and increased cortisol need; treat with IV glucose and hydrocortisone or vasopressors), secondary insufficiency caused by excess cortisol replacement

E. Congenital adrenal hyperplasia (CAH)
1. Enzymatic defect in synthesis of cortisol, resulting in decreased cortisol, reactive increase in ACTH production, adrenal hyperplasia, and androgen excess (see Figure 5-6)
2. **17-α-Hydroxylase deficiency**
   a. Deoxycorticosterone overproduction; cortisol, androgen, and estrogen deficiencies
   b. H/P = amenorrhea (women), ambiguous genitalia (men); HTN
   c. Labs = decreased K^+, increased Na^+, decreased androgens, decreased 17-α-hydroxyprogesterone
3. **21-α-Hydroxylase deficiency**
   a. (Usually) partial deficiency of enzyme resulting in excess androstenedione and insufficient cortisol and aldosterone

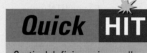
Cortisol deficiency is usually not symptomatic in CAH because hyperplasia can maintain cortisol in the low-normal range despite enzyme deficiency.

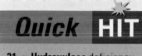
21-α-Hydroxylase deficiency is the **most common** form of CAH.

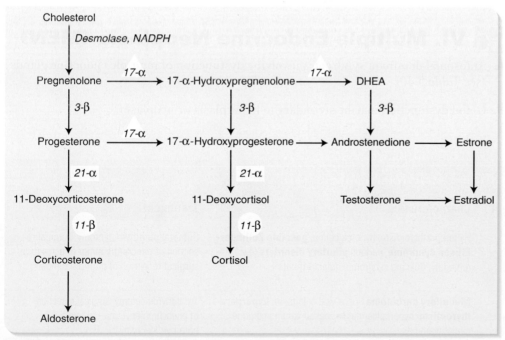

FIGURE
5-6 **Steroid hormone synthesis and causes of congenital adrenal hyperplasia.**
Note the blocks in the pathway from 17-α-hydroxylase deficiency (*triangles*), 21-α-hydroxylase deficiency (*rectangles*), and 11-β-hydroxylase deficiency (*circles*). 3β, 3β-hydroxysteroid dehydrogenase; 11β, 11β- hydroxylase; 17α, 17α-hydroxylase; 21α, 21α- hydroxylase; DHEA, dehydroepiandrosterone; NADPH, nicotinamide adenine dinucleotide phosphate (reduced form).

Endocrine Disorders

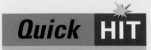

Quick HIT

Pheochromocytoma rule of 10s: 10% malignant, 10% multiple, 10% bilateral, 10% extra-adrenal, 10% children, 10% familial, 10% calcify.

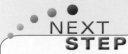

NEXT STEP

Patients with **intermittent tachycardia** and **HTN** with sympathetic symptoms should have a pheochromocytoma workup included in their evaluation.

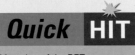

Quick HIT

Mutation of the **RET proto-oncogene** is found in most cases of multiple endocrine neoplasia (MEN) IIa and IIb.

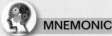

MNEMONIC

Remember MEN type I as **3 Ps: P**arathyroid hyperplasia, **P**ituitary, **P**ancreas. MEN type IIa can be remembered as **1 M and 2 Ps: M**edullary thyroid carcinoma, **P**arathyroid hyperplasia, and **P**heochromocytoma. MEN type IIb can be remembered by the **2 Ms and 1 P: M**ucosal neuromas, **M**edullary thyroid carcinoma, and **P**heochromocytoma.

   b. H/P = ambiguous genitalia (female infants), virilization (women), macrogenitosomia and precocious puberty (men); dehydration and **hypotension** in more severe cases
   c. Labs = **decreased Na$^+$**, **increased K$^+$**, increased androgens
4. **11-β-Hydroxylase deficiency**
   a. Enzyme deficiency resulting in **excess deoxycorticosterone**, deoxycortisol, and androgens and insufficient cortisol and aldosterone
   b. H/P = ambiguous genitalia (female infants), virilization (women), macrogenitosomia and precocious puberty (men); HTN (secondary to deoxycorticosterone)
   c. Labs = increased deoxycorticosterone, increased deoxycortisol, increased androgens
5. **Treatment**
   a. 17-α-Hydroxylase deficiency: cortisol replacement to achieve ACTH suppression; most children raised as females; estrogen-progesterone replacement given to genotypic females at puberty; genotypic males may have reconstructive surgery of genitals
   b. 21-α-Hydroxylase deficiency: cortisol replacement therapy for ACTH suppression; fludrocortisone for mineralocorticoid replacement; reconstructive genital surgery
   c. 11-β-Hydroxylase deficiency: cortisol replacement (hydrocortisone or dexamethasone) for ACTH suppression; anti-HTN may be required for persistent HTN

F. Pheochromocytoma
1. Adrenal medulla tumor that secretes epinephrine and norepinephrine, leading to stimulation of sympathetic nervous system; rarely extra-adrenal in location
2. H/P = sudden palpitations, chest pain, **diaphoresis**, **headache**, anxiety; intermittent **tachycardia**, HTN
3. Labs = increased 24-hr urinary catecholamines and metanephrines; increased plasma-free metanephrines; increased 24-hr urinary vanillylmandelic acid (VMA) (test performed infrequently because of limited sensitivity/specificity)
4. **Treatment** = surgical resection; α- and β-blockers used before and during surgery to control blood pressure; α-blocker must be given **before** β-blocker to avoid hypertensive crisis from unopposed α stimulation

VI. Multiple Endocrine Neoplasia (MEN)

A. Autosomal dominant syndromes involving dysfunction of multiple endocrine glands (*see Table 5-10*)

B. Gland dysfunction may be secondary to hyperplasia or neoplasm

| TABLE 5-10 | Types of Multiple Endocrine Neoplasia (MEN) |

Type	Endocrine Involvement	Characteristics	Treatment
I	Parathyroid adenoma Pancreas (islet cell) or GI endocrine tumors Pituitary adenoma	Hyperparathyroidism, hypercalcemia, **possible Zollinger-Ellison syndrome**, various **pituitary disorders** (e.g., acromegaly, Cushing syndrome, galactorrhea)	Subtotal parathyroidectomy, surgical resection of pancreatic tumor or octreotide, surgical resection of pituitary tumor
IIa	Medullary thyroid cancer Parathyroid hyperplasia Pheochromocytoma	**Medullary carcinoma**, increased calcitonin, **hyperparathyroidism**, hypercalcemia, increased serum and urine catecholamines	Total thyroidectomy, surgical resection of pheochromocytoma, subtotal parathyroidectomy
IIb	Mucosal neuromas Medullary thyroid cancer Pheochromocytoma	**Medullary carcinoma**, increased calcitonin, hypercalcemia, **Marfanoid body habitus**, mucosal nodules	Total thyroidectomy, surgical resection of pheochromocytoma

VII. Pediatric Endocrine Concerns

A. Cretinism

1. Congenital hypothyroidism caused by severe iodide deficiency or hereditary disorder of thyroid hormone synthesis that leads to abnormal mental development and growth retardation
2. **H/P** = frequently asymptomatic if mother has normal thyroid function; poor feeding, lethargy, large fontanelles that remain open, thick tongue, constipation; umbilical hernia, poor growth, hypotonicity, dry skin, hypothermia, jaundice
3. **Labs** = decreased T_4, increased TSH
4. **Radiology** = X-ray shows poor bone development; thyroid scan shows decreased uptake with malformed thyroids and increased uptake with iodide deficiency
5. **Treatment** = levothyroxine started soon after birth to avoid permanent developmental delays

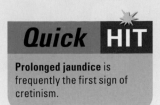

Prolonged jaundice is frequently the first sign of cretinism.

Endocrine Disorders

NEXT STEP

If a patient presents with carbon monoxide poisoning (carbon monoxide displaces O_2 on Hgb, leading to insufficient delivery of O_2 to tissues), administer **100% O_2** via face mask to increase the alveolar concentration of O_2 and decrease the opportunities for carbon monoxide to bind to Hgb.

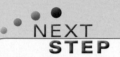

Quick HIT

Carbon monoxide poisoning includes signs of mental status changes, cherry red lips, and hypoxia despite normal pulse oximetry readings.

I. Anemias

A. Red blood cell (RBC) physiology

1. RBCs serve to transport O_2 from the alveoli to tissues via the bloodstream and to transport CO_2 from tissue to lungs.
2. Normal hemoglobin (Hgb) A serves as a binding protein for O_2 and CO_2, and its affinity for O_2 follows the Hgb-O_2 dissociation curve (see Figure 6-1).
   a. **Alkalosis**, decreased body temperature, and increased Hgb F (fetal) shift curve to the left.
   b. **Acidosis**, increased body temperature, **high altitude**, and exercise shift curve to the **right**.
3. Circulating RBCs, myeloid cells, and lymphoid cells all originate from the same pluripotent stem cells in bone marrow (see Figure 6-2).

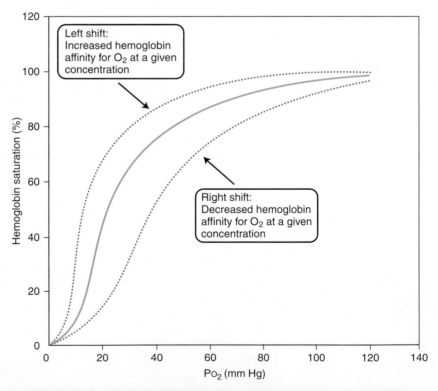

Left shift: Increased hemoglobin affinity for O_2 at a given concentration

Right shift: Decreased hemoglobin affinity for O_2 at a given concentration

Left shift: alkalosis, decreased body temperature, increased Hgb F concentration, ↓CO_2, ↓2,3–DPG
Right shift: acidosis, increased body temperature, high altitude, exercise, ↑CO_2, ↑2,3–DPG

FIGURE 6-1 Hemoglobin–oxygen dissociation curve.

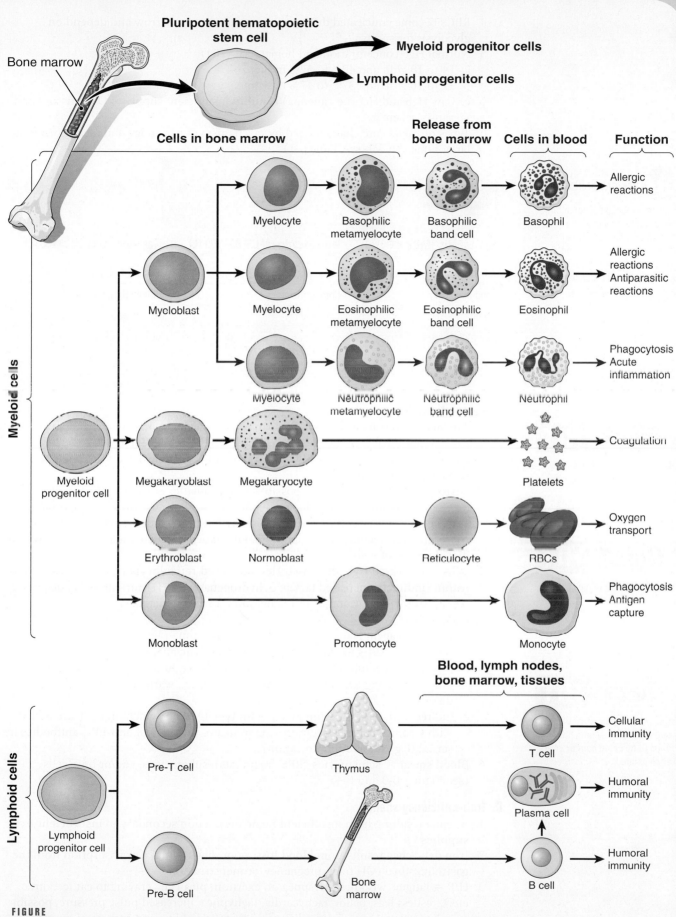

FIGURE 6-2 Development of myeloid and lymphoid cell lines from pluripotent stem cells in bone marrow.

(From McConnell, T. H. [2014]. *The Nature of Disease: Pathology for the Health Professions* [2nd ed., p. 181]. Philadelphia, PA: Lippincott Williams & Wilkins; with permission.)

Hematology and Oncology

4. RBCs become enucleated during maturation in bone marrow and depend on glycolysis for survival.
5. Normal Hgb concentration and hematocrit (Hct):
   a. 14 to 18 g/dL and 42% to 52% in men
   b. 12 to 16 g/dL and 37% to 47% in women
   c. Low Hgb and Hct (i.e., anemia) result in insufficient supply of O_2 to tissues and cause ischemia.
6. Types of anemia are characterized by mechanism of pathology and mean corpuscular volume (MCV) (see Table 6-1).

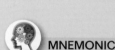

MNEMONIC

Remember the list of common microcytic anemias by the mnemonic **L**ook **F**or **T**hose **S**mall **C**ells: **L**ead poisoning, **F**e (iron) deficiency, **T**halassemia, **S**ideroblastic, **C**hronic disease.

TABLE 6-1	Classification of Anemias by Mean Corpuscular Volume (MCV) and Common Etiologies		
Microcytic (MCV <80 fL)	**Normocytic (MCV 80–100 fL)**	**Macrocytic (MCV >100 fL)**	
Iron deficiency	Hemolytic	Folate deficiency	
Lead poisoning	Chronic disease	Vitamin B_{12} deficiency	
Chronic disease	Hypovolemia	Liver disease	
Sideroblastic		Alcohol abuse	
Thalassemias			

B. Hemolytic anemia

1. Anemia that results when RBC lifespan is shortened and marrow production of RBCs is not capable of meeting demand for new cells (see Table 6-2)
2. Can be caused by defects in RBC membrane, RBC enzyme defects, hemoglobinopathies, or extracellular effects
3. **History and physical (H/P)** = possibly asymptomatic; weakness, fatigue, dyspnea on exertion; **pallor**, tachycardia, tachypnea, increased pulse pressure, possible systolic murmur, **jaundice**; severe cases may have palpitations, syncope, mental status changes, angina, chills, abdominal pain, **hepatosplenomegaly**, and **brownish discoloration of urine**
4. **Labs** = decreased Hgb, decreased Hct, **increased reticulocyte count, increased bilirubin (indirect)**, increased lactate dehydrogenase (LDH), **normal MCV**, decreased serum haptoglobin; Coombs test is helpful for making diagnosis
5. **Coombs test**
   a. Coombs reagent (rabbit IgM directed against human IgG and complement) is mixed with RBCs to aid in diagnosis of hemolytic anemia.
   b. Direct test: Coombs reagent mixed with RBCs; agglutination indicates presence of IgG and complement on RBC membranes (e.g., warm and cold agglutinin disease)
   c. Indirect test: patient serum mixed with type O RBCS which, in turn, are mixed with Coombs reagent; agglutination indicates presence of anti-RBC antibodies in serum (e.g., Rh alloimmunization)
6. **Blood smear** = **schistocytes** (RBC fragments), spherocytes, and/or burr cells (see Figures 6-3 and 6-4)

C. Iron-deficiency anemia

1. Anemia resulting from insufficient heme production secondary to **insufficient iron supplies**
2. Iron deficiency results from **blood loss**, poor dietary intake or absorption from the gastrointestinal (GI) tract, pregnancy, or menstruation.
3. **H/P** = fatigue, weakness, dyspnea on exertion, **pica** (i.e., craving to eat ice, dirt, etc.), restless legs; pallor, tachycardia, tachypnea, increased pulse pressure, possible systolic murmur; **angular cheilitis** (i.e., irritation of lips and corners of mouth), **spooning of nails** in severe cases

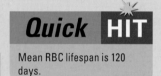

Quick HIT

Mean RBC lifespan is 120 days.

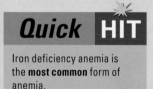

Quick HIT

Iron deficiency anemia is the **most common** form of anemia.

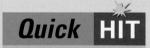

Quick HIT

Consider iron deficiency anemia in **elderly** patients **caused by colon cancer** until such is ruled out.

TABLE 6-2 Types of Hemolytic Anemias

Type	Pathology	Blood Smear	Coombs Test	Other Diagnostic Aids	Treatment
Drug induced	Bind to RBC membrane and cause oxidative destruction, induce production of **antidrug antibodies**, form **immune complexes** that fix complement, or induce **anti-Rh antibodies**	Burr cells, schistocytes	**Direct Coombs+** (unless due to oxidative destruction)	Recent penicillin, methyldopa, quinidine, other drug use	Stop offending agent
Immune	**Anti-RBC antibodies**, autoimmune disease, possibly drug induced	Sphero-cytes (warm agglutinins), RBC aggluti-nation (cold agglutinins)	**Direct Coombs+**	**Warm-reacting antibodies** (IgG) or **cold-reacting antibodies** (IgM)	Corticosteroids, **avoid cold expo-sure** (with cold-reacting antibodies), stop offending agent; splenectomy may be needed in persistent cases
Mechanical	RBCs broken by force or **turbulent flow**	**Schistocytes**	Negative	**Prosthetic heart valve**, HTN, coagulation disorder	Treat underlying cause
Hereditary spherocytosis (see also Figure 6-3)	Genetic **defect of RBC membranes** resulting in spherical RBCs	**Spherocytes**	Negative	**Hepatosplenomegaly**	Splenectomy
G6PD deficiency	Deficiency of G6PD (enzyme required to repair oxidative damage to RBCs); ingestion of oxidant (fava beans, high-dose ASA, sulfa drugs, dapsone, quinine, quinidine, primaquine, nitrofurantoin) causes excessive hemolysis	RBCs with **"bites"** taken out of them, **Heinz bodies** (small densities of Hgb in RBC)	Negative	**Low G6PD** (by indirect measurement); dizziness, fatigue begins within days of ingesting oxidant; mild form in blacks, more severe form in people of Mediterranean decent	Avoid oxidants; transfusion may be needed in severe cases

ASA, aspirin; G6PD, glucose-6-phosphate dehydrogenase; HTN, hypertension; RBC, red blood cell.

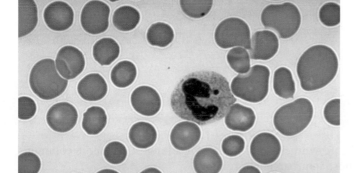

FIGURE 6-3 **Hereditary spherocytosis.**

Blood smear shows numerous spherocytes with decreased diameter, increasing staining, and absence of central pallor.

(From Rubin, R., & Strayer D. S. [2013]. *Rubin's Pathology* [6th ed., p. 964]. Philadelphia, PA: Lippincott Williams & Wilkins; with permission.)

Hematology and Oncology

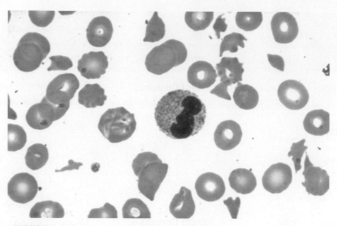

FIGURE
6-4 **Microangiopathic hemolytic anemia demonstrating multiple schistocytes (fragmented red blood cells [RBCs]).**

(From Rubin, R., & Strayer D. S. [2013]. *Rubin's Pathology* [6th ed., p. 971]. Philadelphia, PA: Lippincott Williams & Wilkins; with permission.)

4. **Labs** = decreased Hgb, decreased Hct, decreased MCV, decreased or normal reticulocyte count, **decreased ferritin**, decreased iron, increased transferrin (i.e., total iron-binding capacity), positive stool guaiac possible if secondary to GI losses (see Table 6-3)
5. **Blood smear** = microcytic hypochromic RBCs (see Figure 6-5)
6. **Treatment** = iron supplementation (several months of treatment required to replete stores), determine cause of iron loss

TABLE 6-3 **Laboratory Distinction of Microcytic Anemias**

Type	Serum Iron	Ferritin	TIBC (transferrin)	Iron: TIBC ratio	Blood Smear
Iron deficiency	↓	↓	↑	Low (<12)	Hypochromic, microcytic RBCs
Chronic disease	↓	Normal or ↑	↓	Normal (>18)	Hypochromic, normocytic, or microcytic RBCs
Lead poisoning	Normal or ↑	Normal or ↑	Normal or ↓	Normal	Stippled, microcytic RBCs
Sideroblastic	↑	↑	↓	Normal	Ringed sideroblasts (in **bone marrow**)
Thalassemia	Normal or ↑	Normal or ↑	Normal	↑ in β-thalassemia	Microcytic RBCs, target cells (α), basophilic stippling (β)

MCV, mean corpuscular volume; RBC, red blood cell; TIBC, total iron-binding capacity; ↑, increased; ↓, decreased.

D. Lead poisoning anemia

1. Anemia resulting from heme synthesis inhibition by lead ingestion (more common in **children**, especially those in urban environments)
2. Similar presentation may be seen in anemia caused by alcoholism or isoniazid use.
3. **H/P** = fatigue, weakness, abdominal pain, arthralgias, headache, impaired short-term memory; pallor, mental developmental delays, **gingival lead lines**, **peripheral neuropathy** (e.g., decreased motor control of extremities)
4. **Labs** = decreased Hgb, decreased Hct, decreased MCV, increased serum lead (see Table 6-3)
5. **Blood smear** = microcytic RBCs, **basophilic stippling of RBCs** (see Figure 6-6)

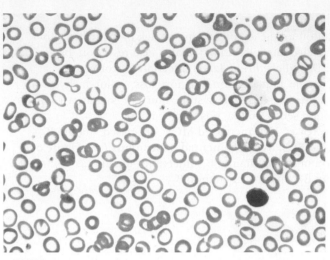

FIGURE 6-5 **Microcytic hypochromic red blood cells (RBCs) characteristic of iron deficiency anemia.**

(From Rubin, R., & Strayer D. S. [2008]. *Rubin's Pathology: Clinicopathologic Foundations of Medicine* [5th ed., p. 865]. Philadelphia, PA: Lippincott Williams & Wilkins; with permission.)

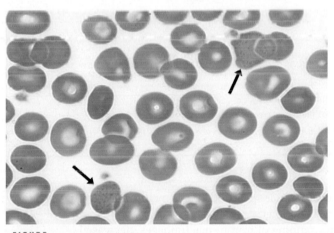

FIGURE 6-6 **Lead poisoning anemia.**

Note the hypochromic red blood cells (RBCs) and basophilic stippling seen in some cells (*arrows*).

(From Anderson, S. C., & Poulsen, K. B. [2014]. *Anderson's Atlas of Hematology* [2nd ed., p. 224]. Philadelphia, PA: Lippincott Williams & Wilkins; with permission.)

6. **Treatment** = remove source of lead; EDTA or dimercaptosuccinic acid (DMSA) if needed for lead chelation (add dimercaprol in children with severe lead intoxication)

E. Folate-deficiency anemia

1. Anemia resulting from inadequate folate intake, increased folate need (e.g., poor nutrition, chemotherapy), or drug-induced folate metabolism defects (e.g., methotrexate, trimethoprim, phenytoin)
2. **H/P** = **poor nutrition**, fatigue, weakness, dyspnea on exertion, diarrhea, **sore tongue**; pallor, tachycardia, tachypnea, increased pulse pressure, possible systolic murmur; **no neurologic symptoms**
3. **Labs** = decreased Hgb, decreased Hct, **increased MCV**, decreased serum folate, decreased red cell folate level, decreased reticulocyte count
4. **Blood smear** = macrocytic RBCs, hypersegmented neutrophils
5. **Treatment** = oral folate supplementation

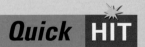

Quick HIT

Folate deficiency is the most common cause of **megaloblastic** anemia.

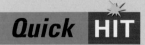

Quick HIT

Inadequate folate intake is seen with **alcoholism** and in the elderly because of poor nutrition.

F. Vitamin B₁₂ deficiency anemia

1. **Pernicious anemia** (i.e., autoimmune anemia owing to lack of intrinsic factor) or anemia resulting from inadequate vitamin B₁₂ intake, ileal resection, bacterial overgrowth in GI tract, or *Diphyllobothrium latum* infection (a worm)
2. **H/P** = fatigue, weakness, dyspnea on exertion, memory loss; pallor, tachycardia, tachypnea, increased pulse pressure, possible systolic murmur, **symmetric paresthesias**, loss of vibration sense, **ataxia**, possible dementia
3. **Labs** = decreased Hgb, decreased Hct, **increased MCV**, decreased vitamin B₁₂
4. **Blood smear** = **macrocytic RBCs, hypersegmented neutrophils** (see Figure 6-7)
5. **Treatment** = monthly intramuscular vitamin B₁₂ injections, dietary supplementation of vitamin B₁₂, intranasal vitamin B₁₂

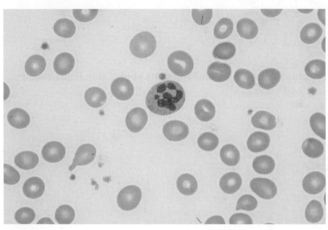

FIGURE
6-7   **Anemia caused by vitamin B₁₂ deficiency.**

Note the macrocytic red blood cells (RBCs) and presence of a hypersegmented neutrophil.

(From Anderson, S. C., & Poulsen, K. B. (2003). *Anderson's Atlas of Hematology*. Philadelphia, PA: Lippincott Williams & Wilkins, Figure IIA3-3; with permission.)

G. Anemia of chronic disease

1. Anemia occurring in patients with neoplasia, diabetes mellitus, autoimmune disorders, or long-standing infections
2. Frequently associated with trapping of iron in macrophages, decreased erythropoietin production, and increased hepcidin levels (inhibitor of iron absorption and mobilization)
3. **H/P** = history of appropriate disease state, fatigue, weakness, dyspnea on exertion; tachycardia, pallor
4. **Labs** = **mildly decreased Hgb and Hct**, normal or decreased MCV, decreased iron, decreased transferrin, normal or increased ferritin (see Table 6-3)
5. **Blood smear** = normocytic RBCs
6. **Treatment** = **treat underlying disorder**; supplemental erythropoietin

H. Aplastic anemia

1. **Pancytopenia** resulting from bone marrow failure
2. Due to **radiation**, drugs (e.g., chloramphenicol, sulfonamides, phenytoin, chemotherapeutics), toxins, viral infection, or idiopathic and congenital causes
3. **H/P** = fatigue, weakness, **persistent infections**, **poor clotting** with possible uncontrolled bleeding, easy bruising, persistent menstruation; pallor, petechiae, tachycardia, tachypnea, systolic murmur, increased pulse pressure
4. **Labs** = decreased Hgb, decreased Hct, decreased white blood cells (WBCs), decreased platelets; bone marrow biopsy shows **hypocellularity** and fatty infiltrate
5. **Treatment** = stop offending agent; transfusions for acute anemia and thrombocytopenia; immunosuppressive agents and bone marrow transplant indicated to improve long-term survival

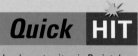

Quick **HIT**

Inadequate vitamin B₁₂ intake is usually only seen in **strict vegetarians** (vegans).

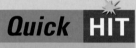

Quick **HIT**

Folate deficiency caused by inadequate dietary intake develops significantly more quickly than vitamin B₁₂ deficiency from inadequate intake.

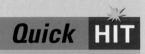

Quick **HIT**

Aplastic anemia in a sickle cell patient is classically caused by **parvovirus B19**.

6. **Complications** = prognosis worsens with increasing age and severity with 5-year survival of 85% in young patients with moderate disease and 20% in elderly patients with severe disease

II. Genetic Disorders of Hemoglobin

A. Sideroblastic anemia

1. Anemia caused by **defective heme synthesis** resulting in decreased Hgb levels in cells
2. Can be a genetic disorder or caused by alcohol, isoniazid, or lead poisoning (patient history is useful for differentiating cause)
3. **H/P** = fatigue, weakness, dyspnea on exertion, angina; pallor, tachycardia, tachypnea, increased pulse pressure, hepatosplenomegaly, possible systolic murmur
4. **Labs** = decreased Hgb, decreased Hct, increased ferritin, increased iron, decreased transferrin, possible decreased MCV (see Table 6-3)
5. **Blood smear** = **multiple sizes of RBCs** with normocytic, **microcytic**, and macrocytic cells possible; **ringed sideroblasts** (RBC precursors) in the bone marrow (see Figure 6-8)
6. **Treatment**
   a. Hereditary cases: vitamin B_6 may normalize Hgb concentrations
   b. Acquired cases: supplemental erythropoietin
   c. Both types: significant iron overload requires therapeutic phlebotomy (mild cases) or chelation with deferoxamine (more severe cases); transfusion may be required in severe cases
7. **Complications** = 10% patients progress to acute leukemia

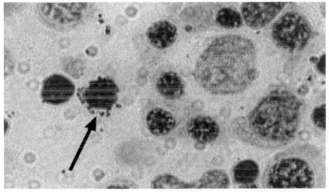

FIGURE
6-8 **Bone marrow in a patient with sideroblastic anemia.**

Note several red blood cells (RBCs) surrounded by rings of iron granules (ring sideroblasts) *(arrow)*.

(From Handin, R. I., Lux, S. E., & Stossel, T. P. [2003]. *Blood: Principles and Practice of Hematology* [2nd ed., Color Figure 3-6D]. Philadelphia, PA: Lippincott Williams & Wilkins; with permission of Robert I. Handin, MD.)

B. Thalassemia

1. Hgb defects resulting from abnormal production of heme α-globin or β-globin subunits
2. Disease state arises from **unbalanced production** ratio of α and β chains (see Table 6-4).
3. **Normal Hgb**
   a. Composed of two α chains and two β chains
   b. Four genes determine α-chain synthesis; two genes determine β-chain synthesis.
4. **α-Thalassemia**
   a. More prevalent in people of Asian or African descent
   b. Variants have between one and four defective alleles.

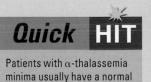

Quick **HIT**

Patients with α-thalassemia minima usually have a normal MCV.

TABLE 6-4	Variants of α- and β-Thalassemias		
Thalassemia Type	**Variant**	**Number of Abnormal Alleles**	**Characteristics**
α	α-Thalassemia minima	1	Generally **asymptomatic**; children of carriers at increased risk for thalassemia, pending genotype of other parent
	α-Thalassemia minor	2	Reduced α-globin production; **mild anemia**; microcytic RBCs and target cells on blood smear
	Hemoglobin H disease	3	Minimal α-globin production; **chronic hemolytic anemia**, pallor, splenomegaly; microcytic RBCs on blood smear; Hemoglobin H in blood; decreased lifespan
	Hydrops fetalis	4	Hemoglobin Bart's (no α-globin production); **fetal death** occurs
β	β-Thalassemia minor	1	Reduced β-globin production; mild anemia; increase in hemoglobin A2; patients can lead normal lives; transfusions may be needed during periods of stress
	β-Thalassemia major	2	No β-globin production; asymptomatic until decline of fetal hemoglobin; growth retardation, developmental delays, bony abnormalities, hepatosplenomegaly, anemia; increase in hemoglobin A2 and F; microcytic RBCs on blood smear; patients die in childhood without transfusions

RBCs, red blood cells.

5. **β-Thalassemia**
   a. More prevalent in patients of Mediterranean descent
   b. Variants have either one or two defective alleles.
6. **Labs = decreased MCV**, increased reticulocyte count, increased hemoglobin Bart (i.e., Hgb that binds O_2 but is unable to release it to tissues in hydrops fetalis), increased hemoglobin A_2 or F in β-Thalassemia; Hgb electrophoresis can detect genetic abnormalities and severity of defects (see Table 6-3)
7. **Blood smear**
   a. α-Thalassemia: abnormally shaped microcytic RBCs, target cells (see Figure 6-9)
   b. β-Thalassemia: RBCs in variable size and shape (including microcytic cells) with target cells
8. **Treatment**
   a. α-Thalassemia minor or minima and β-Thalassemia minor frequently are asymptomatic and only require symptomatic treatment during periods of stress.

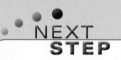

NEXT STEP

If microcytic anemia is found on blood smear, rule out thalassemia before administering supplemental iron to prevent iron overload.

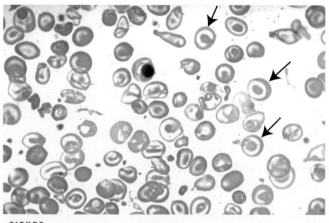

FIGURE 6-9 **Thalassemia.**

The peripheral blood erythrocytes are hypochromic and microcytic and show anisocytosis, poikilocytosis, and target cells (*arrows*).

(From Rubin, R., & Strayer D. S. [2008]. *Rubin's Pathology: Clinicopathologic Foundations of Medicine* [5th ed., p. 871]. Philadelphia, PA: Lippincott Williams & Wilkins; with permission.)

Hematology and Oncology

b. Folate supplementation may be helpful in all symptomatic forms and in mild forms during stress.

c. **Transfusions** are required for more severe variants and may be needed for mild forms during periods of stress.

d. **Iron chelation** may be required in patients receiving chronic transfusions.

e. Bone marrow transplant may be helpful in children with minimal hepatomegaly, no portal fibrosis, and adequate iron chelation therapy.

9. **Complications** = **chronic iron overload** from repeat transfusions causes damage to heart and liver; patients with Hgb H disease and β-Thalassemia major have high childhood mortality without transfusion therapy; children of asymptomatic parents with defective genes are still at risk for developing disease, depending on inherited alleles

C. Sickle cell disease

1. Autosomal recessive defect in β-globin chain of Hgb, leading to production of **abnormal Hgb S** that is poorly soluble when deoxygenated

2. Acidosis, hypoxia, and dehydration cause Hgb S molecules to polymerize and distort RBCs into a **sickle shape** that is **more susceptible to hemolysis** and **vascular clumping** than normal cells.

3. More common in people of African heritage

4. **H/P** = frequently asymptomatic between crises; stressful events (e.g., infection, illness, trauma, hypoxia) induce **sickle cell crisis** characterized by **deep bone pain**, chest pain, new stroke onset, painful swelling of hands and feet, dyspnea, priapism (i.e., painful, prolonged erection); growth retardation, splenomegaly, jaundice, fever, tachypnea, leg ulcers seen on examination

5. **Labs**
   a. Decreased Hct, increased reticulocyte count, increased polymorphonuclear (PMN) cells, decreased serum haptoglobin, increased bilirubin (indirect)
   b. Hemoglobin electrophoresis detects Hgb S without normal Hgb A; Hgb F may be increased.
   c. Sickledex solubility test can detect Hgb abnormalities but cannot differentiate between carrier trait and homozygous disease state.

6. **Radiology** = "codfish" vertebrae; lung infiltrates in acute chest syndrome (radiologic findings in setting of chest pain and dyspnea)

7. **Blood smear** = target cells, nucleated RBCs; **deoxygenation of blood produces sickle cells** (see Figure 6-10)

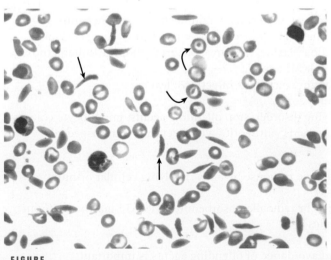

FIGURE 6-10 Sickle cell anemia.

Sickled cells (*straight arrows*) and target cells (*curved arrows*) are evident.

(From Rubin, R., & Strayer D. S. [2008]. *Rubin's Pathology: Clinicopathologic Foundations of Medicine* [5th ed., p. 874]. Philadelphia, PA: Lippincott Williams & Wilkins; with permission.)

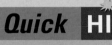

β-Globin defects:
- In sickle cell disease, causes production of **defective β chains.**
- In β-thalassemia, causes **decreased production of normal β chains.**

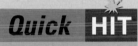

Heterozygous **carriers** of sickle cell defect (sickle cell trait) are **asymptomatic** and carry **improved resistance to malaria.**

Quick HIT

Presence of fetal Hgb in newborns delays presentation of sickle cell symptoms until after 6 months of age, when fetal Hgb levels have decreased.

Hematology and Oncology

8. Treatment
   a. **Hydration, supplemental O₂,** and **analgesics** (frequently narcotics required) **during sickle cell crises**
   b. Hydroxyurea (increases Hgb F production) and avoidance of crisis stimuli decrease frequency of crises.
   c. Pneumococcal vaccine reduces risk of infection in asplenic patients; prophylactic penicillin should be given until 5 years of age to help prevent pneumococcal infection in asplenic children.
   d. Chronic transfusions may help keep the level of Hgb S as low as possible.
   e. Hematopoietic stem cell transplantation and gene therapy show future promise as potential cures.
9. Complications
   a. Chronic anemia, pulmonary hypertension, heart failure, **aplastic crisis** (usually secondary to parvovirus B19 infection), **acute chest syndrome** (i.e., acute pneumonia, pulmonary infarction, and embolus)
   b. Autosplenectomy, stroke, osteonecrosis, and multiple organ ischemia (particularly kidney, heart, retina) can result secondary to **vascular occlusion**.
   c. Increased risk of infection by **encapsulated organisms**

III. Leukocyte Disorders and Hypersensitivity

A. Lymphopenia without immune deficiency
1. Decreased lymphocyte count seen in diseases with **increased cortisol** levels or after **chemotherapy**, radiation, or lymphoma; antibody production not affected
2. **H/P** = repeated infections with possible recent history of chemotherapy or radiation
3. **Labs** = decreased WBCs, especially B and T lymphocytes
4. **Treatment** = if possible, stop offending agents; bone marrow transplant may be needed

B. Eosinophilia
1. Abnormally high levels of eosinophils seen in Addison disease, neoplasm, asthma, allergic drug reactions, collagen vascular diseases, transplant rejection, and parasitic infections
2. **H/P** = **asymptomatic**; history of predisposing condition
3. **Labs** = increased eosinophil count
4. **Treatment** = treat underlying disorder; stop offending agent

C. Neutropenia
1. Decreased neutrophil count seen with some viral infections (e.g., hepatitis, human immunodeficiency virus [HIV], Epstein-Barr virus), drugs (e.g., clozapine, antithyroid medications, sulfasalazine, methimazole, trimethoprim-sulfamethoxazole), chemotherapy, and aplastic anemia
2. **H/P** = weakness, chills, fatigue, **recurrent infections**; fever
3. **Labs** = decreased neutrophil count
4. **Treatment** = treat underlying disorder, stop offending agents, granulocyte colony-stimulating factor, corticosteroids; antibiotics whenever infection suspected

D. Hypersensitivity reactions
1. Allergen-induced immunologic response by body involving cellular or humoral mechanisms (see Table 6-5)
2. **Labs** = skin allergen testing or radioallergosorbent test (RAST) may be useful in determining specific allergies
3. Treatment
   a. **Contact prevention** and **avoidance** of offending agents is important.
   b. Type I: antihistamines, leukotriene inhibitors, bronchodilators, and corticosteroids may improve symptoms after reaction; desensitization may be considered to avoid recurrent reactions; if anaphylaxis is a concern, epinephrine injections should be kept readily available

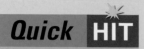

Patients with sickle cell disease are particularly susceptible to *Salmonella* **osteomyelitis** and **sepsis** by **encapsulated organisms** (*Streptococcus pneumoniae, Haemophilus influenzae, Neisseria meningitidis, Klebsiella*).

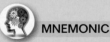

MNEMONIC

Remember the types of hypersensitivity reactions by the mnemonic **ACID: A**naphylactic, **C**omplement mediated, **I**mmune complex mediated, and **D**elayed.

TABLE 6-5	Types of Hypersensitivity Reactions		
Type	Mediated By	Mechanism	Examples
I	IgE antibodies attached to mast cells	Antigens react with antibody to cause **mast cell degranulation** and histamine release	Allergic rhinitis, asthma, **anaphylaxis**
II	IgM and IgG antibodies	Cellular antigens react with antibodies to initiate **complement cascade** and cell death	**Drug-induced or immune hemolytic anemia**, hemolytic disease of the newborn
III	IgM and IgG immune complexes	Antibodies bind to soluble antigens to form **immune complexes**, which are then deposited in tissue and initiate complement cascade	Arthus reaction, serum sickness, glomerulonephritis
IV	T cells and macrophages	**T cells** present antigens to macrophages and secrete lymphokines that induce macrophages to destroy surrounding tissue	Transplant rejection, **allergic contact dermatitis**, PPD testing

PPD, purified protein derivative.

c. Type II: anti-inflammatories or immunosuppressive agents, possibly plasmapheresis
d. Type III: anti-inflammatories
e. Type IV: corticosteroids or immunosuppressive agents

E. Anaphylaxis

1. Severe type I hypersensitivity reaction after re-exposure to allergen (penicillins, insect stings, latex, eggs, nuts, and seafood are common causes)
2. H/P = symptoms and signs typically occur 5 to 60 minutes after exposure; tingling in skin, itching, cough, chest tightness, **difficulty swallowing and breathing** (secondary to angioedema), syncope; tachycardia, wheezing, urticaria, hypotension, arrhythmias
3. Labs = skin testing or RAST can confirm allergic response, increased histamine and tryptase
4. **Treatment = subcutaneous epinephrine, intubation** (if closed airway), antihistamines, bronchodilators, recumbent positioning, intravenous (IV) hydration; vasopressors may be needed for severe hypotension; avoidance of stimuli is key to prevention; elective desensitization therapy may be appropriate following an episode, depending on allergen, to avoid future incidents

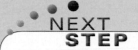

NEXT STEP

Epinephrine should be given **immediately** to a person having an anaphylactic reaction without waiting for additional tests.

IV. Clotting Disorders

A. Normal clotting function

1. Platelets
   a. Circulate in plasma
   b. Important in **primary control** of bleeding
   c. Cause local vasoconstriction and form platelet plug at site of vascular injury in response to adenosine diphosphate (ADP) secreted by injured cells
   d. Bleeding time can be used to assess platelet function but is poorly reproducible and time consuming.
2. Coagulation cascade
   a. Responsible for formation of **fibrin clot** at site of injury (see Figure 6-11)
   b. **Intrinsic pathway** induced by exposure to negatively charged foreign substances; measured by partial thromboplastin time (**PTT**)
   c. **Extrinsic pathway** induced by tissue factor exposed at site of injury; measured by prothrombin time (**PT**)

Hematology and Oncology

Hematology and Oncology

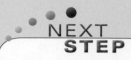

NEXT STEP

Monitor **heparin** anticoagulation with **PTT**.

Quick HIT

Low molecular weight heparins (LMWH) do **not** require monitoring by PTT.

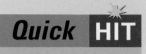

NEXT STEP

Monitor **warfarin** anticoagulation with a normalized PT (i.e., **international normalized ratio [INR]**) to track relative effect on the extrinsic pathway.

Quick HIT

Do not start warfarin therapy for a thrombus until after starting LMWH or until PTT is therapeutic on unfractionated heparin because warfarin inhibits proteins C and S to cause a short period of **hypercoagulability** immediately after therapy is initiated.

Quick HIT

vWF and factor VIII are the only clotting factors not synthesized exclusively by the liver and remain at normal levels, whereas other factor levels decrease in liver failure.

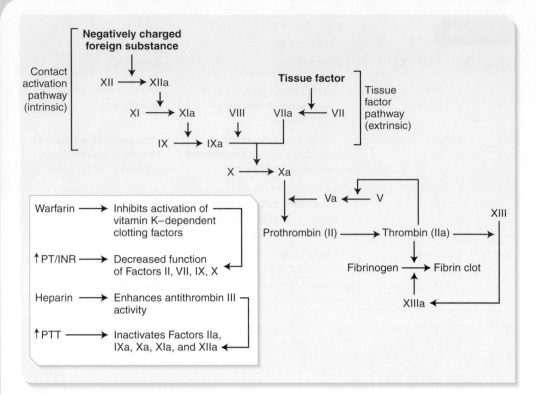

FIGURE
6-11 **Coagulation cascade.**

INR, international normalized ratio; PT, prothrombin time; PTT, partial thromboplastin time.

3. **Antithrombotic drugs**
   a. Used to prevent or treat pathologic clot (thrombus) formation (e.g., deep vein thrombosis [DVT], thromboembolic stroke, mural thrombus, pulmonary embolism [PE], postsurgical or traumatic thrombus, etc.)
   b. Can affect platelet function, intrinsic pathway, or extrinsic pathway (see Table 6-6)

B. Thrombocytopenia
1. Decreased number of platelets (<150,000) leading to increased risk of hemorrhage
2. May be idiopathic, autoimmune, or result from external causes (e.g., drugs, infection, nutrition) (see Table 6-7)
3. **H/P** = possibly asymptomatic; mucosal bleeding, petechiae, purpura, multiple ecchymoses
4. **Labs** = platelets <150,000/μL, increased bleeding time
5. **Blood smear** = may show low platelet numbers, small platelets, abnormal platelet granules, or neutrophilic granules depending on etiology

C. von Willebrand disease
1. Autosomal dominant disease with deficiencies of **von Willebrand factor** (vWF) and sometimes **factor VIII**, leading to abnormal clotting and platelet function
2. **H/P** = easy bruising, mucosal bleeding (nose, gums), menorrhagia; multiple sites of bruising and mucosal bleeding on examination; antiplatelet drug administration can induce bleeding
3. **Labs** = **increased PTT, increased bleeding time**, decreased factor VIII antigen, decreased vWF antigen, decreased ristocetin cofactor activity
4. **Treatment** = desmopressin during minor bleeding, vWF concentrate and factor VIII concentrate before surgery or during major bleeding, avoidance of aspirin (ASA)

TABLE 6-6	**Common Anticoagulant Drugs**		
Drug	**Mechanism**	**Role**	**Adverse Effects**
ASA	Inhibits platelet aggregation by inhibiting cyclooxygenase activity to suppress thromboxane A_2 synthesis	Decreases thrombus risk in CAD and post-MI; decreases postoperative thrombus risk	Increased risk of hemorrhagic stroke, **GI bleeding**
Thienopyridines (e.g., clopidogrel, ticlopidine)	Block ADP receptors to suppress fibrinogen binding to injury and platelet adhesion	Decreases risk of repeat MI or stroke in patients with prior MI, stroke, or PVD; decreases thrombus risk in postvascular intervention patients	Increased risk of hemorrhage, **GI bleeding**
GP IIb/IIIa inhibitors (e.g., abciximab, tirofiban, eptifibatide)	Inhibit platelet aggregation by binding to platelet GP IIb/IIIa receptors	Reduce risk of thrombus in unstable angina or following coronary vessel intervention	Increased risk of hemorrhage, nausea, back pain, hypotension
Adenosine reuptake inhibitors (e.g., dipyridamole)	Inhibit activity of adenosine deaminase and phosphodiesterase to inhibit platelet aggregation	Used in combination with ASA in patients with recent stroke or with warfarin following artificial heart valve replacement	Dizziness, headache, nausea
Heparin	Binds to **antithrombin** to increase activity and prevent clot formation	Postoperative prophylaxis for DVT and PE, dialysis, decreases post-MI thrombus risk, safer than warfarin during pregnancy	Hemorrhage, hypersensitivity, **thrombocytopenia**, narrow therapeutic window
Low molecular weight heparin (e.g., enoxaparin, dalteparin)	Binds to **factor Xa** to prevent clot formation	Postoperative prophylaxis for DVT and PE, safest option during pregnancy	Hemorrhage, fever, rare thrombocytopenia
Direct thrombin inhibitors (e.g., lepirudin, argatroban)	Highly selective inhibitors of thrombin to suppress activity of factors V, IX, and XIII and platelet aggregation	Alternative anticoagulation in patients with history of heparin-induced thrombocytopenia (HIT)	Hemorrhage, hypotension
Direct factor Xa inhibitors (e.g., apixaban, rivaroxaban)	Highly selective inhibition of factor Xa without activity against thrombin	DVT prophylaxis, anticoagulation following acute DVT or PE	Hemorrhage, fever, anemia, edema, rash, constipation
Warfarin	Antagonizes vitamin K-dependent carboxylation of factors II, VII, IX, and X	**Long-term** anticoagulation post-thrombotic event or in cases of increased thrombus risk (postsurgery, Afib, artificial valves)	Hemorrhage, numerous **drug interactions, teratogenicity**

ADP, adenosine diphosphate; ASA, aspirin; Afib, atrial fibrillation; CAD, coronary artery disease; DVT, deep vein thrombosis; GI, gastrointestinal; MI, myocardial infarction; PE, pulmonary embolism; PVD, peripheral vascular disease.

D. Vitamin K deficiency
1. Inadequate vitamin K supply because of poor intake, malabsorption, or eradication of vitamin K-producing GI flora (secondary to prolonged antibiotic use)
2. Vitamin K is required in synthesis of factors II, VII, IX, and X.
3. **H/P** = easy bruising, mucosal bleeding, melena, hematuria, delayed clot formation
4. **Labs** = increased PT, increased INR
5. **Treatment** = oral or intramuscular vitamin K, fresh frozen plasma (FFP)

E. Hemophilia
1. X-linked recessive disease with deficiency of either factor VIII (hemophilia A) or factor IX (hemophilia B)
2. **H/P** = **uncontrolled bleeding** occurring spontaneously or after minimal trauma, excessive bleeding following surgical or dental procedures; **hemarthroses** (i.e., bleeding in joints), intramuscular bleeding, and GI or genitourinary bleeding may be evident on examination

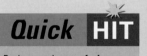

Patients using **warfarin** can present with a clinical picture similar to that of vitamin K deficiency.

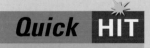

Hemophiliacs tend not to develop significant bleeds unless they have **<5%** clotting activity.

Hematology and Oncology

TABLE 6-7	Causes of Thrombocytopenia		
Cause	**Pathology**	**Diagnosis**	**Treatment**
Impaired production (drugs, infection, aplastic anemia, folate/vitamin B_{12} deficiency, alcohol, cirrhosis)	**Absent** or **reduced** megakaryocytes caused by offending agent or **abnormal megakaryocytes** because of metabolic deficiency	Findings consistent with precipitating condition; bone marrow biopsy helpful for diagnosis	Stop offending agent, treat underlying disorder, bone marrow transplantation
Abnormal pooling	**Splenic platelet sequestration**	Splenomegaly, normal bone marrow biopsy, 90% platelets may be sequestered	May not be required; splenectomy if symptomatic
Heparin-induced thrombocytopenia (HIT)	Development of antiplatelet antibodies that cause widespread platelet destruction in response to heparin therapy	Diffuse thrombus formation, sudden decrease (>50%) in platelet level, positive serotonin release assay, positive heparin-induced platelet aggregation assay	Stop all heparin use; direct thrombin inhibitors for thrombi
Immune thrombocytopenia (ITP)	**Autoimmune** B-cell directed production of antiplatelet antibodies	Other explanations for thrombocytopenia ruled out, **platelets commonly <50,000**	Self-limited in children; adults require corticosteroids, delayed splenectomy, intravenous (IV) immunoglobulin, plasmapheresis, or recombinant factor VIIa
Thrombotic thrombocytopenic purpura-hemolytic uremic syndrome (TTP-HUS)	Diffuse platelet aggregation due to autoantibodies against a preventative enzyme; associated with endothelial injury and *Escherichia coli* O157:H7 infection	**Hemolytic anemia, acute renal failure, thrombocytopenia** without severe bleeding, neurologic sequelae, ± fever	Corticosteroids, plasmapheresis, FFP
Antiphospholipid syndrome	Development of antiphospholipid antibodies during pregnancy leading to arterial and venous thrombosis	During pregnancy, presence of antiphospholipid or lupus anticoagulant antibodies	Anticoagulation with heparin and warfarin, hydroxychloroquine
HELLP syndrome	Sequela of eclampsia associated with elevated liver enzymes and hemolytic anemia	During pregnancy, HTN, increased LFTs, decreased Hgb, schistocytes on blood smear	Induce delivery if fetus >34 wk gestation; anti-HTN drugs and corticosteroids to speed fetal lung maturity if preterm

FFP, fresh frozen plasma; HELLP, hemolysis, elevated liver enzymes, and low platelet counts; HTN, hypertension; LFTs, liver function tests.

MNEMONIC

Remember the signs of thrombotic thrombocytopenic purpura-hemolytic uremic syndrome (TTP-HUS) by the mnemonic **N**asty **F**ever **T**orched **H**is **K**idneys: **N**eurologic deficits, **F**ever, **T**hrombocytopenia, **H**emolytic anemia, **K**idney failure.

3. **Labs = increased PTT, normal PT, normal bleeding time**, decreased factor VIII or IX antigen
4. **Treatment = factor VIII or IX replacement**, desmopressin (may increase factor VIII production in hemophilia A), transfusions frequently needed in cases of large blood loss; hemarthroses and intracranial bleeds require aggressive factor replacement
5. **Complications** = death from severe, uncontrolled bleeding; arthropathy from recurrent hemarthroses frequently requires eventual joint replacement

F. **Disseminated intravascular coagulation (DIC)**
   1. Widespread abnormal coagulation caused by sepsis, severe trauma, neoplasm, or obstetric complications
      a. Initial coagulopathy with widespread clot formation occurs because of extensive activation of the clotting cascade by endothelial tissue factor released during bacteremia.
      b. Deficiency in clotting factors results from extensive clotting.
      c. Abnormal bleeding results from clotting factor deficiencies.

2. **H/P** = appropriate history of precipitating condition; uncontrolled bleeding from wounds and surgical sites, hematemesis, dyspnea; jaundice, digital cyanosis, hypotension, tachycardia, possible neurologic or renal insufficiency signs, possible shock
3. **Labs** = decreased platelets, increased PT, increased PTT, decreased fibrinogen, **increased fibrin split products, increased D-dimer**, decreased Hct
4. **Blood smear** = schistocytes, few platelets
5. **Treatment** = **treat underlying disorder**; platelets, FFP, cryoprecipitate; heparin may be needed for chronic thrombi
6. **Complications** = poor prognosis without early treatment; thrombi cause numerous infarcts

V. Hematologic Infections

A. Sepsis

1. Bacteremia with an associated **excessive systemic inflammatory response** leading to global tissue hypoxia and possibly organ dysfunction
2. Diagnostic criteria for systemic inflammatory response syndrome (SIRS) are two of the following:
   a. Temperature $>38.3°C$ or $<36°C$
   b. Heart rate >90 beats/min
   c. Respiratory rate >20 breaths/min or $PaCo_2$ <32 mm Hg
   d. WBC $>12,000$ cells/mm^3 or $<4,000$ cells/mm^3, or $>10\%$ immature (band) forms
3. Common community-acquired pathogens include *Streptococcus*, *Staphylococcus*, *Escherichia coli*, *Klebsiella*, *Pseudomonas*, and *Neisseria meningitidis*.
4. Common nosocomial pathogens include *Staphylococcus*, gram-negative bacilli, anaerobes, *Pseudomonas*, and *Candida* species.
5. **H/P** = malaise, chills, nausea, vomiting; fever or hypothermia, mental status changes, tachycardia, tachypnea; may progress to **septic shock** with hypotension, cool extremities (initially warm), and petechiae
6. **Labs** = increased ($>12,000$/mL) or decreased ($<4,000$/mL) WBCs; positive urine, blood, or sputum cultures needed to diagnose infection; labs may detect signs of DIC
7. **Radiology** = chest X-ray may show infiltrates and pneumonia
8. **Treatment**
   a. Secure airway, supply adequate oxygenation (may require intubation and ventilation)
   b. Hydration, vasopressors, inotropes, and transfusions to maintain tissue perfusion
   c. Glucocorticoids may be beneficial in select patients.
   d. Broad-spectrum antibiotics **initially**, then pathogen-specific antibiotics when agent identified by culture; remove (or change) possible routes of infection (Foley catheter, IV, etc.)
   e. Maintain glycemic control (glucose 140 to 180 mg/dL)
9. **Complications** = septic shock, DIC

B. Malaria

1. Parasitic infection by ***Plasmodium*** spp. (*P. vivax*, *P. falciparum*, *P. ovale*, *P. malariae*) transmitted by *Anopheles* mosquito
2. **H/P** = **chills**, diaphoresis, headache, myalgias, fatigue, nausea, abdominal pain, vomiting, diarrhea; **periodic fever** at approximately 1- to 3-day intervals, splenomegaly; *P. falciparum* infection can include decreased consciousness, pulmonary edema, and renal insufficiency
3. **Labs** = polymerase chain reaction (PCR) for *Plasmodium* is highly sensitive
4. **Blood smear** = Giemsa stain shows *Plasmodium* spp. (see Figure 6-12)
5. **Treatment** = **antimalarials** (e.g., chloroquine, primaquine, quinine); atovaquone-proguanil or mefloquine used in chloroquine-resistant *P. falciparum*

C. Infectious mononucleosis

1. Infection by **Epstein-Barr virus** (EBV) affecting B cells and oropharyngeal epithelium
2. Transmitted by **intimate contact** (e.g., kissing, intercourse)

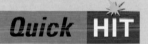
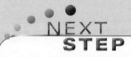
Hematology and Oncology

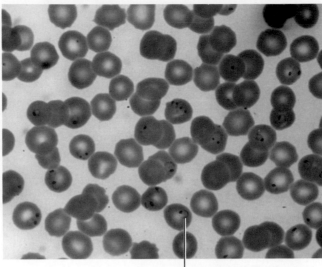

Malaria parasite

FIGURE 6-12 Peripheral blood demonstrating *Plasmodium* infection (malaria).

(From McConnell, T. H. [2007]. *The Nature of Disease: Pathology for the Health Professions* [p. 245]. Philadelphia, PA: Lippincott Williams & Wilkins; with permission.)

3. H/P = **fatigue**, sore throat, malaise; **lymphadenopathy**, splenomegaly, fever, tonsillar exudates
4. **Labs** = positive heterophile antibodies (i.e., Monospot test), positive EBV serology, elevated LFTs, increased WBCs, hemolytic anemia, thrombocytopenia
5. **Blood smear** = increased number of lymphocytes (some with abnormal appearance)
6. **Treatment** = self-limited; supportive care
7. **Complications** = splenic rupture is rare, but patients should refrain from contact sports for 1 month after symptom onset; rare aplastic anemia; disseminated intravascular coagulation; thrombotic thrombocytopenic purpura; fulminant liver failure

D. Human immunodeficiency virus (HIV)

1. RNA retrovirus (HIV-1 and HIV-2 are most common strains) that infects CD4 lymphocytes (**helper T cells**) and destroys them, eventually leading to **acquired immunodeficiency syndrome (AIDS)**
   a. Both strains transmitted in same manner; they share same risks for opportunistic infections and are treated in same manner.
   b. Compared with HIV-1, HIV-2 progresses more slowly, is less infectious in early disease, is more infectious in late disease, and is less common in the United States.
   c. Serologic tests for the two strains are slightly different and do not cross-react consistently.
2. Virus uses reverse transcriptase to incorporate genetic material into host cell genome and produce copies of DNA.
3. Transmitted via **bodily fluids** (e.g., blood, semen, vaginal secretions, breast milk)
4. **Risk factors** (United States) = homosexual or bisexual males, intravenous drug abuse (IVDA), blood transfusions before the mid-1980s (e.g., hemophiliacs), multiple sexual partners, heterosexual partners of other high-risk individuals, infants born to infected mothers, accidental exposure to bodily fluids (e.g., needle sticks, fluid splashes) among health care workers (low probability but possible); higher prevalence among black and Latino populations
5. **Acute H/P** = **flulike symptoms** (e.g., myalgias, nausea, vomiting, diarrhea, fatigue), sore throat, weight loss; **mucosal ulcers**, fever, lymphadenopathy, viral rash; symptoms typically develop 2 to 4 weeks after exposure and last 2 weeks
6. Following acute infection, patient enters **latent phase** with few or no symptoms and low viral load that lasts months to years (time increases with treatment).
7. **Late H/P** (i.e., AIDS) = **opportunistic infections** and **AIDS-defining illnesses** begin to present; weight loss, night sweats, dementia (see Table 6-8)

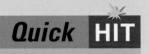

Quick HIT

Symptoms of mononucleosis do not appear until 2–5 weeks after infection with EBV.

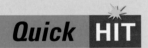

Quick HIT

HIV infection has greatest prevalence in sub-Saharan Africa, where transmission is typically through heterosexual contact.

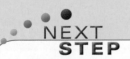

NEXT STEP

Although the rate of HIV transmission through needle sticks (i.e., health care workers) is very low (0.3%), prophylactic tenofovir, emtricitabine, and raltegravir should be started immediately if there is an appreciable risk of transmission; HIV antibody tests should be performed immediately, 6 weeks, 3 months, and 6 months after exposure to determine if transmission occurred; treatment should be continued for 4 weeks.

Hematology and Oncology

| TABLE 6-8 | Common Opportunistic Infections, Neoplasms, and Complications Seen in Acquired Immunodeficiency Syndrome (AIDS) |

Condition/Infection	When Seen	History/Physical	Diagnosis	Treatment
Herpes zoster/simplex	CD4 <500	Shingles, oral or genital lesions	Tzanck smear, viral culture	Acyclovir, valacyclovir foscarnet
Kaposi sarcoma	CD4 <250	**Purple subcutaneous nodules** on face, chest, or extremities	Biopsy of lesions	Topical alitretinoin, chemotherapy, laser therapy, radiation
Parasitic diarrhea (*Isospora, Strongyloides, Cryptosporidium*)	CD4 <500	Prolonged diarrhea, malaise, weight loss, abdominal pain	Stool culture, parasite evaluation	Antiretroviral therapy, metronidazole, TMP-SMX, paromomycin
Wasting syndrome	CD4 <100	Weight loss >10% baseline weight, chronic diarrhea, chronic weakness, fever	Clinical diagnosis, EMG suggests peripheral nerve dysfunction	Exercise, corticosteroids
Coccidioidomycosis	CD4 <250	Cough, fever, dyspnea	Bilateral reticulonodular infiltrates on CXR, positive antibody screen	Fluconazole, itraconazole, or amphotericin B
AIDS dementia	CD4 <200	Confusion, mental status changes, **generalized neurologic symptoms**, including tremor	History of declining mental function, generalized neurologic symptoms, elevated β_2-microglobulin in CSF, cerebral atrophy on CT or MRI	May improve with antiretroviral therapy
Bacterial pneumonia (*Streptococcus pneumoniae, Haemophilus influenzae, Nocardia*)	CD4 <200	**Rapid onset**, productive cough, high fevers	Gram stain, lobar consolidation on CXR	Cephalosporins, β-lactams, or macrolides
Candida esophagitis	CD4 <200	Dysphagia, **odynophagia**	Endoscopy with biopsy, Gram stain on lesion scrapings	Topical or oral fluconazole or ketoconazole
Cervical cancer	CD4 <200	History of human papilloma virus	Detected by screening Papanicolaou (Pap) smear, biopsy confirms diagnosis	Resection, topical 5-flurouracil, radiation therapy, chemotherapy
Pneumocystis jirovecii pneumonia (PCP)	CD4 <200	**Gradual onset, nonproductive cough**, dyspnea on exertion, fever	Bilateral infiltrates on CXR, increased LDH, sputum Gram stain	TMP-SMX, corticosteroids
Tuberculosis	CD4 <200, high-risk groups/ prisons	Cough, night sweats, weight loss, fever	**Acid-fast bacilli**, cavitary defects and hilar adenopathy on CXR, positive PPD (must be checked with anergy test)	Isoniazid, rifampin, pyrazinamide, ethambutol
Histoplasmosis	CD4 <150	Abdominal pain, GI bleeding, skin lesions, dyspnea, meningitis	Bilateral infiltrates on CXR, positive antigen test	Long-term amphotericin B or itraconazole
Cerebral toxoplasmosis	CD4 <100	Headache, confusion, possible **focal neurologic symptoms**	**Positive *Toxoplasma* IgG antibody**, ring-enhancing lesions on CT or MRI	Pyrimethamine, sulfadiazine, clindamycin (**chronic treatment may be needed**)
Lymphoma (CNS or non-Hodgkin)	CD4 <100	Headache, confusion, possible **focal neurologic symptoms**	CT or MRI shows lesion, biopsy confirms diagnosis	Chemotherapy, radiation
Progressive multifocal leukoencephalopathy (JC virus)	CD4 <100	Ataxia, motor deficits, mental status changes	Positive PCR for JC virus DNA	May improve with antiretroviral therapy

(*continued*)

Hematology and Oncology

TABLE 6-8	Common Opportunistic Infections, Neoplasms, and Complications Seen in Acquired Immunodeficiency Syndrome (AIDS) (*Continued*)			
Condition/Infection	**When Seen**	**History/Physical**	**Diagnosis**	**Treatment**
Cryptococcal meningitis	CD4 <50	Headache, neck stiffness, fever, mental status changes	Elevated pressure on lumbar puncture, **yeast seen with India ink** stain of CSF, **positive cryptococcal antigen** in CSF or serum	Amphotericin B, fluconazole
Cytomegalovirus (CMV)	**CD4 <50**	**Vision loss**, esophagitis, diarrhea	Viral titer, yellow infiltrates with hemorrhage on funduscopic exam	Ganciclovir, foscarnet, valganciclovir
Mycobacterium avium complex (MAC)	**CD4 <50**	Fatigue, weight loss, fever, diarrhea, abdominal pain, lymphadenopathy, hepatosplenomegaly	Blood cultures	Clarithromycin, azithromycin, ethambutol, rifabutin, rifampin

CNS, central nervous system; CSF, cerebrospinal fluid; CT, computed tomography; CXR, chest X-ray; EMG, electromyogram; GI, gastrointestinal; LDH, lactate dehydrogenase; MRI, magnetic resonance imaging; PPD, purified protein derivative; TMP-SMX, trimethoprim-sulfamethoxazole.

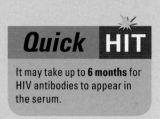

Quick **HIT**

It may take up to **6 months** for HIV antibodies to appear in the serum.

8. **Labs**
   a. Enzyme-linked immunosorbent assay (**ELISA**) detects HIV antibodies and is 99% sensitive; if positive, repeat ELISA performed (see Figure 6-13).
   b. Following two positive ELISAs, **Western blot** (lower sensitivity but high specificity) is performed to rule out false-positive findings.
   c. Rapid serologic tests are being used as initial screening test with increasing frequency, but positive results require standard serologic testing for confirmation.
   d. **CD4 count** is used to track extent of disease progression (AIDS is defined by CD4 count <200).
   e. **Viral load** indicates the rate of disease progression (low during latent phase and high once AIDS is diagnosed) and may be useful in detection of acute infection during presentation with symptoms of seroconversion.
   f. Other nonspecific lab findings include decreased WBCs (during acute infection and again after development of AIDS), increased liver function test (LFT) findings, and mildly decreased Hgb and platelets.

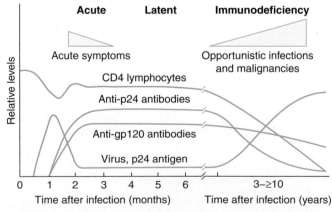

Note: p24 and gp120 are viral proteins that serve as markers for HIV infection.

FIGURE
6-13 Serologic profile of human immunodeficiency virus (HIV) infection.

Note: p24 and gp120 are viral proteins that serve as markers for HIV infection.

(From Mehta, S., Milder, E. A., Mirachi, A. J., & Milder, E. [2006]. *Step-Up: A High-Yield, Systems-Based Review for the USMLE Step 1* [3rd ed., p. 210]. Philadelphia, PA: Lippincott Williams & Wilkins.)

9. **Treatment**
   a. **Antiretroviral therapy** should be initiated for all HIV-infected patients, regardless of CD4 count or viral load.
   b. Utility of starting antiretroviral therapy in acute infection is controversial and currently not universally recommended (performed in health care workers).
   c. Common initial **highly active antiretroviral treatment (HAART)** regimens
      (1) Start with two nucleoside reverse transcriptase inhibitors and either a protease inhibitor or non-nucleoside reverse transcriptase inhibitor (three antiretroviral drug minimum) (see Table 6-9).
      (2) Low-dose ritonavir can be added to the initial regimen to increase protease inhibitor activity.
      (3) Combination therapy (i.e., multiple drugs combined in one pill) will decrease number of pills taken at one time and help avoid dosing schedule mishaps.
   d. Compliance with therapy is vital to delaying disease progression; significant side effects associated with antiretroviral drugs is a major deterrent to good compliance.
   e. Indications for changing antiretroviral regimen include failure to keep viral load <50/mL, drug toxicity, poor compliance, and suboptimal regimen.
      (1) Patients with virologic failure should be tested for viral drug resistance, reviewed for drug interactions, and considered for drug substitution or addition of another drug.
      (2) Drug toxicity may be amenable to changing drugs.
      (3) Poor compliance can be approached by decreasing complexity of regimen (i.e., using combination pills) or enlisting family or friends to assist patient.
      (4) Suboptimal regimens can be improved with drug substitution.
   f. Antibiotic prophylaxis for opportunistic infections is started as below:
      (1) Trimethoprim-sulfamethoxazole (TMP-SMX) for *Pneumocystis jirovecii* pneumonia (PCP) when CD4 count <200
      (2) Azithromycin for *Mycobacterium avis* complex (MAC) when CD4 count <100
   g. Close following of serology is important for dictating the direction of care.

TABLE 6-9   Antiviral Medications Used in Treatment of Human Immunodeficiency Virus (HIV)

Drug Class	Examples of Drug	Mechanism	Adverse Effects
Nucleoside reverse transcriptase inhibitors	**Abacavir** Emtricitabine Lamivudine **Zidovudine** Tenofovir (nucleotide RTI)	Inhibit production of viral genome, prevent incorporation of viral DNA into host genome through reverse transcriptase inhibition	**Lactic acidosis, lipodystrophy,** pancreatitis, hypersensitivity reactions (abacavir), bone marrow toxicity (zidovudine)
Non-nucleoside reverse transcriptase inhibitors	Efavirenz Etravirine Rilpivirine	Inhibit reverse transcriptase activity to prevent viral replication	**Rash**; efavirenz causes neuropsychiatric effects and is teratogenic
Protease inhibitors	Atazanavir Darunavir Fosamprenavir Lopinavir Ritonavir	Interfere with viral replication to cause production of nonfunctional viruses	**Hyperglycemia, hypertriglyceridemia,** GI toxicity, hyperbilirubinemia (atazanavir)
Integrase inhibitor	Elvitegravir Raltegravir	Inhibit the final step in integration of viral DNA into host DNA	Neutropenia, pancreatitis, hepatotoxicity, hyperglycemia
Fusion inhibitor	Enfuvirtide	Bind to gp41, inhibit viral ability to fuse with CD4 membrane and enter cell	Hypersensitivity reactions, reaction at injection site, bacterial pneumonia
CCR5 antagonist	Maraviroc	Inhibit viral CCR5 coreceptor → block viral entry to host cell	Fever, cough, upper respiratory infections, peripheral neuropathy, dizziness

Hematology and Oncology

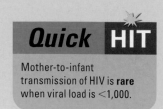

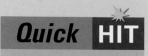

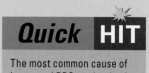

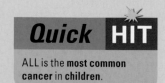

h. Pregnant mothers with HIV should be treated to keep viral load low and should be given zidovudine during labor; newborns to HIV-positive mothers should be given zidovudine for 6 weeks after birth and should be tested for presence of virus (anti-HIV antibodies will always be present in these children) in the initial 6 months of life.

10. **Complications** = opportunistic infections, neoplasms, cardiomyopathy, neuropathy, AIDS dementia complex, arthritis, polymyositis, anemia; although several advancements in treatment have been made, no cure or effective vaccine has been developed

VI. Hematologic Neoplastic Conditions

A. Polycythemia vera

1. Myeloproliferative disorder of bone marrow stem cells leading to **increased production** of RBCS, WBCs, and platelets
2. Tends to occur after age 60 years; many progress to leukemia
3. **H/P** = fatigue, headache, **burning pain in hands or feet, pruritus** (especially after contact with warm water), tinnitus, blurred vision, epistaxis, abdominal pain; **splenomegaly**, hepatomegaly, large retinal veins on funduscopic examination
4. **Labs** = **increased Hgb, increased Hct,** increased RBC mass, increased or normal WBCs and platelets, decreased erythropoietin; biopsy shows hypercellular marrow
5. **Treatment** = serial phlebotomy, antihistamines (for pruritus), ASA (thrombus prophylaxis), hydroxyurea (bone marrow suppression)
6. **Complications** = thrombus formation, **leukemia** (acute and chronic myelogenous), stroke

B. Multiple myeloma

1. Malignant proliferation of **plasma cells**; increased incidence with prior monoclonal gammopathy of undetermined significance (MGUS)
2. Abnormal monoclonal protein (**M protein**) produced from IgG and IgA heavy chains and κ and λ light chains (these light chains are known as **Bence Jones proteins**)
3. **H/P** = **back pain**, radicular pain, weakness, fatigue, weight loss, constipation, **pathologic fractures**, frequent infections; pallor, bone tenderness
4. **Labs** = decreased Hgb, decreased Hct, decreased WBCs, increased blood urea nitrogen (BUN) and creatinine (secondary to renal insufficiency), increased Ca^{2+}; serum protein electrophoresis (SPEP) and urine protein electrophoresis (UPEP) detect high M protein and Bence Jones proteins; bone marrow biopsy shows increased plasma cells
5. **Radiology** = "**punched-out**" lesions in long bones and skull
6. **Treatment** = radiation, chemotherapy, bone marrow transplant, repair of fractures, treat infections
7. **Complications** = renal failure, recurrent infections, hypercalcemia, spinal cord compression; poor prognosis with survival for 2 to 3 years after diagnosis

C. Lymphoma

1. Malignant transformation of lymphocytes primarily in **lymph nodes** that can also involve bloodstream or nonlymphatic organs
2. Categorized as Hodgkin and non-Hodgkin variants (see Table 6-10, Figure 6-14)

D. Leukemia

1. Malignant transformation of myeloid or lymphoid cells involving bloodstream and bone marrow
2. **Acute** leukemia tends to involve immature cells, whereas **chronic** leukemia involves more mature cells.
3. Bone marrow involvement can cause pancytopenia.
4. **Acute lymphocytic leukemia** (ALL)
   a. **Most common in children** (2 to 5 years of age); whites > blacks
   b. Proliferation of cells of **lymphoid** origin (lymphocytes)

TABLE 6-10	Characteristics of Hodgkin and Non-Hodgkin Lymphomas	
Characteristic	**Hodgkin Lymphoma**	**Non-Hodgkin Lymphoma**
Cells of origin	B cells	Lymphocytes (**most commonly B cells**) or natural killer cells
Classification (low to higher grade)	Nodular sclerosis (**most common**, women = men, fibrosis of lymph nodes), mixed cellularity, lymphocyte-rich (rare, best prognosis), lymphocyte-depleted (very rare, worst prognosis)	Many types, common variants include diffuse large B cell (**most common**), follicular small cell (B cells, t[14;18]), small lymphocytic (same disease as CLL), Burkitt (**EBV related**, t[8;14], **"starry sky" pattern**), peripheral (**T cells**)
Risk factors, patient population	Bimodal age distribution (peaks at 20 and 65 yr of age), men > women (except for nodular sclerosis subtype)	EBV, HIV, congenital immunodeficiencies, rheumatic disease
History and physical	Painless lymphadenopathy (**neck**), weight loss, pruritus, night sweats, fever, hepatosplenomegaly	Painless lymphadenopathy (**generalized**), weight loss, fever, night sweats
Labs	Lymph node biopsy shows **Reed-Sternberg cells** (see also Figure 6-14)	Lymph node or bone marrow biopsy shows lymphocyte proliferation (**cleaved cells seen in follicular small cell variant**)
Treatment	Radiation, chemotherapy	Palliative radiation, chemotherapy
Prognosis	**Good**, 80% cure rate unless far progressed	**Poor** (months for aggressive types, years for less aggressive variants), worsens with increasing age

CLL, chronic lymphocytic leukemia; EBV, Epstein-Barr virus; HIV, human immunodeficiency virus.

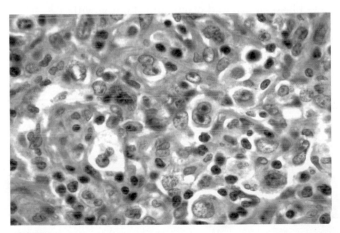

FIGURE 6-14 **Hodgkin disease; histologic section of lymph node demonstrates pathognomonic binucleated Reed-Sternberg cells that resemble owls' eyes.**

(From Rubin, R., & Strayer D. S. [2012]. *Rubin's Pathology* [6th ed., p. 1026]. Philadelphia, PA: Wolters Kluwer/Lippincott Williams & Wilkins; with permission.)

c. **H/P** = **bone pain**, frequent infections, fatigue, dyspnea on exertion, easy bruising; fever, pallor, purpura, hepatosplenomegaly, lymphadenopathy

d. **Labs** = decreased Hgb, decreased Hct, decreased platelets, decreased WBCs, increased uric acid, increased LDH; bone marrow biopsy shows **abundant blasts**; Philadelphia chromosome (i.e., translocation of chromosomes 9 and 22 in *BCR-ABL* genes) found in 15% **adult** cases

e. **Blood smear** = numerous blasts (see Figure 6-15)

f. **Treatment** = chemotherapy (induction followed by maintenance dosing), bone marrow transplant

g. **Complications** = although 5-year survival rates are good (85%) in children, adults have worse prognosis; presence of Philadelphia chromosome carries poor prognosis

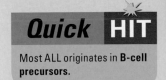

Quick **HIT**

Most ALL originates in **B-cell precursors.**

Hematology and Oncology

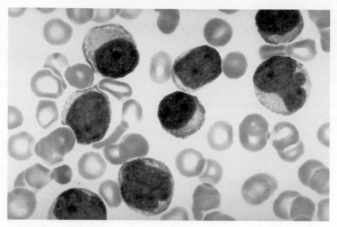

FIGURE

6-15 **Acute lymphocytic leukemia.**

Note lymphoblasts with irregular nuclei and prominent nucleoli.

(From Rubin R., Strayer D. S., & Bubin, E. [2012]. *Rubin's Pathology* [6th ed., p. 1026]. Philadelphia, PA: Lippincott Williams & Wilkins with permission.)

5. **Acute myelogenous leukemia** (AML)
   a. Proliferation of **myeloid** cells; both children and adults affected
   b. **H/P** = fatigue, easy bruising, dyspnea on exertion, frequent infections, arthralgias; fever, pallor, hepatosplenomegaly, mucosal bleeding, ocular hemorrhages
   c. **Labs** = decreased Hgb, decreased Hct, decreased platelets, decreased WBCs; bone marrow biopsy shows **blasts** of myeloid origin and staining with **myeloperoxidase**
   d. **Blood smear** = large myeloblasts with **notched nuclei** and **Auer rods** (see Figure 6-16)
   e. **Treatment** = chemotherapy (regimen guided by cytogenetic analysis), bone marrow transplant
   f. **Complications** = relapse common, DIC; long-term survival is poor despite frequently successful remissions
6. **Chronic lymphocytic leukemia** (CLL)
   a. Proliferation of **mature B cells** in patients >65 years of age

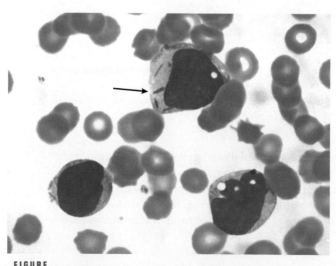

FIGURE

6-16 **Acute promyelocytic leukemia** (a subtype of AML).

Prominent Auer rods are seen (*arrow*)

(From Rubin, R., & Strayer, D. S. [2008]. *Rubin's Pathology: Clinicopathologic Foundations of Medicine* [5th ed., p. 903]; Philadelphia, PA: Lippincott Williams & Wilkins; with permission.)

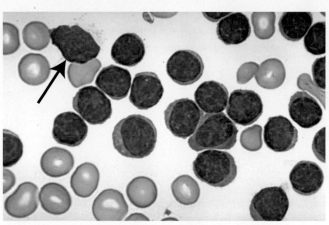

FIGURE
6-17 **Chronic lymphocytic leukemia.**

Note small lymphocytes of comparable size to nearby red blood cells (RBCs) and presence of smudge cells (fragile lymphocytes disrupted during smear preparation) in upper portion of image.

(From Rubin, R., & Strayer, D. S. [2008]. *Rubin's Pathology: Clinicopathologic Foundations of Medicine* [5th ed., p. 916]. Philadelphia, PA: Lippincott Williams & Wilkins; with permission.)

b. **H/P** = fatigue, frequent infection (secondary to no plasma cells), night sweats; fevers, lymphadenopathy, hepatosplenomegaly

c. **Labs** = **increased WBCs** (may be >100,000/μL); bone marrow shows lymphocyte infiltration

d. **Blood smear** = numerous small lymphocytes, **smudge cells** (see Figure 6-17)

e. **Treatment** = supportive therapy, chemotherapy, radiation for bulky lymphoid masses, splenectomy for splenomegaly

f. **Complications** = malignant B cells may form autoantibodies, leading to severe hemolytic anemia; course of disease tends to be either indolent (>10-year survival) or aggressive with high mortality within 4 years

7. **Chronic myelogenous leukemia (CML)**

a. Proliferation of **mature myeloid** cells seen in middle-aged adults; can be associated with **radiation exposure**

b. Follows stable course for several years before progressing into **blast crisis** (i.e., rapid worsening of neoplasm) that is usually fatal

c. **H/P** = possibly asymptomatic before progression; fatigue, weight loss, night sweats; fever, splenomegaly; blast crisis presents with worsening symptoms and bone pain

d. **Labs** = **increased WBCs** (>100,000/μl) with high proportion of neutrophils, decreased leukocyte alkaline phosphatase; bone marrow shows granulocyte hyperplasia; cytogenetic analysis demonstrates **Philadelphia chromosome** (t[9;22]) or *BCR-ABL* fusion gene

e. **Treatment** = chemotherapy (imatinib is promising agent), bone marrow transplant in younger patients

f. **Complications** = blast crisis signals rapid progression and is usually fatal

8. **Hairy cell leukemia**

a. Proliferation of B cells most frequently in middle-aged men

b. Similar in appearance to CLL (but better prognosis); now considered an indolent type of non-Hodgkin lymphoma

c. **H/P** = fatigue, frequent infections, abdominal fullness, no night sweats; no fever, **massive splenomegaly, no lymphadenopathy**

d. **Labs** = decreased Hgb, Hct, platelets, and WBCs (rarely, WBCs increased); bone marrow biopsy shows lymphocyte infiltration

e. **Blood smear** = numerous lymphocytes with "**hairy**" projections (irregular cytoplasmic projections) (see Figure 6-18)

f. **Treatment** = chemotherapy once patients develop symptomatic cytopenia

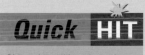

Quick HIT

CLL and small lymphocytic lymphoma are considered to be the same disease process in different stages of evolution.

Quick HIT

Patients with CLL are asymptomatic 25% of the time and may be diagnosed following a workup for an abnormal CBC performed for an unrelated reason.

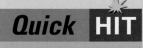

Quick HIT

The Philadelphia chromosome (t[9;22]) or *BCR-ABL* gene is almost always seen in CML but may also be seen in about 5% of ALL cases and rarely in AML.

Hematology and Oncology

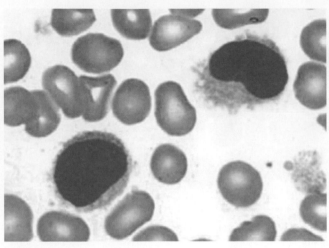

FIGURE
6-18 **Hairy cells typical of hairy cell leukemia.**

Note the numerous cytoplasmic projections giving the cell its name.

(From Rubin, R., & Strayer, D., [2012]. *Rubin's Pathology: Clinicopathologic Foundations of Medicine* [6th ed., p. 1017]. Philadelphia, PA: Lippincott Williams & Wilkins.)

 # VII. Oncologic Therapy

A. Treatment strategy

1. **Eradication** of neoplastic cells is the ultimate goal.
2. When eradication is not possible, therapy seeks to **delay disease progression** or to serve a **palliative** role.
3. Mass effect of tumors and paraneoplastic syndromes can cause effects that are treated with surgery, radiation, or chemotherapy to relieve symptoms even when overall prognosis is bleak.

B. Cancer surgery

1. Performed to **reduce mass** of solid tumors or **remove** well-contained tumors
2. Resection of surrounding tissue frequently performed to increase chances of removing microscopic extensions of tumor
3. Many procedures carry significant morbidities and prolonged recoveries because of size of surgery or organ removal (e.g., Whipple procedure for pancreatic cancer, gastrectomy for gastric cancer).

C. Radiation therapy

1. Performed to **necrose** tumor cells and **decrease tumor size**
2. May be curative in some cancers (some head and neck tumors); serves palliative role in several cases (e.g., Pancoast tumor)
3. Adverse effects include impaired surgical wound healing, fibrosis of tissue, skin irritation, esophagitis, gastritis, pneumonitis, neurologic deficits, bone marrow suppression, and **radiation-induced malignancies** (e.g., thyroid, CML, sarcomas).

D. Chemotherapy

1. Aims to eradicate smaller populations of neoplastic cells and destroy cells not removed through surgery or radiation (see Table 6-11)
2. Can sensitize neoplastic cells to radiation therapy (i.e., radiosensitizers)
3. Can be primary treatment modality in certain cancers particularly receptive to pharmacologic therapy
4. **Multiple drugs** with different cell cycle–specific targets are frequently combined to increase neoplastic cell death while minimizing toxicity to normal tissues, to have an effect against a broader range of cells, and to slow development of resistance.
5. Adverse effects include bone marrow suppression, alopecia, GI upset, infertility, neurotoxicity, hepatotoxicity, skin changes, pulmonary fibrosis, cardiomyopathy, and renal toxicity.

TABLE 6-11	Mechanisms and Classes of Chemotherapeutic Drugs	
Mechanism	**Drug Class**	**Examples**
Free radical production causing cytotoxic alkylation of DNA and RNA	Nitrogen mustard alkylating agents Nitrosourea alkylating agents Alkyl sulfonate alkylating agents Ethyleneimine or methylmelamine alkylating agents Triazene alkylating agents	Cyclophosphamide, chlorambucil, ifosfamide, mechlorethamine Carmustine, streptozocin Busulfan Thiotepa, hexamethylmelamine Dacarbazine
Inhibition of spindle proteins to stop mitosis or cause cytotoxic polymerization	Vinca alkaloids Taxanes	Etoposide, vinblastine, vincristine Paclitaxel, docetaxel
Inhibition of DNA and RNA synthesis	Antibiotics Monoamine oxidase inhibitors	Bleomycin, dactinomycin, daunorubicin, doxorubicin, mitomycin Procarbazine
Interference with enzyme regulation or DNA and RNA activity	Antimetabolites Platinum analogues	Cytarabine, 5-flurouracil, methotrexate, mercaptopurine Carboplatin, cisplatin
Modulation of hormones to cause tumor remission	Steroid hormones and antagonists	Prednisone, tamoxifen, estrogens, leuprolide

VIII. Other Pediatric Hematologic and Oncologic Concerns (Not Addressed in Other Sections)

A. Hemolytic disease of the newborn

1. If Rh⁺ fetal cells enter circulation of Rh⁻ mother, **anti-Rh antibodies** may develop.
2. Antibodies do not affect pregnancy with initial Rh interaction but cause severe fetal RBC hemolysis in subsequent pregnancies with Rh⁺ fetuses (i.e., fetal hydrops).
3. **Risk factors** = Rh⁻ mother with any history of fetal–maternal hemorrhage (e.g., abortion, amniocentesis, third-trimester bleeding)
4. Hemolysis will likely cause death of fetus.
5. **Treatment** = administration of Rho(D) immune globulin (**RhoGAM**) within 72 hr of delivery of initial Rh⁺ fetus or at any time maternal and fetal blood may have mixed will prevent development of anti-Rh antibodies and protect future pregnancies by suppressing maternal formation of anti-Rh antibodies; intrauterine fetal transfusion may be required if condition develops in utero.

B. Fanconi anemia

1. Autosomal recessive disorder associated with **bone marrow failure**, pancytopenia, and increased risk of leukemia
2. **H/P** = fatigue, dyspnea on exertion, frequent infections; frequently associated with **short stature, abnormal skin pigmentation** (café-au-lait spots or hypopigmented areas), horseshoe kidney, and thumb abnormalities
3. **Labs** = decreased Hgb, Hct, platelets, and WBCs; increased serum α-fetoprotein; bone marrow biopsy shows hypocellularity; chromosome analysis detects multiple strand breakage
4. **Treatment** = antibiotics, transfusions, bone marrow or hematopoietic stem cell transplantation, hematopoietic growth factors; androgens and corticosteroids can increase bone marrow activity
5. **Complications** = death in childhood is common from bone marrow failure or leukemia

C. Diamond-Blackfan anemia

1. Congenital **pure RBC anemia** likely caused by a defect in erythroid progenitor cells
2. **H/P** = fatigue, dyspnea, cyanosis, and pallor detected early in life; craniofacial abnormalities, thumb abnormalities, heart murmurs, mental retardation, hypogonadism

3. **Labs** = decreased Hgb, decreased Hct, decreased reticulocyte count, increased MCV; bone marrow biopsy shows decreased activity but increased presence of erythropoietin
4. **Treatment** = transfusions, corticosteroids, bone marrow transplant

D. Neuroblastoma

1. Tumors of neural crest cell origin that may arise in adrenal glands or sympathetic ganglia
2. **Risk factors** = neurofibromatosis, tuberous sclerosis, pheochromocytoma, Beckwith-Wiedemann syndrome, Turner syndrome, low maternal folate consumption
3. **H/P** = abdominal distention and pain, weight loss, malaise, bone pain, diarrhea; abdominal mass, HTN, possible Horner syndrome, proptosis, movement disorders, hepatomegaly, fever, periorbital bruising
4. **Labs** = possible increased vanillylmandelic and homovanillic acids in 24-hr urine collection
5. **Radiology** = computed tomography (CT) may locate adrenal or ganglion tumor
6. **Treatment** = surgical resection, chemotherapy, radiation
7. **Complications** = poor prognosis if presenting after 1 year of age; metastasizes to bone and brain

E. Rhabdomyosarcoma

1. Tumor of striated muscle in children
2. **H/P** = painful soft tissue mass with swelling; large tumors frequently cause mass effect on nearby structures
3. **Labs** = biopsy is diagnostic
4. **Radiology** = CT or magnetic resonance imaging (MRI) shows extent of tumor
5. **Treatment** = surgical debulking, radiation, chemotherapy

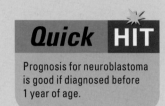

Prognosis for neuroblastoma is good if diagnosed before 1 year of age.

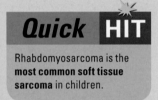

Rhabdomyosarcoma is the **most common soft tissue sarcoma** in children.

Hematology and Oncology

EMERGENCY MEDICINE

I. Accidents and Injury

A. Burns

1. Injury to epithelial surface and deeper tissues caused by exposure to significant heat, radiation, caustic chemicals, or electrical shock
2. Classified by depth of involvement
   a. **1st degree**: epidermis only involved
   b. **2nd degree**: partial-thickness dermal involvement
   c. **3rd degree**: full-thickness dermal and possibly deeper tissue involvement
   d. **4th degree**: additional involvement of muscle and bone
3. Extent of burns is estimated by "rule of 9s" (see Figure 7-1).
4. **History and physical (H/P)** = dependent on degree:
   a. First- and 2nd-degree burns are erythematous and painful; blisters are also seen in 2nd-degree burns.

> **Quick HIT**
>
> Burns secondary to **electrical shock** are sometimes called 4th-degree burns because they may involve muscles, bones, and other internal structures.

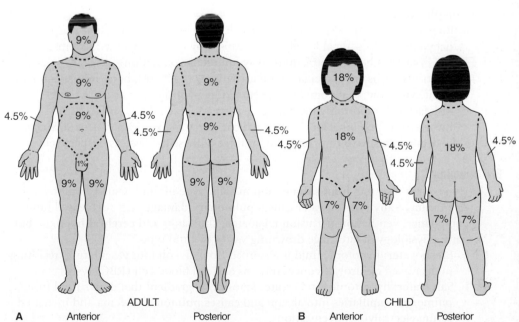

9%

9%

4.5%   9%   4.5%

1%

9%   9%

9%

9%

4.5%
4.5%

9%   9%

18%

18%

4.5%

7%   7%

18%

4.5%
4.5%

7%   7%

4.5%

ADULT   **CHILD**

A Anterior   Posterior   **B** Anterior   Posterior

FIGURE 7-1 **"Rule of 9s" for calculating extent of burns.**

(**A**) The surface anatomy of the adult is divided into sections of 9% body surface area (genitals are considered 1% surface area). Note that the distribution considers both the front and back of the head and arms as one contribution. (**B**) Because of its greater relative size, the contribution of the head is increased in the child. Note that the front and back for the head, arms, and legs are considered as one contribution.

b. Third-degree burns are painless and skin appears charred, leathery, or gray.

c. Electrical burns may appear similar to 4th-degree burns, show severe damage at entrance and exit sites of electrical current, and have cardiac and neurologic symptoms (e.g., ventricular fibrillation, seizures, loss of vision).

5. Treatment

a. Remove any burning agents to prevent further injury (e.g., burning or soaked clothing); caustic chemicals should be diluted or neutralized.

b. **Outpatient** treatment is sufficient for **1st-degree** and minor 2nd-degree burns (e.g., cooling and cleansing, bandaging, topical antimicrobials).

c. **Inpatient** treatment (e.g., intravenous [IV] hydration, wound care, possible escharotomy) is required for **2nd-degree** burns >10% body surface area, **3rd-degree** burns >2% body surface area, or 2nd- and 3rd-degree burns affecting face, hands, genitalia, or major skin flexion creases.

d. Second- and 3rd-degree burns >25% body surface area or involving the face require **airway management** (frequently intubation), IV fluids, and careful control of body temperature (increased risk of hypothermia).

e. Patients with significant **smoke inhalation** (diagnosed by increased carboxyhemoglobin levels) should receive high-flow O_2 and close monitoring for respiratory compromise requiring intubation.

f. Cardiac and neurologic issues in **electrical** burns should be managed to decrease mortality.

g. Nasogastric tube should be placed when there is gastrointestinal (GI) involvement (ileus will frequently develop).

h. Generous use of analgesics and/or regional anesthesia for **pain control**

i. **Antimicrobial agents** (e.g., topical silver sulfadiazine or bacitracin) should be used in dressings to decrease risk of infection, and tetanus toxoid should be administered if immunization status is unknown or not up to date.

j. Nonadherent bandaging or biologic dressings should be applied directly to severe burns; dressings should not be wrapped around affected areas because of potential swelling and constriction.

k. Surgical debridement and exploration should be performed to remove necrotic tissue and to determine extent of deeper tissue involvement; plastic reconstructive surgery with skin grafting may be needed.

6. Complications

a. **Infection** (especially *Pseudomonas,* sepsis), stress ulcers (Curling type), aspiration, dehydration, ileus, renal insufficiency (caused by rhabdomyolysis), compartment syndrome, epithelial contractions (may limit range of motion)

b. Electrical burns are associated with arrhythmias, seizures, bony injury, compartment syndrome, rhabdomyolysis, acute kidney injury.

c. Risk factors for **mortality** include age >60 years, >40% body surface area involvement, and inhalation injury; patients carry a 0.3%, 3%, 33%, or 90% chance of death if they have zero, one, two, or three of these risk factors, respectively.

B. Drowning

1. Hypoxemia resulting from **submersion** in some type of fluid, usually water

2. Aspiration of **any type** of water causes **pulmonary damage** (e.g., decreased lung compliance, ventilation-perfusion mismatch, shunting) and **cerebral hypoxia**, but pathophysiology of late-stage drowning varies by fluid type.

a. **Fresh water**: hypotonic fluid is absorbed from alveoli into vasculature, resulting in decreased electrolyte concentrations and red blood cell (RBC) lysis.

b. **Salt water**: hypertonic fluid creates an osmotic gradient that draws fluid from pulmonary capillaries into alveoli and causes **pulmonary edema** and increased serum electrolyte concentrations.

3. **H/P** = prolonged submersion in liquid (pools, bathtubs, and buckets are frequent sites); cyanosis, decreased consciousness; patient may not be breathing or may have cardiac arrest

4. **Treatment** = secure airway and perform resuscitation; **supplemental O_2**, nasogastric tube placement, maintenance of adequate body temperature; any symptoms

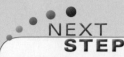

NEXT STEP

Determine IV fluid resuscitation need in 2nd-degree (and higher) burns with the **Parkland formula**: lactated Ringer's solution given in total volume of [(4 mL) × (kg body mass) × (% body surface area burned)]. Half of volume is given during the initial 8 hr, and the remaining half is given over the following 16 hr.

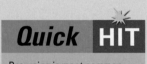

***Quick* HIT**

Drowning is most common in **children <5 years of age** and in **males** between 15 and 25 years of age.

of hypoxia following aspiration require inpatient admission for neurovascular monitoring and possible diuresis and bronchodilator therapy

5. **Complications** = correlate with degree and length of hypoxemia and include brain damage and hypothermia

C. Choking

1. **Aspiration of foreign body** into trachea or bronchi preventing normal gas exchange
2. Food is a common cause in all ages; toys, coins, and other small objects are common in children.
3. H/P = patient eating or child playing with small objects; gagging, coughing, or wheezing that progresses to stridor with increased severity of obstruction
4. Radiology = chest X-ray (CXR) may be useful in identifying item and determining location; bronchoscopy may visualize item
5. Treatment
   a. Actively coughing patients should be encouraged to remain calm and to keep coughing to dislodge object.
   b. Patients unable to breathe should be given the **Heimlich maneuver**.
   c. Emergent tracheotomy may be required in a patient with continued obstruction.
   d. Rigid bronchoscopy may be required to remove objects.
   e. Administration of IV corticosteroids before extraction attempt may ease removal by decreasing bronchial inflammation.
6. **Complications** = atelectasis, pneumonia, lung abscess; hypoxemia can cause complications similar to those seen with drowning

D. Heat emergencies

1. **Hyperthermia** (can be associated with **physical exertion** or comorbid medical condition) that occurs because of failure of thermoregulation
2. Categorized as heat stroke or heat exhaustion (see Table 7-1)

E. Hypothermia

1. Body temperature **<95°F/35°C** from cold exposure
2. Risk factors = alcohol intoxication, elderly
3. H/P = lethargy, weakness, severe shivering, confusion; decreased body temperature, possible arrhythmias, hypotension
4. **Electrocardiogram (ECG)** = **J waves**, possible ventricular tachycardia (Vtach) or ventricular fibrillation (Vfib) (see Figure 7-2)
5. **Treatment** = warm patient externally (e.g., warm bed, bath, blankets) or internally (e.g., warm IV fluids or ingested fluids); treat arrhythmias and hypotension as appropriate (see Chapter 1, **Cardiovascular Disorders**)

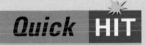

Quick HIT

The right mainstem bronchus is the most common location of aspirated items that pass beyond the trachea because of its greater vertical orientation compared with the left main bronchus.

Quick HIT

In the final stage of hypothermia, the patient will stop shivering, be unable to maintain body temperature, and will undergo a fatal increase of blood viscosity.

ER, ICU, and Surgery

TABLE 7-1	Heat Emergencies	
Disorder	**Heat Exhaustion**	**Heat Stroke**
Symptoms	Weakness, headache, substantial sweating	Confusion, blurred vision, nausea, no or little sweating
Body temperature	Slightly increased	Substantially elevated
Labs	Usually normal	Increased WBC, increased BUN, increased creatinine
Treatment	Hydration (oral unless progressive symptoms), electrolyte replacement	Evaporative cooling (spray naked patient with lukewarm water and then fan); benzodiazepines if seizures are present; antipyretics are **not** effective
Complications	Progression to heat stroke	Rhabdomyolysis, seizures, brain damage, death

BUN, blood urea nitrogen; WBC, white blood cell count.

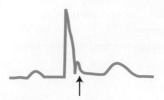

FIGURE
7-2 Diagram of electrocardiogram demonstrating a J wave (*arrow*), a characteristic finding in hypothermia.

F. **Bites and stings** (*see Table 7-2*)
   1. Injection of venom from bite or sting of snakes (e.g., in United States: rattlesnake, copperhead, water moccasin, coral snake), spiders (e.g., black widow, brown recluse), or other animals (e.g., scorpion)
   2. Venom contains neurotoxins, cardiotoxins, or proteolytic enzymes that can potentially be fatal.

TABLE 7-2	Common Types of Bites and Stings		
Type of Bite	**Symptoms**	**Treatment**	**Complications**
Snake (rattlesnake, copperhead, water moccasin, coral snake)	Pain and swelling at bite, progressive dyspnea, toxin-induced DIC	Immobilize extremity and cleanse wound; **antivenin** likely required	Effects more severe in children; increased mortality without prompt treatment
Scorpion	Severe pain and swelling at site of sting, increased sweating, vomiting, diarrhea	Antivenin, atropine, phenobarbital	Acute pancreatitis, myocardial toxicity, respiratory paralysis
Spider Black widow	Muscle pain and spasms, localized diaphoresis, abdominal pain, autonomic stimulation	Local wound care, benzodiazepines, antivenin	Ileus, cardiovascular collapse Hemolytic anemia, DIC, rhabdomyolysis
Brown recluse	Increasing pain at site, possible ulceration and necrosis	Local wound care, dapsone to prevent tissue necrosis	
Mammals	Pain and swelling at bite, penetrating trauma, depending on size of bite	Saline irrigation, debridement, tetanus and rabies prophylaxis, antibiotics for infection	Infection (staphylococci, *Pasteurella multocida*, rabies virus)
Human	Pain and swelling at bite, tender local lymphadenopathy	Saline irrigation, broad coverage antibiotics, debridement, thorough documentation	High incidence of infection with primary closure or delayed presentation

DIC, disseminated intravascular coagulation.

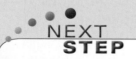

NEXT
STEP

Beware of alcohol abusers who come into the emergency department **fictitiously** saying that they have ingested ethylene glycol and need ethanol for treatment; check for sweet breath and a toxin screen before giving ethanol.

II. Toxicology

A. **General principles**
   1. Initial evaluation must focus on **determining type of poison ingested**; patient history, witness input, and clues found near patient (e.g., empty bottles of medications, other medications, etc.) help in making diagnosis.
   2. The sooner treatment is begun after toxic exposure, the better the outcome.
   3. Types of poisoning therapy (see Table 7-3)
      a. Induced vomiting: only useful in initial 1 to 2 hr after ingestion and only for noncaustic agents; **rarely** performed
      b. **Charcoal**: blocks absorption of poisons; repeat doses every few hours; not useful for alcohols or metals

TABLE 7-3 Common Poisons and Antidotes

Substance	Symptoms	Treatment
Drugs		
Acetaminophen	Nausea, hepatic insufficiency	N-acetylcysteine
Anticholinergics	Dry mouth, urinary retention, QRS widening on ECG	Physostigmine
Benzodiazepines	Sedation, respiratory depression	Flumazenil
β-Blockers	Bradycardia, hypotension, hypoglycemia, pulmonary edema	Glucagon, calcium, insulin, and dextrose
Calcium channel blockers	Bradycardia, hypotension	Glucagon, calcium, insulin, and dextrose
Cocaine	Tachycardia, agitation	Supportive care
Cyanide	Headache, nausea, vomiting, altered mental status	Nitrates, hydroxocobalamin
Digoxin	Nausea, vomiting, visual changes, arrhythmias	Digoxin antibodies
Heparin	Excessive bleeding, easy bruising	Protamine sulfate
Isoniazid	Neuropathy, hepatotoxicity	Vitamin B_6
Isopropyl alcohol	Decreased consciousness, nausea, abdominal pain	Supportive care
Methanol	Headache, visual changes, dizziness	Ethanol, fomepizole, dialysis
Opioids	Pinpoint pupils, respiratory depression	Naloxone
Salicylates	Nausea, vomiting, tinnitus, hyperventilation, anion gap, metabolic acidosis	Charcoal, dialysis, sodium bicarbonate
Sulfonylureas	Hypoglycemia	Octreotide and dextrose
Tricyclic antidepressants	Tachycardia, dry mouth, urinary retention, QRS widening on ECG	Sodium bicarbonate, diazepam
Warfarin	Excessive bleeding, easy bruising	Vitamin K, FFP
Industrial chemicals		
Caustics (acids, alkali)	Severe oropharyngeal and gastric irritation or burns, drooling, odynophagia, abdominal pain, gastric perforation symptoms	Copious irrigation (do not induce emesis or attempt neutralization), activated charcoal
Ethylene glycol	Ataxia, hallucinations, seizures, sweet breath	Ethanol, dialysis
Organophosphates (insecticides, fertilizers)	Diarrhea, urination, miosis, bronchospasm, bradycardia, excitation of skeletal muscle, lacrimation, sweating, and salivation	Atropine, pralidoxime, supportive care
Metals		
Iron	Nausea, constipation, hepatotoxicity	Deferoxamine
Lead	Peripheral neuropathy, anemia	Succimer, dimercaprol, EDTA
Mercury	Renal insufficiency, tremor, mental status changes	Dimercaprol

ECG, electrocardiogram; EDTA, ethylenediaminetetraacetic acid; FFP, fresh frozen plasma.

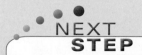

ER, ICU, and Surgery

c. Gastric lavage: usually reserved for intubated patients within initial hour after ingestion

d. **Antidotes**: reverse or inhibit poison activity; use depends on identification of agent

e. Diuretics: may help in cases where increased urination helps remove toxin (e.g., salicylates, phenobarbital)

f. Dialysis or exchange transfusion: used in cases of severe symptoms or when other treatments are unsuccessful

4. Supportive care includes airway protection, IV hydration, cardiac support (e.g., treatment for hypertension, hypotension, arrhythmias); control of seizures is an important adjunct to management of the poison itself.

B. Ingested poisons

1. Poisoning through oral ingestion of a particular toxin

2. Can occur in children from accidental ingestion of cleaning products, medications, or personal care products

NEXT STEP

Organophosphates can also be absorbed through the **skin**, so all contaminated clothing must be removed from patients with this type of poisoning.

3. Can occur in elderly patients from accidental repeat dosing of usual medications
4. Can be intentional (i.e., suicide attempt)

C. Carbon monoxide poisoning

1. Hypoxemia that results from inhalation of carbon monoxide from car fumes, smoke, or paint thinner
2. Carbon monoxide displaces O_2 on hemoglobin (Hgb) and prevents O_2 delivery to tissues.
3. **H/P** = sufficient exposure, headache, dizziness, nausea, myalgias; cherry red lips, mental status changes, possible hypotension
4. **Labs** = increased carboxyhemoglobin on blood gas analysis; **normal pulse oximetry**
5. **Treatment** = 100% O_2 (displaces carbon monoxide from Hgb) or **hyperbaric O_2** therapy; patients with smoke inhalation may require intubation secondary to upper airway edema

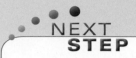

NEXT STEP

Any patient with significant **thermal burns**, burns of the **face**, or exposure to large quantities of **smoke** (e.g., house fires) requires a workup for **carbon monoxide poisoning** and **thermal airway injury**.

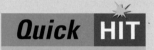
Quick HIT

Pulse oximetry may appear **normal** in carbon monoxide poisoning.

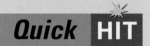
Quick HIT

Cardiac arrest lasting >10 min without cardiac output is generally considered consistent with severe brain injury or brain death.

III. Cardiovascular Emergencies

This section discusses only emergent cardiovascular conditions that require resuscitation and immediate treatment—refer to Chapters 1 and 8 on Cardiovascular and Neurologic Disorders for additional information regarding MI, arrhythmias, and stroke.

A. Cardiac arrest

1. Cessation of cardiac function resulting in acutely insufficient cardiac output
2. Requires immediate treatment to prevent systemic ischemic morbidity and death (see Figure 7-3)
3. Treatment of **Vfib** and **Vtach** requires alternating attempts at electrical and pharmacologic cardioversion (see Figure 7-4).
4. **Pulseless electrical activity** (PEA) consists of detectable cardiac electrical conduction with the absence of cardiac output (see Figure 7-5).
5. **Asystole** is the absence of cardiac activity (see Figure 7-5).

B. Acute stroke (*see Figure 7-6*)

1. Initial workup differentiates between embolic and hemorrhagic types.
2. Appropriateness for anticoagulation and thrombolysis should be considered.

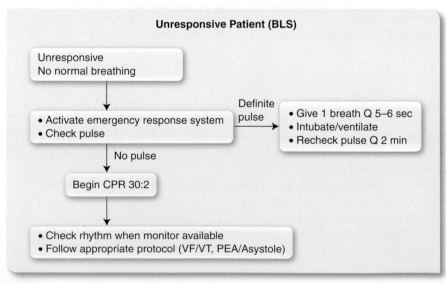

FIGURE 7-3 **Initial treatment protocol for the unresponsive patient.**

CPR, cardiopulmonary resuscitation; PEA, pulseless electrical activity; VF, ventricular fibrillation; VT, ventricular tachycardia.

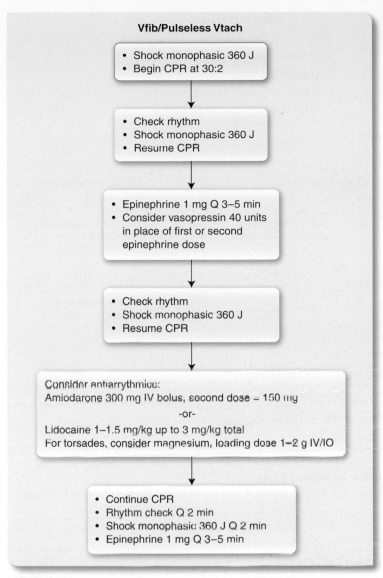

Vfib/Pulseless Vtach

- Shock monophasic 360 J
- Begin CPR at 30:2

↓

- Check rhythm
- Shock monophasic 360 J
- Resume CPR

↓

- Epinephrine 1 mg Q 3–5 min
- Consider vasopressin 40 units in place of first or second epinephrine dose

↓

- Check rhythm
- Shock monophasic 360 J
- Resume CPR

↓

Consider antiarrythmics:
Amiodarone 300 mg IV bolus, second dose = 150 mg
-or-
Lidocaine 1–1.5 mg/kg up to 3 mg/kg total
For torsades, consider magnesium, loading dose 1–2 g IV/IO

↓

- Continue CPR
- Rhythm check Q 2 min
- Shock monophasic 360 J Q 2 min
- Epinephrine 1 mg Q 3–5 min

FIGURE 7-4 Treatment protocol for ventricular fibrillation or pulseless ventricular tachycardia.

CPR, cardiopulmonary resuscitation; IO, intraoral; IV, intravenous.

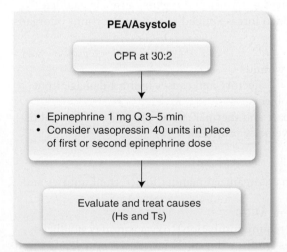

PEA/Asystole

CPR at 30:2

↓

- Epinephrine 1 mg Q 3–5 min
- Consider vasopressin 40 units in place of first or second epinephrine dose

↓

Evaluate and treat causes
(Hs and Ts)

FIGURE 7-5 Treatment protocol for pulseless electrical activity and asystole.

CPR, cardiopulmonary resuscitation.

ER, ICU, and Surgery

Quick **HIT**

Do not resuscitate (DNR) status should be documented for any inpatient; documentation can be provided by a close relative or primary care provider to guide potential resuscitation attempts.

MNEMONIC

Remember the common causes of PEA by the **Hs** and **Ts:** **H**ypovolemia, **H**ypoxia, **H**yperkalemia, **H**ypokalemia, **H**ypothermia, **H**ydrogen ions (acidosis), **T**amponade, **T**ension pneumothorax, **T**hrombosis (myocardial infarction or pulmonary embolism), **T**ablets/toxins (drugs).

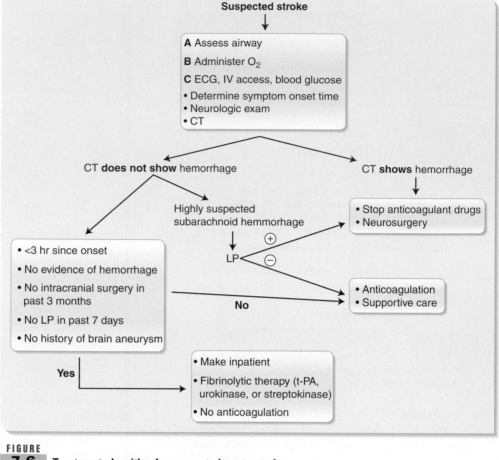

FIGURE
7-6 Treatment algorithm for suspected acute stroke.

CT, computed tomography; ECG, electrocardiogram; IV, intravenous; LP, lumbar puncture; t-PA, tissue plasminogen activator.

IV. Traumatology

A. Mechanisms of injury

1. Acceleration-deceleration injuries
   a. Seen in falls, blunt trauma, and **motor vehicle accidents**
   b. Injury secondary to shearing forces in tissues and organs caused by sudden changes in momentum and sudden forces applied to tethered portions of organs (e.g., aortic arch, mesentery)
2. Penetrating injuries
   a. Include **gunshot wounds, stab wounds**
   b. Missile damages tissue in path of trajectory and causes indirect damage from fragmented bone and external objects.
   c. Shock wave from projectile impact and thermal effects can cause additional tissue damage (particularly high-velocity projectiles).

B. Trauma assessment

1. Patient assessment is performed in an organized manner to detect all injuries and judge their severity.
2. Initial assessment focuses on patient **ABCs**.
3. Secure **a**irway is established (may require intubation), oxygenation is stabilized (**b**reathing), adequate **c**irculation is confirmed, venous access is secured, and bleeding is controlled.
4. Secondary assessment consists of a highly detailed examination to detect all wounds, fractures, signs of internal injury, and neurologic insult.

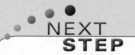

NEXT STEP

Count and pair all entrance and exit gunshot wounds to suggest a number of insulting bullets and to deduce a path for each bullet.

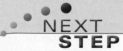

NEXT STEP

Address the ABCs and secondary survey **in order**. Do not proceed to the next step of the examination until the current segment has been addressed.

TABLE 7-4	Glasgow Coma Scale[a]	
Category	**Condition**	**Points**
Eye opening	Spontaneous	4
	To voice	3
	To pain	2
	None	1
Verbal response	Oriented	5
	Confused	4
	Inappropriate words	3
	Incomprehensible	2
	None	1
Motor response	Obeys commands	6
	Localizes pain	5
	Withdraws from pain	4
	Flexion with pain	3
	Extension with pain	2
	None	1

[a]Total score is calculated by adding component score for each category.
12+: minor brain injury with probable recovery
9–11: moderate severity requiring close observation for changes
8 or less: coma; ≤8 after 6 hr associated with 50% mortality

5. The Glasgow Coma Scale (GCS) is used to objectify injury severity (see Table 7-4).

C. Head trauma

1. Head trauma can result in cerebral or subarachnoid hemorrhage (see Chapter 8, **Neurologic Disorders**).
2. Cerebral damage can be at the point of insult (i.e., **coup**) or on the opposite side of the head (i.e., **contrecoup**).
3. **H/P** = evaluation should assess **level of consciousness**, sensation, motor activity, bowel and bladder continence, **pupil responsiveness to light** (nonresponsiveness or unequal response suggests cerebral injury), presence of skull fracture (e.g., discoloration over mastoid, blood draining from ears or nose), and intracranial pressure
4. **Radiology** = **head** computed tomography (CT) should be performed for any unconscious patient to detect intracranial hemorrhage; cervical CT or X-rays (anteroposterior, lateral, open-mouth odontoid) should be performed to detect skull or cervical fractures
5. **Treatment** = maintain cerebral perfusion; decrease high intracranial pressure by elevating head of bed, IV mannitol, or hyperventilation; refer any intracranial injury to neurosurgery for possible decompression

D. Spinal cord trauma (see Chapter 8, Neurologic Disorders)

1. Neurologic injury in any segment of the spinal cord from trauma resulting from direct injury, compression, or inflammation
2. **H/P** = thorough **neurologic examination must** be performed to detect any deficits in sensation, motor activity, or autonomic function
3. **Radiology** = imaging should examine all cervical vertebrae and other vertebral sections of spine considered at risk for injury; **CT** is replacing X-ray as the standard tool for assessing bony injury of the spine; magnetic resonance imaging (MRI) should be performed in any patient with a normal CT scan and abnormal neurologic examination or central spine pain to rule out ligamentous injury or cord edema

ER, ICU, and Surgery

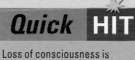

Quick HIT

Loss of consciousness is considered caused by **head trauma** until ruled out.

Quick HIT

Hypertension with bradycardia is suggestive of increased intracranial pressure (Cushing phenomenon).

NEXT STEP

Rule out **cervical fracture** and **spinal cord injury** before performing any examination requiring head movement.

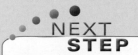

Quick HIT

The spine is considered **unstable** in any **unconscious** patient and should not be moved until neurologic injury has been ruled out with examination and radiology.

4. **Treatment** = spine must be stabilized until injury ruled out; give IV corticosteroids for 24 hr if presenting within initial 8 hr following injury (unless pregnant, isolated cauda equina injury, or child); injuries should be referred to orthopedic surgery or neurosurgery for definitive treatment

E. Neck trauma

1. Neck is divided into **zones** based on anatomic site of injury; injury can involve trachea, esophagus, vascular structures, cervical spine, or spinal cord (see Figure 7-7)
2. **H/P** = examination should focus on cervical neurologic deficits and signs of vascular damage in neck (e.g., hematoma, worsening mental status)
3. **Radiology** = potential studies include cervical X-ray, CT of cervical spine, carotid Doppler ultrasound, esophagogastroduodenoscopy (EGD), angiography, or bronchoscopy (particularly zones I and III)
4. **Treatment**
   a. Penetrating trauma with stable vital signs may be treated **conservatively**.
   b. Exploration of zones I and III is difficult and should be carried out only if vascular injury is suspected.
   c. Intubation is frequently required because of airway occlusion.
   d. Prophylactic antibiotics may be indicated because of increased risk of contamination by oropharyngeal flora.

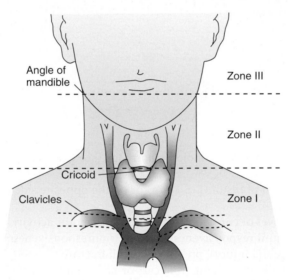

FIGURE 7-7 Zones of the neck used to determine treatment for traumatic injury.

F. Chest trauma

1. Can result in injury to lungs, heart, or GI system
2. Aortic rupture (caused by sudden acceleration and deceleration), tension pneumothorax, hemothorax, and cardiac tamponade are potentially fatal injuries.
3. **H/P** = examination should look for signs of pneumothorax (e.g., hyperresonance, decreased breath sounds), flail chest (e.g., multiple rib fractures), **tamponade** (e.g., decreased breath sounds, jugular venous distention, and pulsus paradoxus), and aortic rupture (e.g., unstable vital signs); ECG and central venous pressure are useful in assessing cardiac function
4. **Radiology**
   a. CXR and neck X-rays may show pneumothorax, hemothorax, cardiac hemorrhage, aortic injury, or rib fractures.
   b. **Chest CT** is important to assess for air leaks, hematoma formation, and pulmonary collapse.

c. EGD and bronchoscopy are used to assess injury to esophagus and bronchi.

d. Angiography can detect vascular injury.

5. **Treatment** = urgent **thoracotomy** for thoracic cavity **hemorrhage; pericardiocentesis** for suspected cardiac **tamponade;** chest tube for pneumothorax or hemothorax; ventilatory support may be required for multiple rib fractures (flail chest)

G. Abdominal trauma

1. Can cause injury to any abdominal organ or severe bleeding from the aorta, aortic branches, mesentery, spleen, or liver

2. Penetrating trauma requires exploratory laparotomy; blunt trauma may be treated conservatively in the absence of signs of an acute abdomen.

3. H/P

   a. In cases where exploratory laparotomy is not automatically performed, examination must look for signs of **abdominal bleeding** (e.g., decreased blood pressure, cyanosis, anxiety, flank discoloration, severe abdominal tenderness, abdominal rigidity, shock).

   b. **Peritoneal lavage** (i.e., saline infused by catheter into abdominal cavity and then removed and examined) is useful for detecting presence of blood or fecal matter in uncertain cases.

4. Radiology

   a. CT is sensitive for detecting abdominal fluid.

   b. Focused abdominal sonography for trauma **(FAST)** is a quick and sensitive means of determining the presence of free abdominal fluid and solid organ injury and has become the primary test performed for evaluation of blunt abdominal trauma at most trauma centers.

   c. Abdominal X-ray may detect free air or large collections of blood but is of less utility than CT or FAST.

5. Treatment

   a. All **penetrating abdominal trauma** needs **exploratory laparotomy.**

   b. Diagnosed **intra-abdominal bleeding** or visceral damage from blunt trauma requires **laparotomy** for repair if the patient is hemodynamically unstable.

   c. **Retroperitoneal hematomas** in the **upper** abdomen (pancreas, kidneys) require laparotomy for repair.

   d. **Low retroperitoneal bleeding** should be treated with **angiography** and **embolization** if caused by blunt trauma and **laparotomy** if from penetrating trauma.

H. Genitourinary and pelvic trauma

1. Injury can result from initial insult or indirectly from fracture of the pelvis.

2. H/P

   a. Examination should look for blood at the **urethral meatus** or hematuria (indicative of urologic injury), "high-riding" prostate on rectal examination (urethral injury in men), or scrotal or penile hematoma.

   b. Pelvic examination should be performed in women.

   c. Patients with a **pelvis fracture** should be given a thorough **neurovascular examination.**

3. Radiology

   a. Intravenous pyelogram (IVP) can detect renal pelvis injury.

   b. **Retrograde urethrogram** or cystogram can detect urethral or bladder injury.

   c. X-ray can detect pelvis fracture.

   d. **CT** can detect renal damage and pelvic blood collections.

4. Treatment

   a. **Penetrating** injuries need **surgical exploration.**

   b. Urethral, intraperitoneal bladder, and renal pelvis injuries require cystoscopy and surgical repair; **extraperitoneal bladder** and **renal parenchymal** injuries may be treated **nonoperatively.**

   c. Pelvic fractures may be treated nonoperatively if stable and with open reduction and internal fixation when unstable.

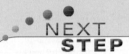

***Quick* HIT**

Sites of significant (**>1,500 mL**) blood loss frequently not found by physical examination include blood left at the **injury scene, pleural cavity** bleeding (seen with CXR), **intra-abdominal** bleeding (seen with CT or ultrasound [US]), **pelvic** bleeding (seen with CT), and bleeding into the **thighs** (seen on X-ray).

NEXT STEP

The **hemodynamically unstable** patient with blunt trauma should be taken to the **operating room** and not to radiology, if FAST sonogram is not available in the emergency department.

ER, ICU, and Surgery

***Quick* HIT**

A Foley catheter should **never** be placed in a patient with a **suspected urethral rupture** (e.g., blood seen at the urethral meatus, high-riding prostate on rectal examination) to avoid further urologic injury unless performed under cystoscopic guidance.

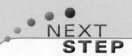

NEXT STEP

Perform a **fasciotomy** in any patient with a combined bone and neurovascular extremity injury because of the high risk of **compartment syndrome**.

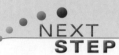

NEXT STEP

Serial neurovascular examinations should be performed following any type of treatment for an extremity to detect an evolving or iatrogenic neurologic injury.

Quick HIT

Criteria that should be met in post-traumatic pregnant women before discharge are **contractions no more frequent than every 10 minutes, no vaginal bleeding, no abdominal pain**, and a **normal fetal heart tracing**.

Quick HIT

Injuries suggestive of child abuse include multiple simultaneous facial injuries, bruises in patterns of objects, bruises over trunk and abdomen, multiple burns (especially in shape of object), rib or skull fractures, long bone fractures in nonambulatory children.

Quick HIT

A physician who has reason to suspect child abuse but does not report it or act to protect the child **may be held liable** for subsequent injury or mortality.

I. Extremity trauma

1. Injury can involve **bones**, **vasculature**, **soft tissues**, or **nerves** in extremities.
2. H/P = a thorough **neurovascular examination** must be performed; gross deformities are indicative of fracture.
3. **Radiology** = X-ray or CT detects fractures; angiography can detect vascular injury; MRI may be required to detect soft tissue injuries
4. **Treatment**
   a. Superficial or soft tissue wounds require irrigation and approximation (e.g., sutures, Steri-Strips, dermatologic adhesive).
   b. Bone injury alone is treated with immobilization, if stable and internal, or external fixation, if unstable.
   c. Combined bone, vessel, and nerve injuries are treated by fracture repair **followed** by vascular and neurologic repair.
   d. Large wounds frequently require debridement or amputation.

J. Trauma during pregnancy

1. Leading cause of **nonobstetric** maternal death
2. Anatomic differences
   a. Inferior vena cava (IVC) compression by the uterus makes pregnant women more susceptible to **poor cardiac output** following injury.
   b. Decreased risk of GI injury from lower abdominal trauma because of **superior displacement of bowel** by the uterus (but greater risk of GI injury from upper abdominal or chest trauma)
3. Low risk of fetal death with minor injuries (high risk in life-threatening injuries)
4. Trauma increases the risk of **placental abruption**.
5. **H/P** = immediate assessment of cardiovascular stability, mother should be evaluated for injury **before** the fetus, examination should be performed with mother in **left lateral decubitus position** to minimize IVC compression, obstetric assessment performed following maternal stabilization
6. **Treatment** = needs of **mother** are **prioritized**; caesarian section should be performed for fetuses >24 weeks of gestation that are in **distress** or in any mother with **cardiovascular compromise** not responsive to early cardiopulmonary resuscitation (CPR); mother should be monitored for 4 to 48 hr (based on severity of trauma) to detect fetal distress; **RhoGAM** should be given to any Rh⁻ mother with bleeding

V. Abuse and Sexual Assault

A. Abuse

1. Most frequently seen in children, spouses or partners (especially women), and the elderly
2. Abuse can be physical, emotional, sexual, or exploitative; neglect
3. **Child** abuse
   a. Neglect, the most prevalent form of child abuse, constitutes the **failure to provide** the physical, emotional, educational, and medical needs of a child.
   b. **H/P** = several red flags should raise suspicion in **history** (e.g., inconsistent with injury, vague details, changes in story, blame placed on others, implausibility), **parental actions** (e.g., aggressive nature, delay in seeking treatment, lack of emotional attachment or concern), and **physical examination** (e.g., injuries inconsistent with history, multiple injuries at various stages of healing, pathognomonic injuries, signs of neglect, abnormal behavioral responses to being examined)
   c. **Treatment** = physician has **obligation** to report any suspected cases of abuse to child protective services
   d. Suspected cases should be **well documented**.

4. Spousal or partner abuse
   a. H/P = similar red flags as for child abuse; presentation to physician frequently for a vague symptom (e.g., chronic abdominal pain, headaches, depression, recurrent sexually transmitted diseases); **history** may be **inconsistent** with **injury**; partner may be very attentive or vigilant during visit
   b. Patient should be interviewed **without** partner present.
   c. **Treatment** = initial approach should focus on safety of patient; provide victim with information on safety plans, escape strategies, legal rights, and shelters; care should be taken not to force victim into any action; reporting of abuse is typically nonmandatory (unless it involves child abuse)
5. Elder abuse
   a. Abuse in a patient >60 years of age occurring at the hands of a caregiver (e.g., family, friends, institution)
   b. H/P = red flags as seen with child and domestic abuse; multiple bruises or fractures, malnutrition, depression, or **signs of neglect**
   c. **Treatment** = placement in a safe facility; facilitate contact with social services that can help facilitate safe care; physician has **obligation** to report suspected cases to an official state agency

B. Sexual assault

1. **Nonconsensual** sexual activity with physical contact; forced intercourse is **rape**
2. Victims can be children or adults.
3. H/P
   a. **Detailed history** must be collected and thoroughly documented in cases where patient reports assault.
   b. Examination should focus on the entire body, with particular attention to genitals, anus, and mouth to look for signs of assault.
   c. Patients who have not admitted to being assaulted may appear depressed or very uncomfortable with examination.
4. Labs
   a. Collect oral, vaginal, and penile cultures to test for sexually transmitted diseases.
   b. In cases of rape, all injuries must be well documented and vaginal fluid and pubic hair should be collected for evidence (i.e., rape kit).
   c. Pregnancy testing should be performed to look for incidental conception occurring during assault.
5. **Treatment** = careful and well-documented collection of all details and evidence important to future follow-up and legal action; referral to **social support systems** and **counseling** is very important; appropriate treatment should be given for infections

BASIC CRITICAL CARE

 ## I. Issues in the Intensive Care Unit (ICU)

A. Role of the ICU
1. Provides intensive nursing care for **critically ill patients**
2. Patients may require intubation, ventilation, **invasive monitoring**, **vasoactive** and antiarrhythmic medications, and close nursing supervision.

B. Pulmonary concerns
1. **Intubation** and **ventilation** required when a patient is at risk for airway obstruction or needs support in breathing
2. Ventilator support is required in patients to maintain respiratory effort or in poor-oxygenation states (see Chapter 2, **Pulmonary Disorders**).

ER, ICU, and Surgery

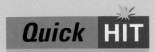

C. Invasive monitoring

1. **Arterial line** (A-line)
   a. Placed in either radial, femoral, axillary, brachial, or dorsalis pedis artery
   b. Used to record more accurate blood pressure than blood pressure cuff
2. **Pulmonary artery catheter** (Swan-Ganz catheter)
   a. Catheter inserted through subclavian or jugular vein; runs through heart to pulmonary artery
   b. Measures pressures in **right atrium** and **pulmonary** artery; balloon can be inflated at catheter tip to fill pulmonary artery lumen and measure wedge pressure (equivalent to **left atrium pressure**)
   c. Also may measure **cardiac output**, mixed venous O_2 saturation, systemic vascular resistance

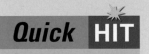

II. Hemodynamic Stability

A. Transfusions

1. Infusion of blood products to treat insufficient supply of a given blood component (see Table 7-5)
2. **ABO blood groups**
   a. Blood is defined by **A** and **B** antigens and antibodies to absent antigens.
   b. Blood with **both** antigens **will not have antibodies** to either antigen in plasma (i.e., AB blood type).
   c. Blood with **neither** antigen will have **antibodies to both** antigens in plasma (i.e., O blood type).
   d. Transfusions must be matched for each patient's particular ABO blood type.
3. **Rh blood groups**
   a. Patient are either Rh antigen positive (Rh^+) or negative (Rh^-).
   b. **Rh^-** patients have **antibodies to Rh factor** in plasma.
   c. Transfusions must be matched for each patient's Rh factor.
4. **Transfusion reactions**
   a. Reaction that occurs when incompatible blood is infused into a patient
   b. Types
      (1) **Nonhemolytic febrile:** most common reaction (3% of transfusions); caused by cytokines generated by cells in the blood component to be transfused while in storage; onset 1 to 6 hours after transfusion; fevers, chills, rigors, malaise; treated with acetaminophen; recurrence is uncommon
      (2) **Acute hemolytic:** 1 in 250,000 transfusions; caused by **ABO incompatibility**; onset during transfusion; fever, chills, nausea, flushing, tachycardia, tachypnea, hypotension; severe destruction of donor RBCs; requires aggressive supportive care
      (3) **Delayed hemolytic:** caused by antibodies to Kidd or D (Rh) antigens; onset 2 to 10 days after transfusion; slight fever, falling H/H, mild increase in **unconjugated bilirubin**; no acute therapy needed but determine responsible antibody type to help prevent future reactions
      (4) **Anaphylactic:** 1 in 50,000 transfusions; rapid onset of shock and hypotension; some cases may be caused by anti-IgA IgG antibodies (in patient with IgA deficiency) that bind IgA on the surface of donor RBCs and trigger mast cell degranulation; requires epinephrine, volume maintenance, and airway maintenance
      (5) **Minor allergic reactions:** 3% of transfusions; caused by plasma present in donor blood; urticaria; treated with diphenhydramine
      (6) **Post-transfusion purpura:** thrombocytopenia developing 5 to 10 days after transfusion; occurs primarily in women sensitized by pregnancy; treated with IVIG or plasmapheresis
   c. H/P = occurs in patient receiving transfusion; pain in vein receiving transfusion, chills; flushing, pruritus; fever, jaundice

TABLE 7-5 Types of Blood Products Used in Transfusions

Blood Product	Definition	Indications
Whole blood	Donor blood not separated into components (full volume blood)	Rarely used except for massive transfusions for severe blood loss
Packed RBCs	RBCs separated from other donor blood components (2/3 volume of transfusion unit is RBCs)	Product of choice for treatment of low Hct due to blood loss or anemia
Autologous blood	Blood donated by patient before elective surgery or other treatment Blood is frozen until needed by patient	Elective surgery or chemotherapy
FFP	Plasma from which cellular components have been separated	Warfarin overdose, clotting factor deficiency, DIC, TTP
Cryoprecipitate	Clotting factor and vWF-rich precipitate collected during thawing of FFP Same indications as FFP	Smaller volume than FFP Preferable to FFP in cases where large transfusion volume is unwanted
Platelets	Platelets separated from other plasma components	Thrombocytopenia not due to rapid platelet destruction
Clotting factors	Concentrations of a specific clotting factor pooled from multiple donors	Specific clotting factor deficiencies (e.g., hemophiliac)

DIC, disseminated intravascular coagulation; FFP, fresh frozen plasma; Hct, hematocrit; RBCs, red blood cells; TTP, thrombotic thrombocytopenic purpura; vWF, von Willebrand factor.

   d. **Labs** = both patient's and donor's blood should be rechecked and retyped
   e. **Treatment** = **acetaminophen, diphenhydramine**, stop transfusion; mannitol or bicarbonate may be required in severe reactions to prevent hemolytic debris from clogging vessels; vasopressors may be required if significant hypotension develops

B. Vasoactive medications

1. Drugs used to **maintain hemodynamic stability** by increasing blood pressure (i.e., vasopressors) and cardiac output (i.e., inotropes) or decreasing blood pressure and cardiac output (i.e., vasodilators and negative inotropic agents)
2. Vasopressors frequently used in cases of shock and insufficient cardiac output (see Table 7-6)
3. Vasodilators reduce vascular tone; negative inotropic drugs decrease cardiac contractility (see Chapter 1, **Cardiovascular Disorders**).

TABLE 7-6 Vasopressors and Inotropes Commonly Used in the Intensive Care Unit

Drug	Mechanism	Effects	Indication
Phenylephrine	Agonist for α-adrenergic receptors ($\alpha_1 > \alpha_2$)	Vasoconstriction, reflex bradycardia	Sepsis, shock
Norepinephrine	Agonist for α_1- and β_1-adrenergic receptors	Vasoconstriction, mildly increased contractility	Shock
Epinephrine	Agonist for primarily β_1 and, to a lesser extent, α_1- and β_2-adrenergic receptors; α effects (vasoconstriction) predominate at high doses	Increased contractility (increased CO), vasodilation at low doses; increased contractility and vasoconstriction at higher doses	**Anaphylactic** shock, septic shock, post-bypass hypotension
Dopamine	Agonist for β_1-adrenergic receptors (low dose) and α-adrenergic receptors (high dose)	Increased heart rate and contractility (increased CO), vasoconstriction (high dose only)	**Shock**
Dobutamine	Agonist for β_1-adrenergic receptors	Increased heart rate and contractility (increased CO), mild reflex vasodilation	**CHF**, cardiogenic shock
Isoproterenol	Agonist for β_1- and β_2-adrenergic receptors	Increased heart rate and contractility (increased CO), vasodilation	Contractility stimulant in cardiac arrest
Vasopressin	ADH analogue with weak pressor effect	Vasoconstriction	Resistant septic shock, second vasopressor

ADH, antidiuretic hormone; CHF, congestive heart failure; CO, cardiac output.

ER, ICU, and Surgery

BASIC SURGICAL CONCERNS

Most surgical issues are discussed in the chapters concerning the appropriate systems. The following sections reflect concerns not addressed elsewhere.

I. Preoperative and Postoperative Issues

A. Preoperative risk assessment

1. In elective surgery, a patient must be assessed before operation to determine if he or she will tolerate a procedure and what the likelihood is of an adverse cardiopulmonary event.

2. **Cardiac risk**
   a. Cardiac function (i.e., ejection fraction, rate, rhythm), exercise capacity, cardiac disease (e.g., congestive heart failure, CAD, recent MI), and age assessed before surgery
   b. Young, healthy patients may be cleared with a normal ECG by a primary care physician.
   c. Other patients should be cleared by a cardiologist and/or following appropriate cardiac functional testing.
   d. Findings consistent with high surgical risk for a cardiac event
      (1) **Age**: >70 years
      (2) **Pulmonary**: forced expiratory volume in 1 second (FEV_1)/forced vital capacity (FVC) <70% expected, Pco_2 >45 mm Hg, pulmonary edema
      (3) **Cardiac**: MI within past 30 days, poorly controlled nonsinus arrhythmia, pathologic Q waves on preoperative ECG, severe valvular disease, decompensated congestive heart failure with poor ejection fraction
      (4) **Renal**: creatinine (Cr) >2 or 50% increase from baseline
      (5) **Surgery type**: vascular, anticipated high blood loss
   e. Patients determined to be at **high risk** for cardiac complications should **not be operated on** until cardiac function is stabilized unless surgical need is emergent.
   f. Minimally invasive techniques may be appropriate in high-risk patients.
   g. Postoperative noninvasive cardiac monitoring is frequently recommended for patients determined to have increased cardiac risk.

3. **Pulmonary concerns**
   a. **Smoking** increases risk of infection and postoperative ventilation.
   b. Smoking should be stopped before surgery; nicotine replacement may help patients stop smoking 8 weeks before surgery.
   c. Patients with chronic obstructive pulmonary disease (COPD) should be given preoperative antibiotics if showing signs of infection.
   d. A preoperative **CXR** is an important screening tool in any patient age >50 years, a history of pulmonary disease, or anticipated surgical time >3 hr.
   e. Patients with respiratory concerns (e.g., smokers, COPD, myasthenia gravis) should have pulmonary function tests performed to assess their respiratory capacity and to anticipate the need for lengthy ventilation and tracheostomy placement.
   f. **Incentive spirometry**, deep breathing exercises, pain control, and **physical therapy** are all very important postoperatively to help prevent **atelectasis**, **pneumonia**, and **pulmonary embolism**.
   g. Bronchodilators and inhaled steroids may be beneficial in postoperative patients with preexisting disease.

4. **Renal concerns**
   a. Patients with renal insufficiency may have electrolyte abnormalities, anemia, or poor immune function.
   b. **Dialysis** may be required before surgery in some patients with renal insufficiency.
   c. **N-Acetylcysteine** may be used as a renal protectant in patients with renal insufficiency who are expected to receive intraoperative contrast.

5. **Hepatic concerns**
   a. Mortality increases with increased bilirubin, decreased albumin, prolonged prothrombin time (PT), and encephalopathy.

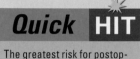

Quick HIT

The greatest risk for postoperative MI is **within the initial 48 hr** after surgery.

ER, ICU, and Surgery

b. Electrolyte disorders, coagulopathy, and encephalopathy should be corrected before operation.

c. Surgery should be avoided (unless emergent) in patients with significant hepatitis, cirrhosis, or extrahepatic manifestations of liver disease.

6. **Diabetes mellitus (DM)**

a. **Diabetic** patients have increased infection risk, worse wound healing, increased cardiac complication risk, and increased postoperative mortality.

b. Blood sugar levels should be well controlled via subcutaneous insulin sliding scale and frequent glucose checks; glycemic fluctuations can increase postoperatively and may require greater insulin administration than at baseline.

7. **Coagulation concerns**

a. A history of **abnormal bleeding** or **easy bruising** should raise concerns for a coagulopathy (increased risk of bleeding complications intraoperatively and postoperatively).

b. Patients taking **warfarin** before surgery should **stop** their warfarin use **3 to 4 days** before surgery; international normalized ratio (INR) should be kept <1.5 for any surgery with significant bleeding risk.

c. Fresh frozen plasma (FFP) and vitamin K may be used for rapid reversal of warfarin therapy.

d. Patients with **recent thromboembolism** should be anticoagulated with **heparin** or **low molecular weight heparin** (LMWH) after stopping warfarin use until surgery and then restarted on warfarin postoperatively; heparin or LMWH should be restarted 12 hr postoperatively and continued until a therapeutic INR (>2.0) is reached.

e. Patients not on prior warfarin therapy may be anticoagulated with **aspirin**, **antiplatelet drugs**, or **LMWH** per surgeon's preference.

f. In general, warfarin, heparin, and LMWH are associated with a **lower risk** of postoperative **thromboembolism** than aspirin or antiplatelet medications but carry a **greater risk** of **postoperative bleeding complications**.

B. Postoperative fever

1. Fever develops postoperatively from pulmonary, infectious, vascular, or pharmacologic causes (see Table 7-7, Figure 7-8).

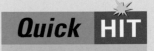

Quick HIT

LMWH should not be restarted for at least 2 hr after removal of an epidural catheter to avoid formation of an epidural hematoma.

ER, ICU, and Surgery

TABLE 7-7	Causes of Postoperative Fever		
Cause	**When Seen**	**Diagnosis**	**Treatment**
Pneumonia	**After** 3rd postoperative day	**Productive** cough, positive sputum Gram stain or culture, infiltrates or consolidation on CXR	Antibiotics, bronchoscopy
Urinary tract infection	**3–5** days postoperatively	Urine Gram stain or culture, urine nitrates, presence of **Foley catheter**	Antibiotics, remove Foley
Wound/IV catheter infection	**5–8** days postoperatively	Red, warm surgical wound; drainage from wound (possibly purulent)	Antibiotics, irrigation and drainage, surgical debridement
Deep vein thrombosis	Any time postoperatively	Lower extremity warmth and tenderness; US demonstrates noncompressible vein	Anticoagulation, IVC filter
Pulmonary embolism	Any time postoperatively	Dyspnea, tachycardia, pleuritic chest pain, **increased A-a gradient, V/Q mismatch**	Anticoagulation, IVC filter
Medications	Any time postoperatively	Onset linked to new medication; antibiotics are frequent cause	Stop offending agent
Transfusion reaction	Any time postoperatively	Begins after initiation of transfusion; confirmed by donor/recipient blood compatibility workup	Acetaminophen and diphenhydramine, stop transfusion if symptoms persist

A-a, alveolar-arterial; CXR, chest X-ray; IVC, inferior vena cava; US, ultrasound; V/Q, ventilation-perfusion.

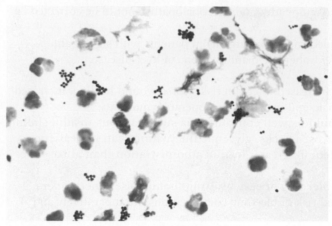

FIGURE 7-8 Gram stain for a patient with staphylococcal bacteremia.

Note organization of bacteria in grapelike clusters.
(From McClatchey, K. D. [2002]. *Clinical Laboratory Medicine* [2nd ed., Figure 51-1]. Philadelphia, PA: Lippincott Williams & Wilkins; with permission.)

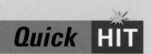

Quick HIT

Postoperative fevers are caused by the 5 Ws:
Wind (pneumonia)
Water (urinary tract infection)
Wound (wound infection)
Walking (deep vein thrombosis, pulmonary embolism)
Wonder drugs (medications)

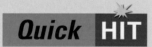

Quick HIT

Atelectasis is no longer considered to be a cause of postoperative fever.

2. Any postoperative fever should be evaluated with a **CXR**, complete blood count (CBC), and urinalysis; **urine** and **blood cultures** should also be performed for any fever beyond the first postoperative day.

C. Wounds and healing

1. **Types of wounds**
    a. **Clean**: surgical incisions through disinfected skin; no GI or respiratory entry; 1% to 3% infection risk
    b. **Clean-contaminated**: similar to clean wounds but with GI or respiratory entry; 2% to 8% infection risk
    c. **Contaminated**: gross contact of wound with GI or genitourinary contents; traumatic wounds; 6% to 15% infection risk
    d. **Dirty**: established infection in tissue before incision; continued infection following procedure, including debridement; ranges from 7% to 40% infection risk
2. **Wound approximation and healing**
    a. **Primary intention**: low risk of infection (clean and clean-contaminated wounds or contaminated wounds with good clean-up in healthy patient); full closure of tissue and skin performed
    b. **Secondary intention**: higher risk for infection; wound left open and allowed to heal through epithelialization
    c. **Delayed primary closure**: heavily contaminated wounds; left open for a few days and cleaned before wound closure
    d. **Skin grafts**: portion of epidermis and dermis from other body site transferred to wounds that are too large to close by themselves; large deeper grafts with revascularization are called flaps
3. Closed wounds require dressings for **initial 48 hr** after closure.
4. Open wounds require debridement and specialized dressings.
5. Wound healing can be inhibited by malnutrition, corticosteroids, smoking, hepatic or renal failure, or DM.

II. Surgical Emergencies

A. Acute abdomen

1. **Severe abdominal pain** and rigidity lasting up to several hours that requires **prompt** treatment (see Table 7-8)
2. H/P = **abdominal pain** (severe or crampy, rapidly or gradually progressive), nausea, vomiting, possible history of recent surgery; fever, abdominal tenderness

TABLE 7-8	Causes of Acute Abdomen		
Condition	**History and Physical**	**Diagnosis**	**Treatment**
Obstruction/ strangulation (from adhesions, hernias, tumors)	**Previous surgery**, abdominal distention, crampy pain, nausea, vomiting, high-pitched bowel sounds	CT or AXR shows distended loops of bowel and air-fluid levels; barium studies may locate site of obstruction	**Surgical lysis of adhesions**, hernia repair, surgical excision of tumors
Diverticulitis	**Left lower quadrant** pain (may progress over several days), blood in stool	CT or AXR may show free air from perforation; increased WBC	Surgical repair
Massive GI hemorrhage (perforation)	Sudden severe pain, **hematemesis**, **hematochezia**, hypotension	Colonoscopy or EGD visualizes lesion; technetium scan may detect smaller bleeding sources	Octreotide, **angiography with embolization**, surgical repair of detectable site of bleeding
Appendicitis	**Right lower quadrant** and **periumbilical** pain, psoas sign, rectal examination tenderness	Increased WBC; thickened appendix or fecalith on CT if unruptured; free air on CT or AXR if perforated	**Appendectomy**
Mesenteric ischemia	Severe abdominal pain **out of proportion to examination**, bloody diarrhea	Bowel wall thickening and air within bowel wall on CT; increased WBC and serum lactate	NPO, antibiotics, resection of necrotic bowel
Pancreatitis	**Upper abdominal** and **back** pain, nausea, vomiting, history of gallstones or alcoholism	CT shows inflamed pancreas; increased amylase and lipase	Nasogastric tube, NPO, analgesics
Ruptured ectopic pregnancy	**Amenorrhea**, lower abdominal pain, possible vaginal bleeding, or palpable pelvic mass	US **unable** to locate intrauterine pregnancy in presence of **positive urine pregnancy test**	Surgical excision
Pelvic inflammatory disease	Lower abdominal pain, vaginal discharge, cervical motion pain	Increased WBC; positive serology for *Chlamydia* or *Neisseria gonorrhoeae*	Antibiotics, treat sexual partners

AXR, abdominal X-ray; CT, computed tomography; EGD, esophagogastroduodenoscopy; GI, gastrointestinal; NPO, nothing by mouth; US, ultrasound; WBC, white blood cell count.

ER, ICU, and Surgery

(with possible **rebound tenderness**, rigidity, **guarding**, spasm, or mass), possible hypotension; pelvic or testicular examination should be performed to rule out gynecologic or testicular condition

3. **Labs** = increased white blood cell count (WBC) in cases of infection or bowel perforation; increased amylase in pancreatitis; increased liver function tests with hepatobiliary dysfunction
4. **Radiology** = abdominal or pelvic CT or abdominal radiograph helpful to recognize bowel gas patterns, air collections, and calcifications; IVP, barium studies, or ultrasound (US) may also be helpful
5. **Treatment** = adequate pain control; **emergent laparotomy** or **laparoscopy** may be needed depending on pathology

B. Malignant hyperthermia

1. Rare genetic disorder in which certain anesthetics (e.g., halothane, succinylcholine) induce hyperthermia (104°F/40°C)
2. **H/P** = symptoms begin after anesthesia use; rigidity, cyanosis, tachycardia, continually rising **body temperature**
3. Uncontrolled hyperthermia can lead to arrhythmias, disseminated intravascular coagulation (DIC), acidosis, cerebral dysfunction, and electrolyte abnormalities.
4. **Labs** = mixed acidosis acutely; abnormal increase in muscle contraction following in vitro treatment with halothane or caffeine (testing performed as outpatient)
5. **Treatment** = evaporative cooling (i.e., patient sprayed with water and placed in front of fans), cold inhaled O_2, cold GI lavage, cool IV fluids, **dantrolene, stop offending agent**

III. Transplantation

A. Indications and selection

1. Organ transplantation is considered in cases of **end-stage organ failure** that are untreatable by other means or are incompatible with survival without treatment by extraordinary means (e.g., frequent dialysis).
2. **Transplant frequency** (see Table 7-9)
   a. Renal transplants are the most common type.
   b. Liver, bone marrow, pancreas, heart, lung, skin, and cornea transplants also performed
   c. Small bowel transplant has been performed on a very limited basis with limited success.
3. **Donor selection**
   a. Donors are most frequently brain-dead or living voluntary donors without cancer, sepsis, or organ insufficiency.
   b. Donors are selected based on **ABO blood group compatibility, crossmatch compatibility** (i.e., presence of antidonor antibodies on recipient T cells), and **HLA antigen matching**.
   c. HLA antigen matching is **more** important for **kidney** and **pancreas** transplants and **less** important for **heart** and **liver**.
4. Transplant rejection can be hyperacute, acute, or chronic (see Table 7-10).
5. Patients must be given **immunosuppressive** agents to reduce risk of rejection (see Table 7-11).
6. Transplant recipients have greater risks of infection (secondary to immunosuppression), **cancer** (e.g., skin, B-cell lymphoma, oral squamous cell, cervical, vaginal), and infertility.

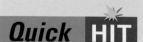

Individuals with a specific infection (e.g., **hepatitis**) may be used as donors for patients with the same infection if no significant donor organ injury is detected.

ER, ICU, and Surgery

TABLE 7-9	Common Types of Organ Transplantation		
Type	**Indications**	**Contraindications**	**Results**
Bone marrow	**Aplastic anemia, induction chemotherapy**, leukemia, lymphoma, hematopoietic disorders	Donor–recipient mismatch, recipient with high risk for developing post-transplant infection	Improved quality of life and long-term survival if surviving >1 yr post-transplant
Heart (may be performed with lung transplant)	Severe heart disease (CAD, congenital defects, cardiomyopathy) with estimated death within 2 yr without transplant	**Pulmonary hypertension, smoking** (prior 6 months), renal insufficiency, COPD, >70 yr of age, terminal illness	Acute rejection common, higher mortality risk in initial 6 months, 70% **5-yr** survival
Lung	**COPD** (particularly α_1-antitrypsin deficiency), primary pulmonary hypertension, **cystic fibrosis**; estimated death within 2 yr	**Smoking** (prior 6 months), poor cardiac function, renal or hepatic insufficiency, terminal illness, >65 yr of age, HIV	Most have at least one episode of acute rejection, pneumonia common, **56% 3-yr** survival, **chronic rejection** common
Liver	Chronic hepatitis B or **C**, alcoholic cirrhosis, primary biliary cirrhosis, primary sclerosing cholangitis, biliary atresia, progressive Wilson disease	Active **alcoholism**, multiple **suicide** attempts (e.g., acetaminophen poisoning), liver cancer, cirrhosis from chronic hepatitis (may receive transplants from donors with hepatitis)	40% acute rejection, success correlates with patient health at time of surgery (generally 60%–70% 5-yr survival)
Renal	**End-stage renal disease** requiring dialysis (glomerulonephritis, DM, polycystic kidney disease, interstitial nephritis, renal hypertension)	Stable health (dialysis is always an option for unstable patients)	Living-donor kidneys have 20% acute rejection and 91% 5-yr survival; cadaver kidneys have 40% acute rejection and 85% 5-yr survival
Pancreas (frequently performed with renal transplant)	**DM type I** with renal failure	Age >60 yr, CAD, PVD, obesity, **DM type II**	80% 3-yr survival, acute rejection common

CAD, coronary artery disease; COPD, chronic obstructive pulmonary disease; DM, diabetes mellitus; HIV, human immunodeficiency virus; PVD, peripheral vascular disease.

TABLE 7-10 Forms of Transplant Rejection

Type	When Seen	Cause	Treatment
Hyperacute	**Initial 24 hr** after transplantation	Antidonor antibodies in recipient	**Untreatable**; should be avoided by proper crossmatching
Acute	**6 days–1 yr** after transplantation	Antidonor T-cell proliferation in recipient	**Frequently reversible** through immunosuppressive agents
Chronic	**>1 yr** after transplantation	Development of multiple cellular and humoral immune reactions to donor tissue	Usually untreatable; immunosuppression may serve some role

TABLE 7-11 Immunosuppressive Drugs to Prevent Transplant Rejection

Drug	Indication	Mechanism	Adverse Effects
Cyclosporine	Rejection prevention	**Helper** T-cell inhibition	**Nephrotoxicity**, androgenic effects, HTN
Azathioprine	Rejection prevention	Inhibits T-cell proliferation	**Leukopenia**
Tacrolimus	Rejection prevention and reversal	Inhibitor of T-cell function	**Nephrotoxicity**, neurotoxicity
Corticosteroids	Rejection prevention and reversal	Inhibits **all leukocyte** activity	Cushing syndrome, weight gain, AVN of bone
Muromonab-D3 (OKT3)	Rejection reversal and **early** rejection maintenance	Inhibitor of T-cell function and depletes T-cell population	Induces **one-time cytokine release** (fever, bronchospasm), leukopenia; limited to **short-term therapy**
Rapamycin	Rejection prevention	Helper T-cell inhibition	Thrombocytopenia, hyperlipidemia
Mycophenolic acid	Rejection prevention	Inhibits T-cell proliferation	**Leukopenia**, GI toxicity
Antithymocyte globulin	Rejection reversal and **early** rejection maintenance	Depletes T-cell population	Limited to **short-term therapy**, serum sickness
Hydroxychloroquine	Chronic graft vs. host disease	Inhibits antigen processing	Visual disturbances
Thalidomide	Chronic graft vs. host disease	Inhibits T-cell function and migration	Sedation, constipation, teratogenic

AVN, avascular necrosis; GI, gastrointestinal; HTN, hypertension.

B. Graft versus host disease

1. Reaction of **donor** immune cells in transplanted bone marrow to host cells
2. Host is immunocompromised to avoid transplant rejection and is unable to prevent attack by donor cells.
3. **Risk factors** = HLA antigen mismatch, old age, donor–host gender disparity, **immunosuppression**
4. **H/P** = **maculopapular rash**, abdominal pain, nausea, vomiting, diarrhea, recurrent infections, easy bleeding
5. **Labs** = increased liver function tests, decreased immunoglobulin levels, decreased platelets; biopsy of skin or liver detects an inflammatory reaction with significant cell death
6. **Treatment** = corticosteroids, tacrolimus, and mycophenolate are useful for decreasing graft response; thalidomide and hydroxychloroquine are used in chronic disease
7. **Complications** = patients without an early response to therapy frequently develop **chronic** disease with skin sclerosis, hepatic insufficiency, GI ulceration, and pulmonary fibrosis

ER, ICU, and Surgery

Quick **HIT**

The anterior communicating artery is the most common site of intracranial aneurysm formation.

I. Normal Neurologic and Neurovascular Function

A. Cerebral vasculature

1. The circle of Willis is a system of collateral vessels that supplies all regions of the brain (see Figure 8-1).
2. Symptoms seen with a stroke can be used to determine the site of insult based on association with a particular region of the brain (see Table 8-1).

A Arteries of the base of the brain and brain stem

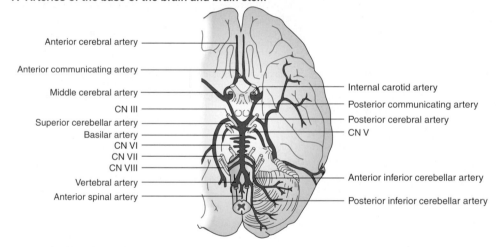

Anterior cerebral artery

Anterior communicating artery

Middle cerebral artery

CN III

Superior cerebellar artery

Basilar artery

CN VI

CN VII

CN VIII

Vertebral artery

Anterior spinal artery

Internal carotid artery

Posterior communicating artery

Posterior cerebral artery

CN V

Anterior inferior cerebellar artery

Posterior inferior cerebellar artery

B Arterial blood supply to the cortex

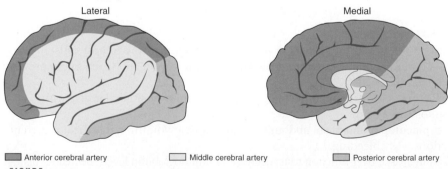

Lateral

Medial

■ Anterior cerebral artery   □ Middle cerebral artery   ■ Posterior cerebral artery

FIGURE
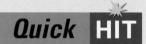
8-1 **Arteries of the brain including the circle of Willis and their anatomic relationship to selected cranial nerves.**

CN, cranial nerve.
(From Mehta, S., Milder, E. A., Mirachi, A. J., & Milder, E. [2006]. *Step-Up: A High-Yield, Systems-Based Review for the USMLE Step 1* [3rd ed., p. 32]. Philadelphia, PA: Lippincott Williams & Wilkins.)

TABLE 8-1 Regions of the Brain Supplied by Vessels in the Circle of Willis

Artery	Region of Brain Supplied
Anterior cerebral artery (ACA)	Medial and superior surfaces and frontal lobes
Middle cerebral artery (MCA)	Lateral surfaces and temporal lobes
Posterior cerebral artery (PCA)	Inferior surfaces and occipital lobes
Basilar artery	Midbrain, brainstem (pons)
Anterior inferior cerebellar artery (AICA)	Brainstem (pons) and parts of cerebellum
Posterior inferior cerebellar artery (PICA)	Brainstem (medulla) and parts of cerebellum

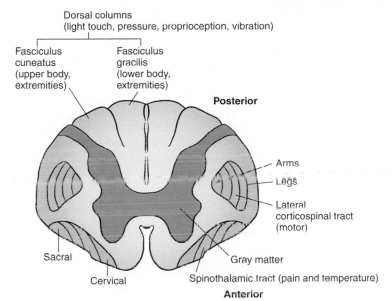

FIGURE 8-2 Primary neuronal pathways of the spinal cord in a thoracic cross section.

TABLE 8-2 Primary Sensory and Motor Tracts of the Spinal Cord

Pathway	Location	First-Order Neurons	Second-Order Neurons	Function
Dorsal columns	Posterior spinal cord	Enter at ipsilateral dorsal horn, ascend in fasciculus gracilis and cuneatus, synapse in nucleus gracilis and cuneatus	Decussate at medulla, ascend as medial lemniscus	**Two-point discrimination**, sense vibration, sense **proprioception**
Spinothalamic tract	Anterior spinal cord	Originate in dorsal root ganglion, synapse in dorsolateral tract of Lissauer	Decussate in ventral white commissure, ascend in lateral spinothalamic tract	**Senses pain**, senses **temperature**
Corticospinal tract	Lateral spinal cord	Descend from internal capsule and midbrain, decussate in medullary pyramids, descend in corticospinal tract, synapse in ventral horn through interneurons	Exit cord through ventral horn	**Voluntary movement** of striated muscle

B. Neurologic organization

1. Sensory and motor neurons are organized into distinct tracts in the spinal cord (see Figure 8-2, Table 8-2).
2. Lesions of the spinal cord cause symptoms that are dependent on the lesion location (see Table 8-3).
3. Cranial nerves (CNs) have distinct functions within the head and neck (see Table 8-4).

TABLE 8-3	Common Lesions of the Spinal Cord	
Condition	**Tracts Affected**	**Symptoms**
Amyotrophic lateral sclerosis (ALS)	Corticospinal tract, ventral horn	Spastic and flaccid paralysis
Poliomyelitis	Ventral horn	Flaccid paralysis
Tabes dorsalis (**tertiary syphilis**)	Dorsal columns	Impaired proprioception, pain
Spinal artery syndrome	Corticospinal tract, spino-thalamic tract, ventral horn, lateral gray matter (**dorsal columns spared**)	Bilateral loss of pain and temperature (one level below lesion), bilateral spastic paresis (below lesion), bilateral flaccid paralysis (level of lesion)
Vitamin B₁₂ deficiency	Dorsal columns, corticospinal tract	Bilateral loss of vibration and discrimination and bilateral spastic paresis affecting legs before arms
Syringomyelia	Ventral horn, ventral white commissure	Bilateral loss of pain and temperature (one level below lesion), bilateral flaccid paralysis (level of lesion)
Brown-Séquard syndrome	**All** tracts on one side of cord	Ipsilateral loss of vibration and discrimination (below lesion), ipsilateral spastic paresis (below lesion), ipsilateral flaccid paralysis (level of lesion), contralateral loss of pain and temperature (below lesion)

TABLE 8-4	Cranial Nerves and Their Functions	
Nerve	**Type**	**Function/Innervation**
Olfactory (CN I)	Sensory	Smell
Optic (CN II)	Sensory	Sight
Oculomotor (CN III)	Motor	Medial, superior, inferior rectus muscles; inferior oblique muscle, ciliary muscle, sphincter muscle of eye
Trochlear (CN IV)	Motor	Superior oblique muscle of eye
Trigeminal (CN V)	Both	Sensation of face; muscles of mastication
Abducens (CN VI)	Motor	Lateral rectus muscle of eye
Facial (CN VII)	Both	Taste (anterior two-thirds of tongue); muscles of facial expression, stapedius muscle, stylohyoid muscle, digastric muscle (posterior belly); lacrimal, submandibular, sublingual glands
Vestibulocochlear (CN VIII)	Sensory	Hearing, balance
Glossopharyngeal (CN IX)	Both	Taste (posterior one-third of tongue), pharyngeal sensation; stylopharyngeus muscle; parotid gland
Vagus (CN X)	Both	Sensation of trachea, esophagus, viscera; laryngeal, pharyngeal muscles; visceral autonomics
Accessory (CN XI)	Motor	Sternocleidomastoid and trapezius muscles
Hypoglossal (CN XII)	Motor	Tongue

CN, cranial nerve.

II. Neurologic Infection

A. Bacterial meningitis

1. Infection of meningeal tissue in brain or spinal cord; common bacterial agents differ depending on patient age (see Table 8-5)
2. Infection is usually caused by hematogenous spread, local extension, or cerebrospinal fluid (CSF) exposure to bacteria (e.g., neurosurgery).
3. **Risk factors** = ear infection, sinusitis, immunocompromise, neurosurgery, maternal group β-streptococci infection during birth
4. **History and physical (H/P)**
   a. Headache, **neck pain**, photophobia, malaise, vomiting, confusion; fever
   b. **Brudzinski** sign (i.e., neck flexion in supine patient prompts reflexive hip flexion) and **Kernig** sign (i.e., painful knee extension occurs with hip flexion in supine patient) are not reliable tests.
   c. Petechiae are seen in *Neisseria meningitidis* infection.
   d. Change in mental status, seizures, decreased consciousness seen with worsening infection
   e. Symptoms in children may be nonfocal.
5. **Labs** = increased white blood cell count (WBC); blood cultures frequently positive; lumbar puncture (LP) useful for differentiating causes of meningitis from each other and from healthy patients; CSF culture may determine exact agent (see Table 8-6)
6. **Radiology** = computed tomography (CT) or magnetic resonance imaging (MRI) may be helpful for ruling out other pathologies
7. **Treatment** = Initially cephalosporins (third generation) until specific agent is identified, then agent-specific antibiotics; close contacts of patient should be given **rifampin or ciprofloxacin for prophylaxis** in cases of *Neisseria* infection (rifampin for *H. influenzae* infection in children without prior vaccination)
8. **Complications** = seizures, increased intracranial pressure (ICP), subdural effusion, empyema, brain abscess, hearing loss, mental impairment

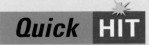

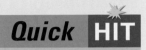

Haemophilus influenzae has been significantly reduced as a cause of meningitis owing to childhood **vaccination**.

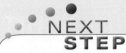

Young children with meningitis frequently have **negative** Brudzinski and Kernig signs.

NEXT STEP

Neurologic examination must be performed before LP. With signs of **increased intracranial pressure (ICP)** (papilledema, focal neurologic deficits, pupil asymmetry), do **not** perform LP because of increased risk of **uncal herniation**.

NEXT STEP

Treat fungal meningitis with amphotericin B, and treat tuberculosis meningitis with the combination of isoniazid, ethambutol, pyrazinamide, and rifampin.

TABLE 8-5 Common Causes of Meningitis by Age Group

Age	Most Common Agent	Other Common Agents
Newborn	Group β-streptococci	*Escherichia coli, Listeria, Haemophilus influenzae*
1 month–2 yr	*Streptococcus pneumoniae, Neisseria meningitidis*	Group β-streptococci, *Listeria, H. influenzae*
2–18 yr	*N. meningitidis*	*S. pneumoniae, Listeria*
18–60 yr	*S. pneumoniae*	*N. meningitidis, Listeria*
60+ yr	*S. pneumoniae*	*Listeria*, gram-negative rods

TABLE 8-6 CSF Findings for Different Causes of Meningitis

Status	WBCs	Pressure	Glucose	Protein
Healthy patient	<5	50–180 mm H$_2$O	40–70 mg/dL	20–45 mg/dL
Bacterial infection	↑↑ (PMNs)	↑↑	↓	↑
Fungal infection or tuberculosis	↑ (Lymphocytes)	↑↑	↓	↑
Viral infection	↑ (Lymphocytes)	↑	Normal	Normal

CSF, cerebrospinal fluid; PMNs, polymorphonuclear cells; WBCs, white blood cells; ↑, mild increase; ↑↑, significant increase.

B. Viral meningitis (aseptic meningitis)

1. Meningitis caused by viral infection by enterovirus, echovirus, herpes simplex virus, lymphocytic choriomeningitis virus, mumps virus
2. **H/P** = nausea, vomiting, headache, neck pain, photophobia, malaise; fever, rash; symptoms generally **milder** than for bacterial meningitis
3. **Labs** = LP helpful for diagnosis; viral culture will confirm etiology
4. **Treatment** = empiric antibiotics may be started until viral cause is confirmed; supportive care usually sufficient for confirmed viral cases

C. Encephalitis

1. Inflammation of brain parenchyma caused by **viral** infection (e.g., varicella-zoster virus, herpes simplex virus, mumps virus, poliovirus, rhabdovirus, Coxsackie virus, arbovirus, flavivirus, measles) or immunologic response to viral infection
2. **H/P**
   a. Malaise, headache, vomiting, neck pain, decreased consciousness; **change in mental status**, focal neurologic deficits (e.g., hemiparesis, pathologic reflexes, nerve palsy), fever
   b. Skin lesions seen with herpes simplex virus
   c. Parotid swelling seen with mumps
   d. Flaccid paralysis with maculopapular rash seen in West Nile virus
3. **Labs**
   a. LP shows increased WBCs and normal glucose.
   b. Culture generally not reliable
   c. Serologic testing may be useful to identify viral cause.
   d. Brain biopsy can provide definitive diagnosis but is generally impractical.
4. **Radiology** = CT or MRI may show inflamed region of brain with effusion
5. **Treatment** = maintain normal ICP, supportive care; herpes simplex virus treated with acyclovir

D. Brain abscess

1. Collection of pus in brain parenchyma resulting from extension of local bacterial infection, head wound, or hematogenous spread of bacteria
2. **H/P** = **headache**, neck pain, nausea, vomiting, malaise; fever, change in mental status, focal neurologic deficits, papilledema, seizures
3. **Labs** = brain biopsy or culture of abscess material performed during surgical drainage can be used to confirm bacterial identity
4. **Radiology** = **MRI** or CT may show "ring-enhancing lesion"; CT-guided biopsy can be performed to collect material for culture
5. **Treatment** = empiric antibiotics until specific agent identified; corticosteroids; **surgical drainage**

E. Poliomyelitis

1. Poliovirus (a picornavirus) infection of brain and motor neurons
2. Nearly eradicated through polio vaccine given in childhood
3. **H/P** = possibly asymptomatic; headache, neck pain, vomiting, sore throat; fever, **normal sensation, muscle weakness** that may progress to paralysis in severe cases
4. **Labs** = **positive polio-specific antibody**; LP consistent with viral meningitis; viral culture helpful for diagnosis
5. **Treatment** = with supportive care, most patients recover fully; assisted respiration may be required if respiratory muscles are affected

F. Rabies

1. Rhabdovirus transmitted to humans by **bite of infected animal**
2. Causes severe encephalitis with neuronal degeneration and inflammation
3. **H/P** = malaise, headache, restlessness, **fear of water ingestion** (secondary to laryngeal spasm); progressive cases exhibit severe central nervous system (CNS) excitability, **foaming at mouth**, very painful laryngeal spasms and **alternating mania and stupor**

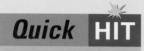

Quick HIT

Common arboviruses include St. Louis and California strains. Common flaviviruses include **West Nile** and Japanese strains.

Quick HIT

In young children, encephalitis may be caused by **Reye syndrome** (reaction in children with viral infection who are given aspirin [ASA]).

Quick HIT

Poliomyelitis may rarely occur after **oral** polio vaccine administration, so inactivated intramuscular polio vaccine is now more commonly used.

Neurologic Disorders

4. Labs
   a. Suspected animal should be caught and tested or observed for signs of rabies.
   b. If the animal appears to be infected, it should be killed and the brain should be tested for presence of virus and **Negri bodies** (i.e., round eosinophilic inclusions in neurons).
   c. Viral testing in humans (CSF, skin, serum) with symptoms is confirmatory of disease.
5. **Treatment** = clean wound area thoroughly; administer rabies immunoglobulin and vaccine to patient if animal was infected or if rabies suspicion is high
6. **Complications** = 100% mortality without treatment

III. Headache (see Table 8-7)

A. Head pain that may be a primary disorder (migraine, cluster, tension) or secondary to other pathology (hemorrhage, encephalopathy, meningitis, temporal arteritis, neoplasm)

B. Trigeminal neuralgia
1. Head and **facial pain** in trigeminal nerve distribution possibly caused by compression or irritation of trigeminal nerve root
2. H/P = sudden severe pain in distributions of maxillary and mandibular branches; "trigger zone" stimulation may induce pain
3. Radiology = MRI may identify lesions related to nerve compression
4. Treatment = **carbamazepine**, baclofen, phenytoin, gabapentin, valproate, clonazepam, or other **anticonvulsants**; surgical decompression of nerve may be helpful

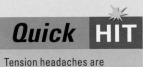

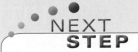

TABLE 8-7 **Primary Headache Disorders**

Variable	Migraine	Cluster	Tension
Patients	10–30 yr of age, **female** > male	Young **men**	Female > male
Pathology	Poorly understood; likely due to neuronal dysfunction	Poorly understood, likely extracerebral cause	Poorly understood
Precipitating factors	Stress, oral contraceptives, **menstruation**, exertion, foods containing tyramine or nitrates (chocolate, cheese, processed meats)	Alcohol, vasodilators	Stress, fatigue
Pain characteristics	Unilateral, throbbing	Severe, unilateral, **periorbital**, recurrent ("in clusters" over time)	**Bilateral**, tightness, occipital or neck pain
Other symptoms	**Nausea, vomiting**, preceding aura (visual abnormalities), photophobia	**Horner syndrome** (ptosis, miosis, anhidrosis), lacrimation, nasal congestion	Anxiety
Duration	4–72 hr	30 min–3 hr	Variable
Treatment	NSAIDs, ergots, sumatriptan; IV antiemetics useful for severe cases; prophylaxis includes tricyclic antidepressants, β-blockers, calcium channel blockers, ergots	100% O$_2$, ergots, sumatriptan; prophylaxis similar to that for migraines	NSAIDs, ergots, sumatriptan, relaxation exercises

IV, intravenous; NSAIDs, nonsteroidal anti-inflammatory drugs.

IV. Cerebrovascular and Hemorrhagic Diseases

A. Transient ischemic attack (TIA)
1. Acute focal neurologic deficits that last <**24 hr** and are caused by temporarily impaired vascular supply to brain (e.g., emboli, aortic stenosis, vascular spasm)
2. **Risk factors** = hypertension (HTN), diabetes mellitus (DM), coronary artery disease (CAD), tobacco, hyperlipidemia, hypercoagulable states

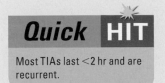

3. H/P
   a. Sudden appearance of focal neurologic deficits, including weakness, paresthesias, brief unilateral blindness (i.e., amaurosis fugax) or other vision abnormality, impaired coordination, vertigo
   b. Carotid bruits suggest carotid atherosclerosis.
   c. Harsh systolic murmur suggests aortic stenosis.

4. **Radiology** = ultrasound (US) may quantify degree of carotid or aortic stenosis; MRI or CT may demonstrate areas of brain ischemia; magnetic resonance angiography (MRA) or CT angiography (CTA) may locate intracranial vascular defects; echocardiography may be useful to determine if septic emboli, mural thrombus, or patent foramen ovale are cause of condition

5. Treatment
   a. Any patient with disease attributable to atherosclerosis should be given **antiplatelet** (e.g., ASA) and **antilipid** (e.g., statins) therapy.
   b. **Carotid endarterectomy or angioplasty** performed for carotid narrowing >60% in asymptomatic men, >50% in symptomatic men, and >70% in symptomatic women
   c. β-Blockers, valvuloplasty, or valve replacement used in treatment of aortic stenosis
   d. Long-term anticoagulation used for arrhythmias
   e. Treat other underlying disorders

B. Stroke [cerebrovascular accident [CVA]]

1. Acute focal neurologic deficit **lasting >24 hr** caused by ischemia of brain via **impaired perfusion** (i.e., ischemic stroke) or **hemorrhage** (i.e., hemorrhagic stroke)
2. Ischemic stroke may be **thrombotic** (i.e., obstruction of supplying artery by clot) or **embolic** (i.e., blockage of supplying artery by embolization of distant thrombus)
3. **Risk factors** = increased age, family history, obesity, DM, HTN, tobacco use, atrial fibrillation (Afib)
4. Area of neurologic deficit is dependent on location of stroke (see Figure 8-3, Table 8-8)

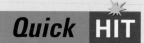

> **Quick HIT**
>
> Atherosclerosis of carotid, basilar, or vertebral arteries is the most common cause of **thrombotic** ischemic stroke.

> **Quick HIT**
>
> The **middle cerebral artery** is the most common artery involved in **embolic ischemic** stroke. Most emboli originate in the heart, aorta, carotid, or intracranial arteries.

Neurologic Disorders

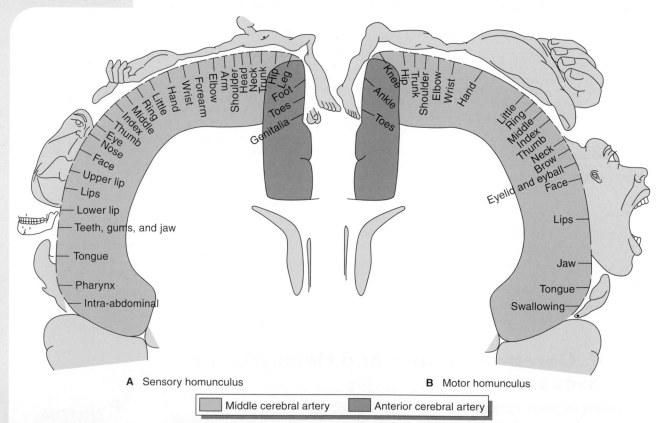

A Sensory homunculus   **B** Motor homunculus

| Middle cerebral artery | Anterior cerebral artery |

FIGURE 8-3 **Motor and sensory cortex and corresponding arterial supply.**

(From Mehta, S., Milder, E. A., Mirachi, A. J., & Milder, E. [2006]. *Step-Up to the Bedside: Clinical Case Review for USMLE Step 1.* [2nd ed.]. Philadelphia, PA: Lippincott Williams & Wilkins.)

TABLE 8-8	Common Stroke Locations and Corresponding Signs and Symptoms
Location of Stroke	**Signs and Symptoms**
ACA	Contralateral lower extremity and trunk weakness
MCA	Contralateral face and upper extremity weakness and decreased sensation, bilateral visual abnormalities, aphasia (if dominant hemisphere), neglect, and inability to perform learned actions (if nondominant hemisphere)
PCA	Contralateral visual abnormalities, blindness (if bilateral PCA involvement)
Lacunar arteries	Focal motor or sensory deficits, loss of coordination, difficulty speaking
Basilar artery	Cranial nerve abnormalities, contralateral full body weakness and decreased sensation, vertigo, loss of coordination, difficulty speaking, visual abnormalities, coma

ACA, anterior cerebral artery; MCA, middle cerebral artery; PCA, posterior cerebral artery.

5. **H/P**
   a. Sudden appearance of focal neurologic deficit lasting >24 hr
   b. Constellation of symptoms depends on location of pathology.
   c. Stable findings indicate stable stroke, but progressive findings indicate evolving stroke.
   d. Thorough serial neurovascular examinations are important to determining region of involvement and evolution.
6. **Radiology** = CT without contrast or MRI useful to differentiate ischemic from hemorrhagic stroke; MRA or CTA may be helpful for locating ischemic cause
7. **Electrocardiogram (ECG)** = detection of new onset arrhythmia or history of Afib seen on prior ECG may be useful in determining cause
8. **Treatment**
   a. Acute treatment of ischemic stroke
      (1) **Thrombolytic therapy** can be administered for ischemic stroke if **within 3 hr** of onset and no contraindications (i.e., evidence of hemorrhage on CT, recent surgery, anticoagulant use, recent hemorrhage, blood pressure >185/110 mm Hg) exist.
      (2) **Antiplatelet therapy** should be started within 48 hr of the event to prevent additional strokes.
      (3) Heparin or low molecular weight heparin (LMWH) may be considered in patients suspected of having progressive thromboembolism causing worsening symptoms.
      (4) Lipid-lowering drugs should be started after the acute stages of stroke in addition to optimization of blood pressure control.
   b. Acute treatment of **hemorrhagic** stroke
      (1) Reversal of anticoagulation, control of blood pressure, and control of ICP (e.g., mannitol, hyperventilation, anesthesia)
      (2) Surgical decompression may be considered for collections causing decreased consciousness.
      (3) Antiplatelet drugs can be restarted 2 weeks after stroke if patient is stable.
   c. Physical therapy is useful in improving persistent functional deficits.
   d. Treatment of underlying disorders is important to **prevent** future strokes.
9. **Complications** = better prognosis for recovery in young patients with greater overall health and limited deficits; some deficits may not improve despite treatment

C. Parenchymal hemorrhage
1. Bleeding within brain parenchyma caused by HTN, arteriovenous malformation (AVM), brain aneurysm, or stimulant abuse
2. **H/P** = headache, nausea, vomiting; change in mental status, focal motor or sensory deficits, possible seizure
3. **Radiology** = CT without contrast used to localize and determine extent of bleeding; MRA or CTA may be useful for locating site of bleed

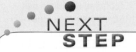

NEXT STEP

Do **not** treat HTN immediately following stroke unless it is extreme (>220/120 mm Hg) or it patient has CAD in order to **maintain cerebral perfusion.**

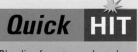

Bleeding from parenchymal hemorrhage can extend into the subarachnoid space.

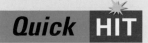

Berry aneurysms are associated with **autosomal dominant polycystic kidney disease** and **Ehlers-Danlos syndrome.**

Neurologic Disorders

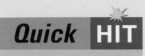

Quick HIT

Patients may describe the headache in SAH as the "**worst headache of my life.**"

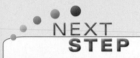

Quick HIT

Patients with imminent rupture of a berry aneurysm may have multiple, although less severe, sentinel headaches in the preceding weeks.

NEXT STEP

If SAH is suspected despite a **negative** CT, perform an LP.

Quick HIT

A **declining red blood cell (RBC) count** over successive collection tubes can occur in a traumatic LP and can help differentiate it from subarachnoid hemorrhage.

Quick HIT

The most common cause of epidural hematoma is damage to the **middle meningeal artery** from blunt trauma.

Quick HIT

An epidural hematoma may appear to cross the brain midline on CT; subdural hematomas do not.

4. **Treatment** = supportive care, maintain normal ICP; surgical decompression for large hemorrhages to reduce risk of herniation; surgical repair of AVMs or aneurysms frequently required
5. **Complications** = significant supratentorial bleeding can cause transtentorial (uncal) herniation (brainstem damage) and CSF flow obstruction (leading to hydrocephalus and brainstem compression); large hemorrhages are frequently fatal

D. Subarachnoid hemorrhage (SAH)

1. Bleeding between the pia and arachnoid meningeal layers because of rupture of **arterial aneurysm** (i.e., berry aneurysm), AVM, or trauma
2. H/P = **sudden severe headache**, neck pain, nausea, vomiting; fever, loss of (or decreased) consciousness, possible seizure
3. **Labs** = LP shows red blood cells, xanthochromia (i.e., yellowish discoloration of CSF), and increased pressure
4. **Radiology** = CT without contrast shows blood in the subarachnoid space; MRA or angiography can localize site of bleeding (see Figure 8-4)
5. **Treatment** = prevent increase in ICP (raise head of bed, administer mannitol), treat HTN, reverse anticoagulation, administer anticonvulsants, perform interventional radiologic or surgical clipping or embolization of aneurysm or AVM
6. **Complications** = recurrence of bleeding, arterial vasospasm, hydrocephalus; permanent neurologic damage or death may result

E. Epidural hematoma

1. Collection of blood between dura and skull caused by arterial hemorrhage
2. H/P = possible initial "**lucid interval**" between start of bleeding and onset of symptoms for a few hours or less with no change in consciousness; severe headache, decreased consciousness, nausea; hemiparesis, hemiplegia, seizures, pupil abnormalities (i.e., "blown" pupil)
3. **Radiology** = CT without contrast shows **convex** hyperdensity compressing the brain at site of injury; adjacent skull fracture may be apparent in traumatic cases (see Figure 8-5)

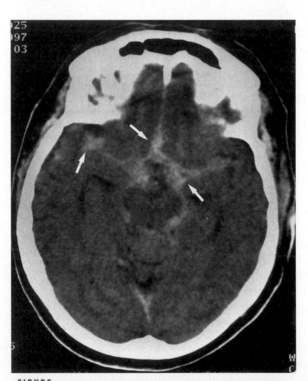

FIGURE 8-4 Subarachnoid hemorrhage seen on computed tomography (CT) scan without contrast; blood is evident in the subarachnoid space (**white arrows**).

(From Daffner, R. H. [2007]. *Clinical Radiology: The Essentials* [3rd ed., p. 477]. Philadelphia, PA: Lippincott Williams & Wilkins.)

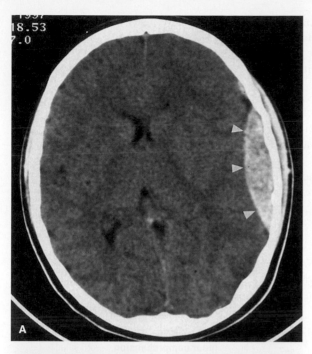

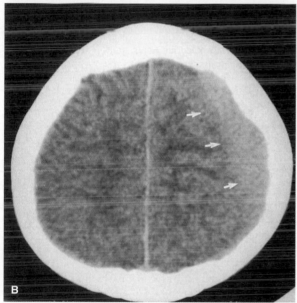

FIGURE
8-5 (A) Epidural hematoma: Note convex hyperdensity caused by blood (*white arrows*).
(B) Subdural hematoma: Note faint concave hyperdensity caused by blood (*white arrows*).

4. **Treatment** = **emergent** drainage of hematoma either under radiographic guidance or by surgical burr hole; stabilization of ICP and blood pressure
5. **Complications** = permanent neurologic injury or death usually results without prompt treatment

F. Subdural hematoma

1. Collection of blood between the dura and arachnoid meningeal layers caused by rupture of bridging veins following trauma
2. H/P
   a. **Slowly progressive** headache (days to weeks); change in mental status, contralateral hemiparesis, increased deep tendon reflexes (DTRs)
   b. Large hematomas can cause transtentorial herniation with decreased consciousness and pupil abnormalities.

NEXT STEP

With mental status changes seen in an elderly patient with a history of **falls**, perform a workup for subdural hematoma.

NEXT STEP

Do **not** perform an LP in patients with **mass lesion or subdural/epidural hematoma** because of increased risk of herniation.

Neurologic Disorders

3. **Radiology** = CT without contrast shows **concave** hyperdensity compressing the brain that does **not** cross midline (see Figure 8-5)
4. **Treatment** = surgical drainage or supportive therapy depending on size of bleed and extent of neurologic deficits

G. Aphasias

1. Disorders in speech caused by injury of specific regions of the brain following stroke or hemorrhage (see Table 8-9)
2. **Broca** and **Wernicke** aphasias are the most common types of aphasia, although other types exist.
3. Speech therapy may be of some benefit in retraining language centers of brain.

TABLE **8-9**	Common Classifications of Aphasias	
Type	**Area Injured**	**Characteristics**
Broca (expressive)	Inferior frontal gyrus, dorsolateral frontal cortex, anterior parietal cortex	Few words, difficulty producing words **(nonfluent); good comprehension**; face and arm hemiparesis, loss of oral coordination
Wernicke (receptive)	Posterior superior temporal gyrus, inferior parietal lobe	Word substitutions, meaningless words, meaningless phrases (**poor comprehension**, "word salad")
Conduction	Supramarginal gyrus, angular gyrus	**Fluent speech**, word substitutions, **frequent attempts to correct words**, word-finding pauses
Global	Large infarcts of left cerebral hemisphere	Difficulty producing words, **nonfluent speech, poor comprehension**, limb ataxia

V. Seizure Disorders

A. Causes of seizures

1. Sudden change in neurologic activity (e.g., behavior, movement, sensation) caused by excessive synchronized discharge of cortical neurons in a limited (focal) or generalized distribution of the brain
2. **Epilepsy** is a condition of **recurrent** seizures.
3. Common causes of seizures vary with age (see Table 8-10).

B. Types of seizures

1. Classified according to electrical activity and extent of brain involvement (see Table 8-11)
2. Electroencephalogram (EEG) used to measure cortical neuron activity and differentiate types of seizures
3. **Treatment**
   a. Anticonvulsants are the mainstay of therapy (see Table 8-12).
   b. One medication used initially, but additional drugs can be added for better control
   c. Drug withdrawal may be considered after an extended seizure-free period, but more than half of patients will have a recurrence.
   d. Surgery is a consideration for resectable sources of abnormal activity (more common in partial seizures).
   e. Vagal nerve stimulation can be considered in a patient failing other therapies.

C. Status epilepticus

1. **Repetitive** or **unremitting seizures** without any period of regained consciousness
2. Caused by withdrawal of anticonvulsants, alcohol withdrawal, trauma, preexisting seizure disorder, metabolic abnormalities
3. **H/P** = uninterrupted seizures lasting **>20 minutes** (frequently several hours) **without** return to normal consciousness

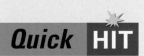

Quick HIT

Generalized seizures involve **the entire cortex**. Partial seizures involve **focal** neurologic deficits and can progress to **secondary** generalization (as distinguished from primary generalized seizures).

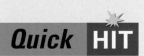

Neurologic Disorders

TABLE 8-10 Common Causes of Seizures by Age Group

Age Group	Causes
Infants	Hypoxic injury Metabolic defects Genetic or congenital abnormality Infection
Children	Idiopathic Infection Fever Trauma
Adults	Idiopathic Metabolic defects Drugs or drug withdrawal Trauma Neoplasm Infection Cerebrovascular disease Psychogenic
Elderly	Stroke or cerebrovascular disease Metabolic defects Drugs or drug withdrawal Infection Trauma Neoplasm

TABLE 8-11 Types of Seizures

Type	Involvement	History and Physical	Electroencephalogram
Simple partial	Focal cortical region of brain	**Focal** sensory (paresthesias, hallucinations) or motor (repetitive or purposeless movement) deficit; **no loss of consciousness**	Distinct focal conductive abnormality
Complex partial	Focal cortical region (most commonly **temporal** lobe)	**Hallucinations** (auditory, visual, olfactory), **automatisms** (repeated coordinated movement), déjà vu, impaired consciousness, postictal confusion	Focal abnormalities in temporal lobe
Generalized convulsive (tonic, clonic, tonic–clonic, myoclonic, atonic)	Bilateral cerebral cortex	Sustained contraction of extremities and back (**tonic**), repetitive muscle contraction and relaxation (**clonic**), brief contraction period followed by repetitive contraction–relaxation (**tonic–clonic**), brief repetitive contractions (**myoclonic**), or loss of tone (**atonic**); loss of consciousness, incontinence, significant postictal confusion, possible unilateral weakness lasting several hours (rarely days) after seizure (Todd paralysis)	**Generalized** electrical abnormalities
Absence	Bilateral cerebral cortex	**Brief** (few seconds) episodes of **impaired consciousness**, normal muscle tone, possible eye blinking, no postictal confusion; more common in **children**	Generalized three-cycle/second **spike-and-wave pattern**

Neurologic Disorders

Neurologic Disorders

TABLE 8-12	Anticonvulsant Medications Used in Epilepsy Treatment	
Drug	**Current Indications**	**Adverse Effects**
Mechanism: Inhibition of voltage-dependent sodium channels		
Carbamazepine	Monotherapy for partial or generalized convulsive seizures	Nausea, vomiting, hyponatremia, Stevens-Johnson syndrome, drowsiness, vertigo, blurred vision, leukopenia
Phenytoin	Monotherapy for partial or generalized convulsive seizures, **status epilepticus**	Gingival hyperplasia, androgenic, lymphadenopathy, Stevens-Johnson syndrome, confusion, blurred vision
Lamotrigine	Partial seizures, second-line drug for tonic–clonic seizures	Rash, nausea, Stevens-Johnson syndrome, dizziness, sedation
Oxcarbazepine	Monotherapy for partial or generalized convulsive seizures	Hyponatremia, rash, nausea, sedation, dizziness, blurred vision
Zonisamide	Second-line drug for partial and generalized seizures	Somnolence, confusion, fatigue, dizziness
Mechanism: Inhibition of neuronal calcium channels		
Ethosuximide	**Absence** seizures	Nausea, vomiting, drowsiness, inattentiveness
Mechanism: Enhanced GABA activity		
Phenobarbital, pentobarbital	Nonresponsive status epilepticus	Drowsiness, general cognitive depression, vertigo, nausea, vomiting, rebound seizures
Benzodiazepines	**Status epilepticus**	Drowsiness, tolerance, rebound seizures
Tiagabine	Second-line drug for partial seizures	Dizziness, fatigue, nausea, inattentiveness, abdominal pain
Mechanism: Inhibition of sodium channels and enhanced GABA activity		
Valproate	Monotherapy or second drug for partial and generalized seizures	Hepatotoxicity, nausea, vomiting, drowsiness, tremor, weight gain, alopecia
Mechanism: Inhibition of NMDA-glutamate receptors and enhanced GABA activity		
Topiramate	Second-line drug for partial and generalized seizures	Weight loss, cognitive impairment, heat intolerance, dizziness, nausea, paresthesias, fatigue
Mechanism: Unknown		
Gabapentin	Monotherapy or second-line drug for partial seizures	Sedation
Levetiracetam	Monotherapy for partial seizures, second-line drug for partial or generalized seizures	Fatigue, somnolence, dizziness

GABA, γ-aminobutyric acid; NMDA, N-methyl-D-aspartate.

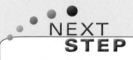

NEXT STEP

Delay CT and EEG during status epilepticus until patient is stabilized.

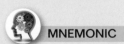

MNEMONIC

Remember the common signs of Parkinson disease by the mnemonic **SMART**:
Shuffling gait
Mask-like facies
Akinesia
Rigidity ("cogwheel")
Tremor (resting)

4. **Labs** = complete blood count (CBC), glucose, electrolytes, toxicology, liver function tests (LFTs), blood urea nitrogen (BUN), and creatinine may be useful to determine underlying cause
5. **EEG** = shows prolonged abnormal electrical activity
6. **Treatment**
   a. Maintain airway, breathing, circulation (ABCs)
   b. **Intravenous (IV) benzodiazepines** used to end seizure activity, phenytoin given to prevent recurrence
   c. Refractive seizure activity can be treated with phenobarbital or pentobarbital.
   d. Treat underlying disorder.
7. **Complications** = >20% mortality if not controlled promptly

VI. Degenerative Neurologic Disorders

A. Parkinson disease
1. Idiopathic dopamine depletion, loss of dopaminergic striated neurons in the substantia nigra, and Lewy body (eosinophilic cytoplasmic inclusions in neurons) formation leading to abnormal cholinergic input to cortex

2. Similar syndrome may be induced by 1-methyl-4-phenyl-1,2,3,6-tetrahydropyridine (MPTP, a side product in illicit opioid production) intoxication.
3. H/P = **resting tremor** (i.e., "pill-rolling" tremor of hands), decreased or slowed voluntary movement (i.e., bradykinesia), masklike facies, **shuffling gait**, involuntary acceleration of gait following initiation, **"cogwheel" rigidity** (i.e., increased tone of agonist and antagonist muscles), memory loss, difficulty initiating movement, postural instability
4. **Treatment**
   a. Dopaminergic agonists (e.g., levodopa, carbidopa, bromocriptine, amantadine), monoamine oxidase type B (MAO-B) inhibitors (e.g., selegiline), anticholinergic agents (e.g., benztropine), amantadine (see Table 8-13)
   b. Deep brain electrical stimulation has emerged as a viable option in disease not responsive to medication alone.

B. Amyotrophic lateral sclerosis (ALS)

1. Progressive loss of UMNs and LMNs in brain and spinal cord, involving degeneration of anterior horn cells and corticospinal tract
2. H/P = asymmetric **progressive weakness** in face (e.g., tongue, dysphagia) and limbs with **normal sensation**, possible change in personality or impaired judgment; increase or decrease in DTRs, spasticity, positive Babinski sign, flaccid paralysis, and fasciculations seen in limbs
3. **Labs** = blood tests used to rule out other pathologies
4. **Electromyogram (EMG)** = demonstrates widespread muscular denervation and motor block
5. **Radiology** = CT or MRI may be helpful to rule out neurologic lesions
6. **Treatment** = riluzole may slow progression; supportive care (e.g., respiratory support, pain control)
7. **Complications** = half of patients die within 3 years of diagnosis secondary to respiratory failure

C. Huntington disease

1. Autosomal dominant disease caused by multiple CAG repeats on chromosome 4; higher numbers of CAG repeats lead to earlier onset of disease
2. Characteristic signs include movement and mental dysfunction starting in middle age.
3. H/P = progressive, rapid irregular involuntary movement of extremities (**chorea**); dementia (e.g., irritability, antisocial behavior); possible seizures

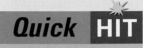

Signs of **UMN** disease include spasticity, increased DTRs, positive Babinski sign. Signs of **LMN** disease include flaccid paralysis, decreased DTRs, fasciculations, negative Babinski sign.

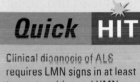

Clinical diagnosis of ALS requires LMN signs in at least two extremities and UMN signs in one region.

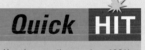

Huntington disease has **100%** genetic penetrance but does not become symptomatic until **middle age.**

TABLE 8-13 Medications Used in Treatment of Parkinson Disease			
Drug	**Mechanism**	**Indications**	**Adverse Effects**
Levodopa	Dopamine precursor	Initial therapy	Nausea, vomiting, anorexia, tachycardia, hallucinations, mood changes, dyskinesia with chronic use
Carbidopa	Dopamine decarboxylase inhibitor that reduces levodopa metabolism	Combined with levodopa to augment effects	Reduces adverse effects of levodopa by allowing smaller dosage
Bromocriptine	Dopamine receptor agonist	Increases response to levodopa in patients with declining response	Hallucinations, confusion, nausea, hypotension, cardiotoxicity
Selegiline	Monoamine oxidase type B inhibitor	Early disease; may help delay need to start levodopa	Nausea, headache, confusion, insomnia
Amantadine	Increases synthesis, release, or reuptake of dopamine	More effective against rigidity and bradykinesia	Agitation, hallucinations
Antimuscarinic agents (e.g., benztropine)	Block cholinergic transmission	Adjuvant therapy	Mood changes, dry mouth, visual abnormalities, confusion, hallucinations, urinary retention

4. **Labs** = genetic analysis will detect chromosome 4 abnormality
5. **Radiology** = CT or MRI shows caudate nucleus atrophy
6. **Treatment** = dopamine antagonists may improve chorea; genetic screening can be used in asymptomatic family members with proper counseling
7. **Complications** = usually fatal in <20 years from diagnosis

D. Multiple sclerosis (MS)

1. Progressive demyelinating disease of brain and spinal cord with possible autoimmune etiology
2. Most patients are **women** 20 to 40 years of age
3. **H/P**
   a. **Variable** initial presentation with multiple neurologic complaints (e.g., vertigo, vision abnormalities, paresthesias, weakness, urinary retention) that are difficult to explain through one cause
   b. Symptoms may progress slowly with several remissions and become worse during stressful events (e.g., infection, childbirth, trauma, heat).
   c. Late symptoms and signs include worsening vision, poor movement control, difficulty speaking (i.e., dysarthria), sensory abnormalities, postural and positional instabilities (i.e., cerebellar signs), spasticity, increased DTRs, and positive Babinski sign.
4. **Labs** = LP shows CSF with increased protein, mildly increased WBCs, oligoclonal bands, increased IgG
5. **Radiology** = MRI shows multiple asymmetric **white matter lesions**
6. Diagnosis is made considering both clinical and radiographic evidence.
7. **Treatment** = corticosteroids, methotrexate, and avoidance of stress may help decrease length of exacerbations; interferon-β and glatiramer acetate decrease frequency of exacerbations; supportive care for worsening neurologic dysfunction
8. **Complications** = progressive neurologic abnormalities with residual deficits; many patients become chronically disabled

E. Syringomyelia

1. Post-traumatic cystic degeneration of spinal cord from an unknown mechanism
2. Syrinx cavity (i.e., centralized channel within spinal cord) expands and compresses adjacent neural tissue.
3. **H/P** = loss of pain and temperature sensation, flaccid paralysis, decreased DTRs, fasciculations
4. **Radiology** = MRI shows syrinx expansion
5. **Treatment** = surgical decompression; shunting may be needed for recurrent cases; supportive care

VII. Peripheral Motor and Neuromuscular Disorders

A. Myasthenia gravis

1. Autoimmune disorder characterized by antibodies that bind to acetylcholine (ACh) receptors at neuromuscular junction and block normal neuromuscular transmission, resulting in easy fatigability
2. Often associated with thymoma and thyrotoxicosis

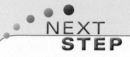

MNEMONIC

Remember that **MS** affects the **M**yelin **S**heath and is more common in **MS** (women) than in MR (men).

NEXT **STEP**

Highly suspect MS in a **young woman** with a confusing constellation of neurologic symptoms. Perform MRI to look for white matter lesions and LP to look for oligoclonal bands.

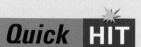

Quick **HIT**

Lambert-Eaton syndrome is a paraneoplastic disorder (e.g., **small cell lung cancer**) with similar presentation to myasthenia gravis. It occurs because of antibodies to presynaptic Ca^{2+} channels and is treated with immunosuppressive agents and plasmapheresis.

Neurologic Disorders

3. Most common in **young adult women**
4. **H/P = periodic weakness** and muscle fatigue that worsens throughout day; ptosis, diplopia (i.e., double vision), dysarthria; in severe cases, patients have dyspnea
5. **Labs = positive ACh receptor antibodies**; when edrophonium is administered, symptoms improve (i.e., Tensilon test); nerve stimulation and EMG are helpful in making diagnosis
6. **Treatment** = anticholinesterase agents (e.g., neostigmine, pyridostigmine), thymectomy, immunosuppressive agents (e.g., prednisone, azathioprine), plasmapheresis, IV immunoglobulin for refractory cases

B. Guillain-Barré syndrome

1. Autoimmune demyelinating disorder of peripheral nerves associated with recent **viral infection**, surgery, or vaccination (rare)
2. **H/P**
   a. Rapidly progressive **bilateral weakness** initially in distal extremities in "stocking-glove" distribution and extending proximally with **decreased sensation** and possible absent DTRs; possible severe neuropathic pain
   b. Recent history of viral infection, vaccination, or surgery
   c. Blood pressure, heart rate, or core temperature may be labile.
   d. Severe cases may include respiratory muscle weakness.
3. **Labs** = LP shows increased protein with normal pressure and glucose
4. **EMG** = consistent with widespread demyelination
5. **Treatment** = self-resolving within 1 month; plasmapheresis or IV immunoglobulin may accelerate resolution; patients must be watched for signs of respiratory failure; adequate analgesia for neuropathic pain
6. **Complications** = respiratory failure requires intubation and ventilation; most patients recover fully

C. Facial nerve palsy (Bell's palsy)

1. Facial weakness (usually unilateral) affecting both the **upper and lower face**; may be due to herpes simplex virus (HSV) reactivation (most common), herpes zoster, Lyme disease, AIDS, sarcoidosis, tumors, diabetes; many "idiopathic" are thought to be due to undiagnosed HSV
2. **H/P** = sudden onset of **unilateral facial muscle weakness**/paralysis (**asymmetrical smile**, drooling, ptosis, inability to close the eye, **inability to raise eyebrow**)
3. **Treatment** = supportive care (artificial tears, patch the eye at night to prevent injury); high-dose **glucocorticoids** (e.g., prednisone) for one week; patients presenting with severe disease may benefit from valacyclovir in addition to prednisone

D. Hyperkinetic disorders

1. Abnormal involuntary movement associated with specific neurologic diseases or other causes
2. Described by pattern of movements (see Table 8-14)

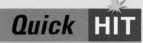

Quick HIT

Edrophonium is a short-acting anticholinesterase agent, making it ideal for myasthenia gravis testing but ineffective for therapy.

NEXT STEP

If myasthenia gravis is diagnosed in a patient, always perform a chest CT to look for a **thymoma**.

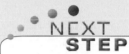

Quick HIT

A peripheral facial nerve palsy will cause paralysis of the upper face, unlike a cortical stroke. The facial nerve nucleus receives bilateral projections from the cortex to control the upper face, so a unilateral cortical stroke will **not** cause paralysis of the upper face.

Neurologic Disorders

TABLE 8-14	Common Hyperkinetic Disorders			
Disorder	**Movement**	**Associated Diseases**	**Treatment**
Essential tremor	Fixed oscillation of hands or head	Idiopathic	β-Blockers, primidone, clonazepam; thalamotomy or deep brain stimulation in refractory cases
Chorea	Rapid **flinching** distal limb and facial movements	**Hyperthyroidism**, stroke, **Huntington disease**, SLE, levodopa use, rheumatic fever	Treat the underlying disorder
Athetosis	Writhing, snakelike movement in extremities	**Cerebral palsy**, encephalopathy, Huntington disease, Wilson disease	Treat underlying disorder
Dystonia	**Sustained** proximal limb and trunk contractions	Wilson disease, **Parkinson disease**, Huntington disease, encephalitis, neuroleptic use (**tardive dyskinesia**)	Carbidopa, levodopa, botulinum toxin, treat underlying disorder
Hemiballismus	**Flinging** of proximal extremities	Stroke (subthalamic nucleus)	Haloperidol
Tics	**Repetitive** brief involuntary movement (blinking, grimacing) or sound (grunting, sniffing, throat clearing)	**Tourette syndrome**, obsessive-compulsive disorder, attention deficit hyperactivity disorder	Fluphenazine, pimozide, tetrabenazine

SLE, systemic lupus erythematosus.

Neurologic Disorders *(sidebar)*

VIII. Neoplasms

A. Primary CNS neoplasms

1. Brain tumors that are not caused by distant metastases; more common in young and middle-aged adults
2. Tumors in **adults** tend to be **above** the tentorium (i.e., fold of dural meninges that separates cerebellum below from cortex above); tumors in children tend to be **below** the **tentorium**.
   a. The three most common primary CNS tumors in adults are glioblastoma, meningioma, and schwannoma.
   b. The three most common primary CNS tumors in children are astrocytoma (benign), medulloblastoma (malignant), and ependymoma (may be malignant).
3. Symptoms result from focal compression (i.e., mass effect) of tumor (e.g., hydrocephalus, increased ICP, venous obstruction).
4. **H/P** = headache, vomiting, lethargy; focal neurologic abnormalities, change in mental status, possible seizures; blown pupil seen if herniation occurs
5. **Labs** = biopsy under CT guidance of detected lesion used for diagnosis
6. **Radiology** = MRI or positron emission tomography (PET) scan detects lesion
7. **Treatment** = surgical resection (if possible), radiation, chemotherapy; corticosteroids may decrease cerebral edema; anticonvulsants used for seizure prophylaxis

B. Metastatic CNS neoplasms

1. Tumors that have metastasized to brain from distant site; lung, renal cell carcinoma, melanoma, breast, and colorectal cancer are most common primary tumors
2. **H/P** = symptoms similar to presentation for primary tumors; headache, vomiting, lethargy; focal neurologic abnormalities, change in mental status, seizures
3. **Labs** = biopsy confirms origin of tumor
4. **Radiology** = MRI is most commonly used tool to detect lesions
5. **Treatment** = treat original tumor; surgical resection for single metastasis, palliative radiation
6. **Complications** = poor prognosis

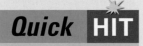

Quick HIT

Glioblastoma is the most common primary brain tumor in **adults**. **Astrocytoma** is the most common brain tumor in **children**. **Medulloblastoma** is the most common *malignant* brain tumor in children.

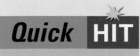

Quick HIT

Metastatic brain tumors are **more common** than primary tumors.

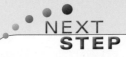

Quick HIT

Most metastases to the brain are **supratentorial**.

NEXT STEP

If an intracranial tumor is the initial lesion detected, workup should include a full search for a source neoplasm (full body CT, blood cancer antigens, etc.).

C. Neurofibromatosis type 1 (von Recklinghausen disease)

1. Autosomal dominant disorder (NF1 gene on chromosome 17) with multiple neurologic tumor and dermatologic manifestations
2. Neurofibromatosis type 2 is a rare autosomal dominant disorder linked to chromosome 22, characterized by the development of bilateral **acoustic neuromas.**
3. At least two of the following required for diagnosis:
   a. >5 **café-au-lait macules** >15 mm diameter
   b. >1 **neurofibromas** or 1 plexiform neurofibroma (i.e., tumors with mix of Schwann cells, fibroblasts, and mast cells)
   c. Axillary or inguinal freckling
   d. Optic glioma (i.e., tumor of optic nerve)
   e. >1 iris hamartomas (i.e., **Lisch nodules**)
   f. Bone lesions (e.g., cortical thinning of long bones, sphenoid dysplasia)
   g. First-degree relative with neurofibromatosis type 1
4. **H/P**
   a. Initial signs are freckling, **café-au-lait spots, Lisch nodules, neurofibromas,** and **bone abnormalities** evident in first few years of life.
   b. Severe functional limitations are seen in movement and gait, caused by nonunion of bone fragments (i.e., pseudoarthrosis) and fractures during development.
   c. Short stature and scoliosis may be evident.
   d. Visual abnormalities may result from compression of optic nerve by glioma.
   e. Possible cognitive impairments, seizures, or peripheral neuropathic signs
5. **Labs** = genetic testing detects abnormal gene
6. **Radiology** = MRI shows multiple areas of increased signal intensity in brain and increased brain volume
7. **Treatment** = therapy directed at maintaining function and treating complications
8. **Complications** = increased risk of malignant CNS tumors, developmental delays, mental retardation, peripheral neuropathy, pheochromocytoma, vision abnormalities, severe bone abnormalities, seizures

IX. Sleep and Loss of Consciousness

A. Sleep

1. Normal sleep cycles
   a. Stage N1 sleep is light sleep with fast θ waves on EEG.
   b. Stage N2 sleep is intermediate sleep with sleep spindles and K-complexes on EEG.
   c. Stage N3 is deep sleep with slow δ waves on EEG.
   d. Rapid eye movement (REM) sleep occurs every 90 to 120 minutes and is characterized by REMs, dreams, and low-voltage, high-frequency EEG pattern.
2. Sleep apnea
   a. Hypoventilation during sleep secondary to pulmonary obstruction or decreased neurologic respiratory drive (see Chapter 2, **Pulmonary Disorders**)
3. Narcolepsy
   a. Persistent excessive daytime sleepiness regardless of prior sleep quality
   b. **H/P** = possible sudden loss of muscle tone (i.e., cataplexy), vivid dreams, sleep paralysis; **hypersomnia** (i.e., sudden occurrence of sleep) may occur suddenly during the daytime
   c. **Labs** = polysomnography may show multiple arousals and decreased latency until REM sleep
   d. **Treatment** = modafinil (preferred), methylphenidate, or pemoline help prevent hypersomnia; tricyclic antidepressants may help prevent cataplexy; establishing regular sleep schedule with short naps improves wakefulness

B. Syncope

1. Acute transient loss of consciousness frequently related to inadequate blood supply to the brain
2. Common causes include **cardiac dysfunction** (e.g., aortic stenosis, bradycardia, decreased stroke volume), vasovagal response, hypotension, **hypoglycemia**, seizures, and cerebrovascular ischemia.

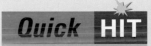

Quick **HIT**

40%–50% of sleep is spent in stage N2. **Benzodiazepines** increase stage N2 sleep, decrease stage N3, and do not reproduce normal sleep architecture.

Neurologic Disorders

3. **H/P** = possible prodrome of lightheadedness, nausea, and weakness preceding loss of consciousness (i.e., fainting); few generalized spasms may be observed; **patient quickly regains consciousness** (although seizure patients may display postictal sleepiness); hypotension, arrhythmias, and neurologic deficits may be detected following the episode

4. **Labs** = glucose levels should be measured; **orthostatics** or tilt testing (i.e., patient response is measured with rapid posture changes), with or without β-blocker infusion, can help diagnose cardiovascular cause; echocardiography or stress testing may be useful

5. **ECG** = useful for diagnosing cardiac causes; ambulatory monitoring may be used to measure extended periods of time

6. **EEG** = useful for detecting epileptic causes

7. **Radiology** = MRI, MRA, or angiography may detect vascular abnormalities

8. **Treatment** = treat underlying cause

C. Coma (*see Figure 8-6*)

1. Condition in which patient is **unresponsive to stimuli** and **unable to be aroused**; associated with bilateral cortical or brainstem reticular activating system dysfunction

2. Can result from cerebral hemorrhage, tumor, abscess, sedating drugs (e.g., alcohol, benzodiazepines, narcotics), hypoglycemia, metabolic dysfunction, hypothermia, hepatorenal failure, or psychogenic causes

3. **H/P** = patient unresponsive to stimuli; pertinent history and physical examination helpful for determining cause; CN examination particularly helpful for determining level of injury

4. **Labs** = CBC, electrolytes, BUN and creatinine, glucose, LFTs, coagulation factors, toxicology, CSF analysis, EEG, or arterial blood gas are helpful for diagnosis

5. **Radiology** = CT or MRI may detect intracranial cause (e.g., hemorrhage, tumor)

6. **Treatment** = maintain ABCs; prevent increase in ICP (hyperventilation, mannitol, elevate head); treat underlying cause

> **Quick HIT**
>
> A patient in a **persistent vegetative state** has normal sleep cycles, an inability to perceive and interact with the environment, and preserved autonomic function for **>1 month**. Recovery is unlikely if these symptoms last **>3 months**.

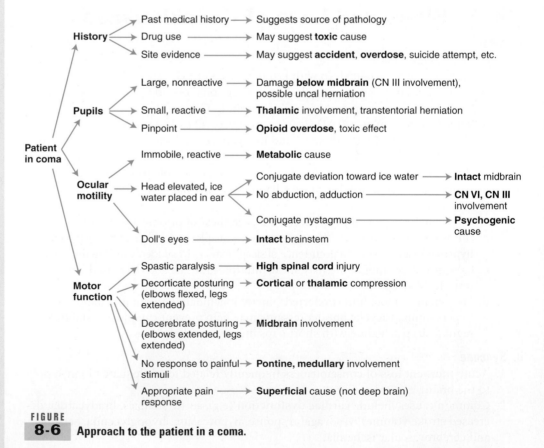

FIGURE

8-6 Approach to the patient in a coma.

X. Pediatric Neurologic Issues

A. Febrile seizures

1. Childhood seizures between 6 months and 6 years of age associated with **fever**
2. Occur in absence of CNS infection or lesion, metabolic abnormality, or history or prior afebrile seizures
3. **H/P** = fever >102°F/38.9°C with rapid rise in temperature; tonic–clonic seizure lasting <15 minutes; atypical seizures can occur at lower temperature and last longer
4. **Labs** = LP should be performed if meningitis suspected or in children <12 months of age
5. **EEG** = usually normal, unless atypical seizure
6. **Treatment** = confirm respiratory stability; **acetaminophen** as antipyretic; atypical seizures should receive more in-depth workup, including blood laboratory studies, EEG, and MRI
7. **Complications**
   a. Thirty-five percent of patients have recurrent febrile seizures, but there is little increase in lifetime risk of epilepsy.
   b. Atypical febrile seizures are more likely to recur, occur over longer periods of time, and carry an increased risk of **epilepsy**.

B. Childhood hydrocephalus

1. Hydrocephalus in children caused by either obstruction of CSF circulation in 4th cerebral ventricle (i.e., **noncommunicating**) or dysfunction of subarachnoid cisterns or arachnoid villi (i.e., **communicating**)
2. **H/P** = **increased head growth**, bulging fontanelles, and dilated scalp veins in infants; lethargy, vomiting, poor appetite, irritability, headache, diplopia, papilledema, poor skull suture fusion in older children
3. **Labs** = LP should be performed if infection is suspected
4. **Radiology** = US, CT, or MRI will show expanded ventricles
5. **Treatment** = acetazolamide or furosemide can be used temporarily to relieve symptoms; surgical shunting usually required for most cases
6. **Complications** = increased risk of epilepsy; increased risk of bacterial infection with shunting; 50% mortality before 3 years of age if untreated

C. Tay-Sachs disease

1. Autosomal recessive disorder caused by absence of hexosaminidase A (i.e., enzyme required for lipid ganglioside metabolism)
2. **Risk factors** = **Ashkenazi Jews**, French Canadians
3. **H/P** = poor development after first few months of life, decreased alertness, hyperacute hearing; **cherry red spots** on **retina** on funduscopic examination, progressive paralysis, vision loss, change in mental status
4. **Labs** = decreased hexosaminidase A activity; DNA analysis confirms diagnosis
5. **Treatment** = supportive care; genetic screening may aid parents with future childbearing decisions
6. **Complications** = death within first few years of life

D. Neural tube defects

1. Failure of neural tube closure during gestation leading to a spectrum of defects involving CNS formation
2. **Types of defects**
   a. **Spina bifida occulta**: most benign type; defect in **closure of dorsal vertebral arches** above spinal cord (usually lumbosacral junction)
   b. **Meningocele**: larger defect with herniation of meninges through dorsal vertebral defect; soft mass may form in midline superficial to defect.
   c. **Myelomeningocele**: severe defect with herniation of meninges and spinal cord through defect; frequent neurologic deficits, including bowel and bladder incontinence, flaccid paralysis, poor sensation, LMN signs, hydrocephalus

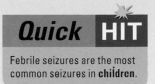

Quick HIT

Febrile seizures are the most common seizures in **children**.

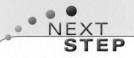

NEXT STEP

Do **not** give ASA to young children as an antipyretic because of risk of Reye syndrome.

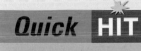

Quick HIT

Arnold-Chiari malformation type II and Dandy-Walker malformations are anatomic defects of the skull and ventricular system associated with hydrocephalus in children.

Neurologic Disorders

    d. **Anencephaly**: severe disorder with failure of cranial neural tube to close; absence of forebrain, meninges, and portions of skull; death occurs within days of birth.

3. **Risk factors** = anticonvulsant use or **poor folate intake** during pregnancy (both result in low maternal serum folate), DM

4. **H/P**
   a. Symptom severity depends on defect severity; patients with mild spina bifida may have tuft of hair over defect and may be asymptomatic.
   b. More severe cases of spina bifida can include delayed motor and mental development.
   c. More severe neural tube defects have more severe neurologic and developmental abnormalities.
   d. Anencephalic neonates have only brainstem function and no upper cortical function.

5. **Labs** = increased amniotic **α-fetoprotein** and **acetylcholinesterase** during gestation (measured in properly timed quadruple screen)

6. **Radiology** = US during pregnancy may detect defects

7. **Treatment**
   a. Surgical repair of all but mild defects needed
   b. Shunting frequently needed for meningocele and myelomeningocele to resolve hydrocephalus
   c. Physical therapy needed for gait abnormalities for patients capable of walking (spina bifida)
   d. Fetal surgery is developing as a potential treatment for lower neural tube defects diagnosed in utero.
   e. Appropriate supportive care for children with more severe neurologic deficits and those involving the genitourinary system
   f. Pregnant women and women trying to conceive should be given folate supplementation to reduce risk of defects.

8. **Complications** = increased risk of urinary tract infection and CNS infection; hydrocephalus in severe defects; children with severe defects may require lifelong care; survival time for anencephaly is typically for only a few days following birth

E. Cerebral palsy (CP)

1. Disorders of motor function resulting from CNS damage during in utero or infantile development; most cases result from **perinatal complications**

2. **Risk factors** = prematurity, intrauterine growth restriction, **birth trauma**, neonatal seizures or cerebral hemorrhage, **perinatal asphyxia**, multiple births, intrauterine infection (chorioamnionitis)

3. Types
   a. **Spastic**: spastic paresis of multiple limbs
   b. **Dyskinetic**: choreoathetoid (see hyperkinetic disorders in this chapter), dystonic, or ataxic movement disorder

4. **H/P**
   a. Patients with spastic CP have multiple limbs with increased tone, increased DTRs, weakness, gait abnormalities, and frequent mental retardation.
   b. Patients with dyskinetic CP have choreoathetoid, dystonic, or ataxic movements that worsen with stress as well as difficulty speaking (i.e., dysarthria).
   c. Both types of CP can include hyperactivity, seizures, or limb contractures.
   d. Some patients may exhibit symptoms of both types.

5. **Radiology** = MRI may be useful for detecting causative lesions

6. **Treatment**
   a. Pharmacologic therapy (e.g., botulinum toxin, dantrolene, baclofen, benzodiazepines), physical therapy, bracing, and surgery can be used to alleviate contractures and improve function.
   b. Speech therapy is useful for dysarthria.
   c. Special education is needed for patients with intellectual disability.
   d. Social and psychological support will be needed to help parents coordinate the many services needed for chronic care.

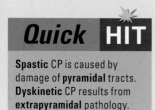

Quick HIT

Spastic CP is caused by damage of **pyramidal** tracts. **Dyskinetic** CP results from **extrapyramidal** pathology.

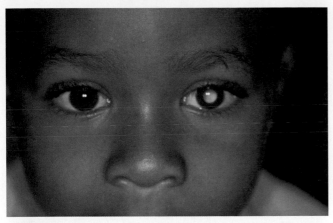

FIGURE
8-7 **Leukocoria in a child with a left-eye retinoblastoma.**

(From Rubin, R., & Strayer D. S. [2012]. *Rubin's Pathology* [6th ed., p. 1413]. Philadelphia, PA: Wolters Kluwer/Lippincott Williams & Wilkins; with permission.)

F. Retinoblastoma

1. Malignant tumor of retina in children and the most common **intraocular** tumor in children
2. Some cases have a genetic link that increases risk of tumor for both eyes
3. **H/P** = rarely, patients experience decrease in vision or eye inflammation; ophthalmologic examination may detect poor red light reflex in affected eye (i.e., **leukocoria**) or white retinal mass (see Figure 8-7)
4. **Labs** = mutation of RBI gene apparent on genetic testing
5. **Radiology** = US and CT detect size and extent of tumor; finding of calcified mass with normal globe size on CT is needed before therapy can be initiated
6. **Treatment**
   a. Enucleation performed for large tumors with no vision potential
   b. Radiation can be used for bilateral tumors or tumors near optic nerve.
   c. Cryotherapy or laser photocoagulation used for smaller tumors
   d. Chemotherapy used for metastases or vision salvage
7. **Complications** = good prognosis if metastasis has not occurred; risk of vision loss is high if tumor is adjacent to cornea

XI. Ophthalmology

A. Normal eye function

1. Retinal artery and vein are vasculature for the retina; vascular pathology affects vision (e.g., occlusion, DM retinopathy).
2. Nerves
   a. Optic nerve (CN II) responsible for vision
   b. Trochlear nerve (CN IV) controls superior oblique muscle (downward medial gaze, inward eye rotation).
   c. Abducens nerve (CN VI) controls lateral rectus muscle (abduction).
   d. Oculomotor nerve (CN III) controls all other eye muscles.
   e. Medial longitudinal fasciculus (MLF) maintains conjugate gaze when one eye abducts.
   f. Specific distortions in vision result from neuronal injury depending on site of insult (see Figure 8-8, Table 8-15).

B. Common vision abnormalities

1. Types of visual irregularity are caused by abnormal eye shape, gaze alignment, or eye focal orientation (see Table 8-16).
2. Usually correctable through lenses, visual training, or surgery

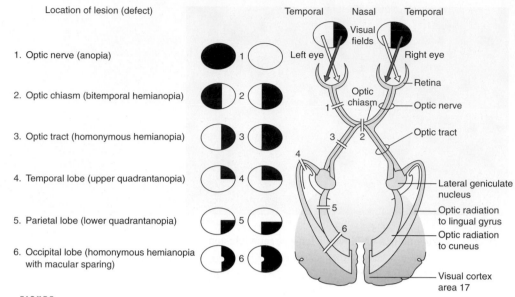

Location of lesion (defect)

1. Optic nerve (anopia)

2. Optic chiasm (bitemporal hemianopia)

3. Optic tract (homonymous hemianopia)

4. Temporal lobe (upper quadrantanopia)

5. Parietal lobe (lower quadrantanopia)

6. Occipital lobe (homonymous hemianopia with macular sparing)

FIGURE 8-8 Visual field defects resulting from neuronal injury.

(From Mehta, S., Milder, E. A., Mirachi, A. J., & Milder, E. [2006]. *Step-Up: A High-Yield, Systems-Based Review for the USMLE Step 1* [3rd ed., p. 40]. Philadelphia, PA: Lippincott Williams & Wilkins.)

TABLE 8-15 Common Pupil and Gaze Abnormalities

Abnormality	Presentation	Cause
Argyll Robertson pupil	Accommodation to near objects, nonreactive to light	Syphilis, SLE, DM
Marcus Gunn pupil	Light in affected pupil causes minimal bilateral constriction, light in normal pupil causes normal bilateral constriction	Afferent nerve defect
Horner syndrome	Ptosis, miosis, anhidrosis	Sympathetic trunk lesion (e.g., Pancoast tumor)
Adie pupil	Minimally reactive dilated pupil	Abnormal innervation of iris
Internuclear ophthalmoplegia	With lateral gaze, there is absent ipsilateral eye adduction	MLF lesion, MS

DM, diabetes mellitus; MLF, medial longitudinal fasciculus; MS, multiple sclerosis; SLE, systemic lupus erythematosus.

TABLE 8-16 Common Vision Abnormalities

Disorder	Cause	History and Physical	Treatment
Myopia	Refracting power of eye is too great, causing image focal point to be anterior to retina	Blurred vision, vision quality worsens as objects move farther away	Corrective lenses, laser correction
Hyperopia	Refracting power of eye is insufficient, causing image focal point to be posterior to retina	Blurred vision, vision quality worsens as objects move closer	Corrective lenses, laser correction
Astigmatism	Asymmetric cornea surface, causing inconsistent refraction of light	Blurred vision	Corrective lenses
Strabismus	Deviation of eye unable to be overcome by normal motor control	Gaze for each eye is in different directions, double vision, progressive blindness	Vision training, surgery frequently required to achieve bilateral alignment
Amblyopia	Developmental defect in neural pathways of eye	Poor visual acuity, spatial differentiation in affected eye	Correct visual acuity in the affected eye, and patch the unaffected eye to encourage use of the affected eye

C. Eye inflammation and infection

1. **Conjunctivitis**
   a. Inflammation of eye mucosa secondary to bacterial (e.g., *Staphylococcus aureus*, *Streptococcus pneumoniae*) or viral infection or allergic reaction
   b. **H/P** = mildly painful eye, **inflamed conjunctiva**, possible lymphadenopathy, pruritic eye when caused by allergy; purulent discharge often seen with bacterial infection (but can also be seen with viral or allergic conjunctivitis)
   c. **Labs** = Gram stain and culture of discharge may indicate bacterial cause
   d. **Treatment** = self-limited; topical sulfonamides or erythromycin reduce duration of bacterial infection; antihistamines improve symptoms caused by allergic reaction; fastidious handwashing decreases community spread of infection

2. **Uveitis**
   a. Inflammation of iris, choroids, and ciliary bodies caused by infectious (e.g., viral, syphilis), autoimmune (e.g., ankylosing spondylitis, **juvenile idiopathic arthritis**), or inflammatory (e.g., ulcerative colitis, Crohn's disease) conditions
   b. **H/P**
      (1) **Anterior uveitis**: pain and photophobia; slit lamp examination shows inflammation of eye and keratin deposits on cornea
      (2) **Posterior uveitis**: mild vision abnormalities; slit lamp examination shows eye inflammation and retinal lesions
   c. **Treatment** = topical antibiotics if caused by infection; topical or systemic corticosteroids if not caused by infection; treat underlying condition

D. Cataracts

1. Clouding of lens leading to progressive vision loss
2. **Risk factors** = trauma (caustic substances), DM, corticosteroid use, age, low education, alcohol use, tobacco use
3. **H/P** = progressive hazy and blurred vision occurring over months to years; examination reveals opacity of lenses and decreased red reflex
4. **Treatment** = lens replacement surgery

E. Glaucoma

1. Increased intraocular pressure (IOP) leading to loss of vision
2. **Open angle glaucoma**
   a. Gradual bilateral increase in IOP
   b. **Risk factors** = increased age, increased IOP, blacks, DM, myopia, family history
   c. **H/P** = initially asymptomatic; gradual loss of visual fields (from **peripheral to central**), halos seen around lights, headache, and poor adaptation to changes in light; **cupping** of optic disc seen on funduscopic examination
   d. **Labs** = IOP testing (i.e., tonometry) shows increased pressure over several tests performed at 2- to 4-week intervals
   e. **Treatment**
      (1) Topical β-blockers (e.g., timolol) and α-adrenergic agonists decrease aqueous humor production; prostaglandin analogues, α-adrenergic agonists, and cholinergic agonists (e.g., pilocarpine) increase aqueous humor removal.
      (2) Laser surgery improves aqueous humor drainage in refractory cases.
      (3) Prevention is important for all at-risk patients, who should receive **regular ophthalmologic examinations**.
   f. **Complications** = progressive, permanent vision loss
3. **Closed angle glaucoma**
   a. **Acute** increase in IOP secondary to narrowing of anterior chamber angle and obstructed drainage of aqueous humor from eye
   b. **Risk factors** = increased age, Asian, hyperopia, dilated pupils (e.g., low-light environments, optometry examination dilation)
   c. **H/P** = severe eye pain, blurred vision, halos seen around lights, nausea, and vomiting; eye is inflamed and **hard** with a **dilated** and nonreactive pupil
   d. **Labs** = tonometry demonstrates increased IOP

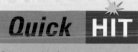

Quick HIT

Conjunctivitis facts:
- Adenovirus is the most common cause.
- Typically highly contagious and can be spread by contact with towels or linens or by close contact
- Can be caused by *Neisseria gonorrhoeae* and *Chlamydia trachomatis* after sexual contact
- Can occur in the perinatal period if mother is infected with *N. gonorrhoeae* or *C. trachomatis*

Neurologic Disorders

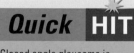

Quick HIT

Open angle glaucoma is the **most common** type of glaucoma.

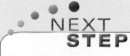

NEXT STEP

Any patient who requires **frequent changes of lens prescriptions** should be suspected of having glaucoma and pressure testing should be performed.

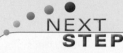

Quick HIT

Closed angle glaucoma is usually **unilateral**.

NEXT STEP

Never induce additional pupil dilation during examination of patient with suspected closed angle glaucoma because it will acutely worsen the condition.

e. Treatment
(1) Timolol, apraclonidine, and pilocarpine eyedrops to lower pressure acutely; oral/IV acetazolamide or IV mannitol may also be given.
(2) Laser iridotomy should be performed to prevent recurrence (frequently performed on unaffected eye as prophylaxis).
f. Complications = rapid permanent vision loss

F. Macular degeneration

1. Atrophic (slow) or exudative (rapid) degeneration of retina, leading to **retinal fibrosis** and **permanent vision loss**
2. **Risk factors** = white, tobacco, family history, increased age, prolonged sunlight exposure, HTN; female > male
3. **H/P** = painless, gradual loss of vision (**central to peripheral**) at all distances; loss of retinal pigmentation (atrophic type) and hemorrhage (exudative type) in macular region and possible retinal detachment seen on funduscopic examination
4. **Radiology** = fluorescein angiography may show neovascular membranes and retina
5. **Treatment** = dietary supplementation with vitamin C, vitamin E, β-carotene, copper, and zinc may slow progression; intravitreal ranibizumab may help treat exudative lesions near the fovea; laser photocoagulation of discrete lesions may delay progression
6. **Complications** = treatment effectiveness is limited; gradual progression to severe vision loss

G. Retinal detachment

1. Separating of retina from adjacent epithelium, leading to acute vision loss
2. **Risk factors** = trauma, cataract surgery, myopia, family history
3. **H/P** = painless acute loss of vision (**"window shade pulled over eye"** or **numerous "floaters"**); pigmented fragments or gray retina floating in vitreous humor seen on funduscopic examination
4. **Treatment** = laser photocoagulation or cryotherapy to halt tear progression and reattachment of retina (may not fully restore loss of vision)

H. Retinal vessel occlusion

1. Occlusion of retinal artery or vein resulting in sudden loss of vision
2. Most commonly caused by atherosclerosis, DM, HTN, **thromboembolic disease** (see Figures 8-9, 8-10, and 8-11)
3. **H/P**
a. Retinal **artery** occlusion: sudden painless loss of vision; funduscopic examination shows **cherry red** spot in fovea and poor arterial filling

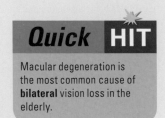

Macular degeneration is the most common cause of **bilateral** vision loss in the elderly.

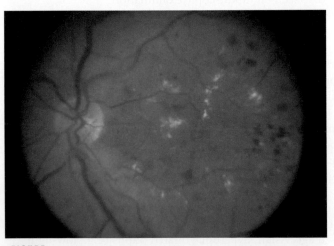

FIGURE 8-9 **Diabetic retinopathy.**

Note yellowish lipid exudates and multiple small retinal hemorrhages.
(From Rubin, R., & Strayer D. S. [2012]. *Rubin's Pathology* [6th ed., p. 1403]. Philadelphia, PA: Wolters Kluwer/Lippincott Williams & Wilkins; with permission.)

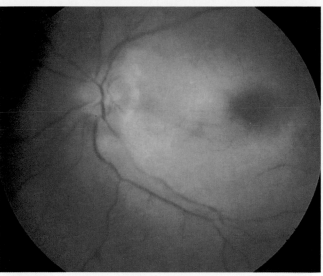

FIGURE

8-10 **Retinal artery occlusion.**

Note generalized retinal edema and presence of cherry red spot.
(From Gold, D. H., & Weingeist, T. A. [2001]. *Color Atlas of the Eye in Systemic Disease* [Figure 75-2]. Philadelphia, PA: Lippincott Williams & Wilkins; with permission.)

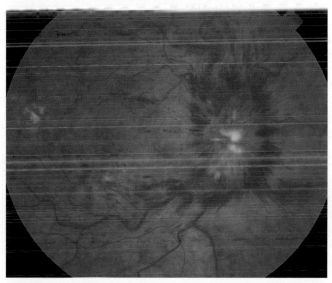

FIGURE

8-11 **Retinal vein occlusion.**

Note edematous retina, retinal hemorrhages, cotton wool spots, and venous dilation.
(From Gold, D. H., & Weingeist, T. A. [2001]. *Color Atlas of the Eye in Systemic Disease* [Figure 29-1]. Philadelphia, PA: Lippincott Williams & Wilkins; with permission.)

Neurologic Disorders

b. Retinal **vein** occlusion: more gradual painless loss of vision; funduscopic examination shows **cotton wool spots**, edema, **retinal hemorrhages**, and dilated veins

4. **Treatment**
   a. Thrombolysis of arterial occlusion should be performed within 8 hr of onset.
   b. Acetazolamide and O_2 administration also used to decrease congestion and increase perfusion for arterial occlusion
   c. Laser photocoagulation may be useful for venous occlusion.
5. **Complications** = without prompt treatment, permanent vision loss results

XII. Audiovestibular Disorders

A. Otitis media

1. Infection of middle ear caused by *Streptococcus pneumoniae*, *Haemophilus influenzae*, *Moraxella catarrhalis*, *S. pyogenes*, or viruses
2. Increased risk in children secondary to shorter and more horizontal ear canal than in adults; pacifier use; hypertrophic tonsillar tissue
3. **H/P** = ear pain, decreased hearing; fever, bulging tympanic membrane with **decreased mobility**, poor light reflex; possible bloody discharge with perforation (i.e., otorrhea)
4. **Treatment**
   a. Initially observation and supportive care
   b. For unresolved cases, amoxicillin for 10 days; resistant strains may require amoxicillin-clavulanic acid or stronger cephalosporins
   c. Recurrent cases may require surgical placement of tympanic tubes to assist in middle ear drainage.
5. **Complications** = mastoiditis, meningitis, hearing loss, sigmoid sinus thrombosis, or brain abscess can occur in untreated cases

B. Otitis externa ("swimmer's ear")

1. Infection of ear canal most commonly caused by *Staphylococcus aureus*, *Pseudomonas*, or *S. epidermidis*; frequently associated with water in ears (e.g., swimming)
2. **H/P** = painful, swollen ear with possible white discharge; **ear canal** is red and **swollen**; tenderness of pinna
3. **Treatment** = topical polymyxin, neomycin, and hydrocortisone; oral cephalosporins or ciprofloxacin can be used for *Pseudomonas* infection or infection that spreads to involved skull; topical drying agents after water exposure to prevent recurrent infection

C. Benign paroxysmal positional vertigo (BPPV)

1. Vertigo (i.e., abnormal feeling of rotational movement leading to poor balance and coordination) caused by a dislodged otolith in the inner ear that interferes with semicircular canal stabilization
2. **H/P**
   a. Brief, episodic vertigo that can occur with certain head movements and is accompanied by nausea and vomiting
   b. Nystagmus may be seen during episodes.
   c. **Dix-Hallpike maneuver** (i.e., moving from sitting to supine while quickly turning head to side) induces symptoms and confirms diagnosis.
3. **Radiology** = CT or MRI can rule out intracranial lesion
4. **Treatment** = physical maneuvers designed to free otolith from semicircular canal can alleviate recurrent episodes

D. Ménière disease (endolymphatic hydrops)

1. Vertigo caused by distension of endolymphatic compartment of inner ear
2. **H/P** = acute vertigo lasting **several hours**, nausea, vomiting, decreased hearing, feeling of ear fullness, tinnitus (ringing in ears)
3. **Labs** = audiometry shows **low-frequency hearing loss**
4. **Treatment** = anticholinergics, antiemetics, and antihistamines improve exacerbations; salt restriction and thiazide diuretics may reduce frequency of episodes; surgical decompression needed in refractory cases
5. **Complications** = progressive hearing loss

E. Acoustic neuroma (acoustic schwannoma)

1. Benign tumor of Schwann cells of CN VIII that can lead to hearing loss secondary to nerve compression
2. **H/P** = hearing loss, dizziness, tinnitus; unilateral facial palsy; decreased sensation may be seen on examination
3. **Labs** = audiometry shows sensorineural hearing loss

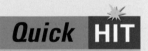

Quick HIT

Conductive hearing loss:
- Pathology occurs along conductive pathway from outer ear to inner ear
- Audiometry shows **preserved bone** conduction, but air conduction shows consistently low hearing threshold (abnormal Rinne test).

Sensorineural hearing loss:
- Pathology in neural pathways from ear to brain
- Audiometry shows both **impaired bone** and **air conduction** (asymmetric Weber test, normal Rinne test)

4. **Radiology** = MRI can localize tumor

5. **Treatment** = surgical excision

6. **Complications** = large tumors can compress cerebellum or brainstem

 # XIII. Dementia and Delirium

A. Alzheimer disease

1. Slowly progressive dementia characterized by neurofibrillary tangles, neuritic plaques, amyloid deposition, and neuronal atrophy; **most common** cause of dementia

2. **Risk factors** = increased age, family history, trisomy 21; female > male

3. **H/P** = progressive **short-term memory loss**, depression, **confusion**, inability to complete complex movements or tasks; severe cases have personality changes and delusions

4. **Labs** = nondiagnostic but can be used to rule out other causes of dementia

5. **Radiology** = CT or MRI shows **cortical atrophy**

6. **Treatment** = cholinesterase inhibitors (e.g., donepezil, rivastigmine, galantamine) may slow progression; memantine may improve symptoms in moderate disease; occupational therapy helpful to prolong independence

7. **Complications** = median survival following diagnosis is 3 years because of comorbidity

B. Frontotemporal dementia (Pick disease)

1. Dementia characterized by intracellular inclusions of tau protein (Pick bodies) plus atrophy of the frontal and temporal lobe

2. H/P
   a. **Behavioral variant** — behavior and personality changes (e.g., inappropriate social behavior and personal conduct) followed by progressive dementia
   b. **Aphasia variant** = dementia plus progressive nonfluent aphasia

3. **Labs** = nondiagnostic

4. **Radiology** = CT or MRI shows bilateral frontal atrophy (especially in the behavioral variant)

5. **Treatment** = SSRIs, trazodone, or atypical antipsychotics may help control the behavioral symptoms; cholinesterase inhibitors are not beneficial

C. Dementia with Lewy bodies

1. Dementia characterized by intracellular cortical inclusions called Lewy bodies (eosinophilic inclusions of the protein α-synuclein)

2. **H/P** = fluctuating cognition, impaired attention, visual hallucinations, syncope, frequent falls; limb rigidity, bradykinesia or akinesia, gait disturbance

3. **Labs** = nondiagnostic

4. **Radiology** — CT and MRI show nonspecific generalized cortical atrophy

5. **Treatment** = behavioral therapy; cholinesterase inhibitors may be beneficial; levodopa-carbidopa can be used for disabling parkinsonian symptoms

D. Normal pressure hydrocephalus

1. Collection of excess CSF in cerebral ventricles and spinal thecal sac; may follow **subarachnoid hemorrhage**, chronic meningitis, or other disease of impaired CSF resorption

2. **H/P** = cognitive impairment, incontinence, gait abnormalities

3. **Labs** = LP shows normal pressure, but removal of CSF can cause improvement in symptoms

4. **Radiology** = MRI shows enlarged cerebral ventricles, white matter lesions, and aqueduct atrophy

5. **Treatment** = ventriculoperitoneal shunting

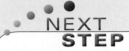

NEXT STEP

Distinguish dementia from Alzheimer disease from that caused by multiple cortical infarcts with MRI. Multiple small lesions or infarcts will be apparent on MRI when the cause is **vascular**.

Neurologic Disorders

Quick HIT

Dementia with Lewy bodies may cause movement symptoms similar to Parkinson disease, which is characterized by Lewy bodies in the substantia nigra and other structures.

 MNEMONIC

Remember the signs of normal pressure hydrocephalus by the **3 Ws:**
Wacky (cognitive impairment)
Wet (incontinence)
Wobbly (gait abnormalities)

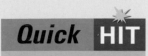

Quick HIT

Elderly patients are particularly susceptible to delirium during inpatient stays.

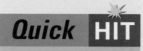

Quick HIT

Delirium differs from "sundowning," the deterioration of behavior during evening hours in patients with dementia, in that it occurs in patients without a history of dementia and can be linked to a medical or substance-related cause.

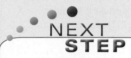

NEXT STEP

Do **not** use benzodiazepines or anticholinergics in the treatment of delirium or dementia-related agitation because they can **worsen** symptoms.

Neurologic Disorders

E. Delirium
1. Altered state of consciousness
   a. Most commonly secondary to:
      1. **Drugs** (e.g., alcohol, corticosteroids, benzodiazepines, antipsychotics, anticholinergics, antihistamines, etc.)
      2. Infection, **hypoxia**, or CNS abnormalities
   b. It is frequently quickly reversible once the underlying cause is identified and treated.
2. H/P
   a. Key features (see Table 8-17)
      1. Altered level of consciousness with inattentiveness and confusion
      2. Change in cognition is not caused by preexisting dementia.
      3. Changes in cognition develop quickly and fluctuate over course of day.
      4. Changes are related to disease, medication, or drug use.
   b. Psychomotor agitation or retardation, disturbance of sleep patterns
   c. Emotional instability
3. Labs = should address potential metabolic or pharmacologic causes
4. Radiology = CT can be used to assess CNS insult
5. Treatment
   a. Treat underlying cause
   b. Reorientation through observation, reassurance, normalization of sleep–wake cycles, and decreasing excess stimuli improves behavior.
   c. Avoid restraints because they frequently exacerbate delirium (use only if patient is at danger of harming self).
   d. Antipsychotics (e.g., haloperidol) can be used to decrease agitation acutely.

Table **8-17**	**Comparison of Delirium and Dementia**	
Characteristics	**Delirium**	**Dementia**
Onset	Acute	Gradual
Daily course	Fluctuating cognitive function and behavior	Generally consistent; sundowning
Level of consciousness	Decreased	Normal
Orientation	Aware of self; impaired for time and place	Generally impaired
Thought production	Disorganized, flight of ideas	Impoverished
Psychotic features	Delusions, hallucinations	Minimal
Memory	Short-term impairment	Short- and long-term impairment
Prognosis	Reversible	Usually irreversible

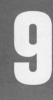

MUSCULOSKELETAL DISORDERS

 I. Common Adult Orthopedic Conditions

A. Carpal tunnel syndrome

1. Syndrome resulting from **median** compression at the wrist (see Figure 9-1)
2. **Risk factors**
   a. Pregnancy, rheumatoid arthritis (RA), diabetes mellitus (DM), acromegaly, hypothyroidism, obesity, **overuse** (activities requiring significant wrist motion, including typing, piano playing, writing, etc.)
   b. Most common in persons 30 to 55 years of age; female > male
3. **History and physical (H/P)**
   a. Wrist pain that radiates up arm and worsens with hand flexion and grasping, decreased hand strength, numbness in thumb and in index and middle fingers; decreased palmar two-point discrimination, except on the radial side of the palm
   b. Positive **Tinel** sign (i.e., tapping over carpal tunnel elicits wrist tingling and pain) and **Phalen** sign (i.e., placing dorsal side of hands together and flexing wrists 90° causes the onset of symptoms within a minute)
   c. Thenar muscle atrophy is seen in long-term cases.
4. **Electromyogram (EMG)** = can be used in addition to nerve conduction studies to evaluate nerve compromise (will show impaired conduction)
5. **Treatment** = wrist splints, **activity modification**, nonsteroidal anti-inflammatory drugs (NSAIDs), corticosteroid injections, surgical release of the transverse carpal ligament

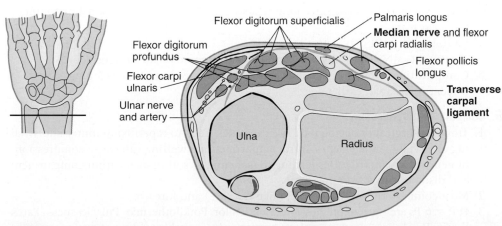

FIGURE 9-1 Tendinous and neurovascular structures superficial and deep to the transverse carpal ligament in the wrist.

(Modified from Moore, K. L., Agur, A. M. R., & Dalley, A. F. [2013] *Clinically Oriented Anatomy* [7th ed.]. Baltimore, MD: Lippincott Williams & Wilkins.)

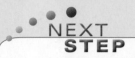

NEXT STEP

Suspect axillary nerve injury in cases of **deltoid** malfunction (inability to extend arm) or shoulder numbness following shoulder dislocation.

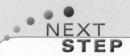

NEXT STEP

An **open** fracture (fracture penetrates skin **and is exposed to outside environment**) requires thorough **irrigation** in the operating room and antibiotics to reduce the risk of **infection**.

Quick HIT

Computed tomography (CT) is generally more useful in the diagnosis of **bone** pathology, whereas **MRI** is more useful for **soft tissue** injuries.

Quick HIT

A medially directed blow to the lateral side of the knee (i.e., a valgus stress) can cause the **unhappy triad**: lateral meniscus tear, **medial collateral ligament** (MCL) tear, and **ACL** tear.

Quick HIT

Young athletes may get an **exertional** compartment syndrome during athletic activity with mild elevation of compartment pressures that **resolves following activity cessation** and carries a **minimal risk** of significant tissue ischemia.

Quick HIT

A painful leg that has a pulse **never** rules out compartment syndrome.

B. Dislocations
1. Shoulder
   a. Most commonly **anterior** (posteriorly directed force on distal humerus or forearm during abduction causes cantilever effect that drives humeral head forward and tears anterior shoulder capsule)
   b. **Posterior** dislocations most frequently occur following **seizures** and **electrical shock** (strong contraction in internally rotated, adducted arm causes humeral head dislocation).
   c. **Treatment** = urgent closed reduction, sling; chronic dislocations may require surgery to improve joint stability
   d. **Complications** = axillary artery and nerve injury, increased risk of future dislocations
2. Hip
   a. Most commonly **posterior** via a posteriorly directed force on an internally rotated, flexed, and adducted hip (e.g., dashboard injury)
   b. **Treatment** = closed reduction, bracing, abduction pillow

C. Fractures
1. Fractures are associated with a particular mechanism of injury and carry different options, depending on location (see Table 9-1).

D. Sprains
1. Injuries to **ligaments** and surrounding soft tissues in a joint; structures are partially or completely torn at ligament–bone interface or within ligament; most common in the ankle and knee
2. H/P = pain in involved joint with weight bearing or movement
3. **Treatment** = RICE: Rest, Icing, Compression of swelling, Elevation of joint; analgesics

E. Ligament tears
1. Occur from excessive stress across joints
2. H/P = pain and swelling that worsens with joint stress, decreased joint range of motion; ligamentous **instability** on joint stress testing
3. **Radiology** = magnetic resonance imaging (MRI) may confirm tear
4. **Treatment** = initially, as for sprains; may require surgical repair

F. Meniscus tears (knee)
1. Result from repetitive microtrauma and degeneration or forceful twisting of a planted knee
2. Frequently associated with anterior cruciate ligament (ACL) injury (especially from blunt trauma or sports injuries)
3. H/P = vague pain inside knee joint, clicking or locking of joint; pain along joint line near tear
4. **Radiology** = MRI may detect tear
5. **Treatment** = NSAIDs, physical therapy, arthroscopic repair or debridement
6. **Complications** = meniscal debridement predisposes knee to developing osteoarthritis at an earlier age

G. Compartment syndrome
1. Trauma (surgical or accidental) in extremities leads to reperfusion injury and swelling of fascial compartments; **intracompartmental swelling** can cause compression of neurovascular structures leading to **ischemia** of soft tissues within compartment and distal to site of compression.
2. Most common in **lower leg** (e.g., tibial fracture) and forearm
3. H/P = 6 Ps are signs of progression (**Pain, Pallor, Poikilothermia, Pulselessness, Paresthesia, Paralysis**); compartment pain with passive stretching is best screening test
4. **Labs** = elevated compartment pressures (needle inserted into compartment and attached to manometer to determine pressures)
5. **Treatment** = **emergent fasciotomy** for pressures >30 mm Hg or for pressures within 20 mm Hg of diastolic blood pressure

TABLE 9-1 Common Fractures, Their Mechanism of Injury, and Appropriate Treatment

Type	Bones Involved	History and Physical	Treatment	Clinical Pearls
Colles	Distal radius ± distal ulna	**Fall on outstretched hand**, distal radius is posteriorly displaced and angulated (forearm profile looks like a **dinner fork**)	Closed reduction Long arm cast Possible surgery	Most common wrist fracture, particularly common in osteoporotic bone
Smith	Distal radius	Fall on flexed wrists, distal radius is anteriorly displaced	Cast Closed reduction Possible surgery	Much less common than Colles fracture
Scaphoid	Scaphoid	"Snuffbox" tenderness, fall on radially deviated outstretched hand	Thumb spica cast Possible surgery	Increased risk of AVN; **not seen on X-ray for 1–2 wk after injury**; most common carpal fracture
Boxer	Fifth-metacarpal neck	Punching hard object or surface with a strong force applied to fifth metacarpal	Closed reduction Ulnar gutter splint Surgical pinning	Beware the **"fight bite"**— open wounds from teeth will need surgical exploration to rule out tendon involvement; antibiotics
Humerus	Humerus	Trauma (motor vehicle accident, blunt trauma, etc.)	Closed reduction splint Possible surgery	With wrist drop or weakened thumb abduction, think **radial nerve injury**
Monteggia	Fracture of proximal one-third of ulna with dislocation of radial head	Fall on outstretched arm with arm hyperpronated	Closed reduction of radial head Surgical repair of ulna	
Galeazzi	Fracture of distal shaft of radius and dislocation of DRUJ	Trauma (direct blow or fall)	Surgical repair Cast forearm in supination to maintain reduction of DRUJ	
Hip	Femoral head or neck	Fall, motor vehicle accident, trauma Injured leg is shortened and externally rotated Frequently occurs from strong axial force (e.g., fall or knee hitting a car dashboard)	Surgical repair May require joint replacement	Increased risk for **AVN** and DVT (should **anticoagulate** patient); particularly common in osteoporotic bone
Femur	Femoral diaphysis	Trauma	Surgical repair	Increased risk of fat embolization
Tibial	Tibia	Trauma	Cast Surgical repair	Increased risk for **compartment syndrome**
Ankle	Medial, lateral, and/or posterior malleoli	Trauma, excessive twist of ankle (most commonly supination and external rotation)	Cast Possible surgical repair	
Rib	Nonfloating ribs	Trauma, pain worse during deep breathing	Pain control Possible splinting	
Pelvic	Pelvis	Major trauma	Pain control surgical repair, if in weight-bearing portion	**High risk of major blood loss**

AVN, avascular necrosis; DRUJ, distal radial ulnar joint; DVT, deep vein thrombosis.

Musculoskeletal Disorders

Musculoskeletal Disorders

❈ II. Spine

A. Back pain
1. Back pain can be caused by musculoskeletal, neurologic, neoplastic, infectious, or rheumatic causes (see Figure 9-2).
2. **Treatment** = NSAIDs, physical therapy, or rest for muscular injuries

B. Degenerative disc disease
1. Vertebral disc is composed of a dense annulus fibrosus and a gelatinous nucleus pulposus.
2. Degenerative changes in disc lead to **herniation** (most frequently, posterior or posterior lateral) of nucleus pulposus and subsequent **nerve impingement**.
3. Herniation is most common in the lumbosacral region (L4–L5, L5–S1 discs) but can also be cervical (see Figure 9-3).
4. **H/P** = pain extending from the nerve root **along path of compressed nerve**; characteristic sensory and motor deficits, depending on nerve root involved; pain worsens with straight leg raises or Valsalva maneuver (see Table 9-2)
5. **Radiology** = MRI confirms diagnosis; CT is helpful for analysis of bone structure

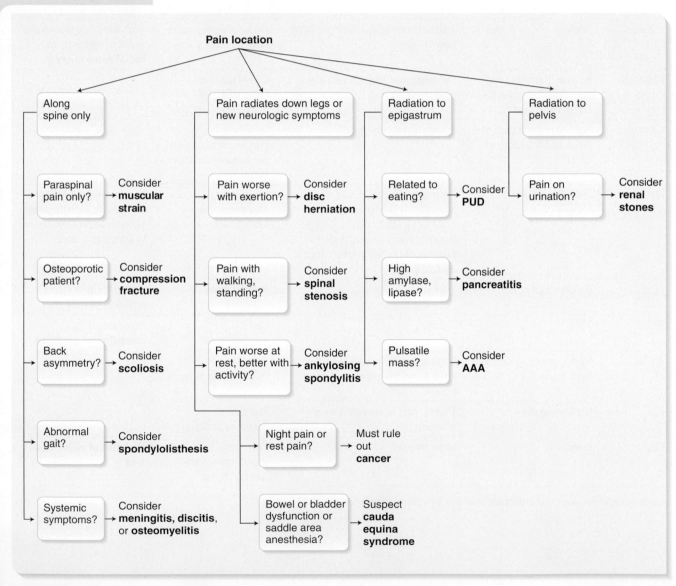

FIGURE
9-2   **Differential diagnosis for back pain.**

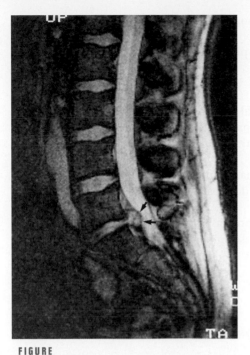

FIGURE 9-3 Magnetic resonance imaging (MRI) of lumbar spine demonstrating herniation of L5–S1 disc (*arrows*) and compression of spinal cord.

(From Daffner, R. H. & Hartman, M. [2013]. *Clinical Radiology: The Essentials* [4th ed., p. 407]. Philadelphia, PA. Wolters Kluwer/Lippincott Williams & Wilkins.)

6. Treatment = disease may be self-limited; NSAIDs, activity modification, epidural injection of anti-inflammatory agents, or surgical decompression can be used, depending on symptom duration and severity

C. Spinal stenosis
1. Generalized narrowing of bony spaces in the spine secondary to arthritic changes, causing nerve compression
2. Most common in middle-aged and older adults
3. H/P = radiating pain that is worse with standing and walking ("pseudoclaudication"), pain relieved when leaning forward while walking or walking uphill

TABLE 9-2 **H/P for Compression of Specific Cervical and Lumbosacral Nerve Roots**

Nerve Root	Reflex	Motor Deficit	Sensory Deficit
C5	Biceps	Deltoid, biceps	Anterior shoulder
C6	Brachioradialis	Biceps, wrist extensors	Lateral forearm
C7	Triceps	Triceps, wrist flexors, finger extensors	Posterior forearm
C8	None	Finger flexors	Fourth and fifth fingers, medial forearm
T1	None	Finger interossei	Axilla
L4	Patellar	Tibialis anterior (foot dorsiflexion)	Medial leg
L5	None	Extensor hallucis longus (first-toe dorsiflexion)	Lateral lower leg, first web space
S1	Achilles	Peroneus longus and brevis (foot eversion), gastrocnemius (foot plantarflexion)	Lateral foot

H/P, history and physical.

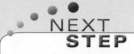

NEXT STEP

Treat **cauda equina syndrome** with **immediate** surgical decompression because it can quickly result in permanent neurologic injury.

MNEMONIC

Remember the organization of the brachial plexus by the mnemonic **R**eal **T**exans **D**rink **C**old **B**eer: **R**oots, **T**runks, **D**ivisions, **C**ords, **B**ranches (proximal to distal).

4. **Radiology** = CT or X-ray confirms diagnosis; MRI may also be helpful to rule out herniation

5. **Treatment** = analgesics (e.g., NSAIDs), physical therapy, epidural injections, surgical decompression

D. Cauda equina syndrome

1. Cauda equina is the extension of the dural-arachnoid sac beyond the inferior tip of the spinal cord and the complex of terminal nerve roots contained within it.

2. Trauma can damage nerves running in the sac; neoplasms can cause nerve compression.

3. **H/P** = **urinary retention** following trauma, change in bowel habits; anesthesia in perineal region (i.e., **saddle anesthesia**), decreased rectal tone or bulbocavernosus reflex

4. **Treatment** = **emergency** surgical decompression of cauda equina; intravenous (IV) corticosteroids commonly given to decrease spinal cord inflammation; radiation used in cases of neoplasm

E. Brachial plexus

1. The brachial plexus is composed of nerve roots C5–T1 and innervates the upper extremity (see Figure 9-4).

2. Brachial plexus disorders are related to specific mechanisms of injury (see Table 9-3).

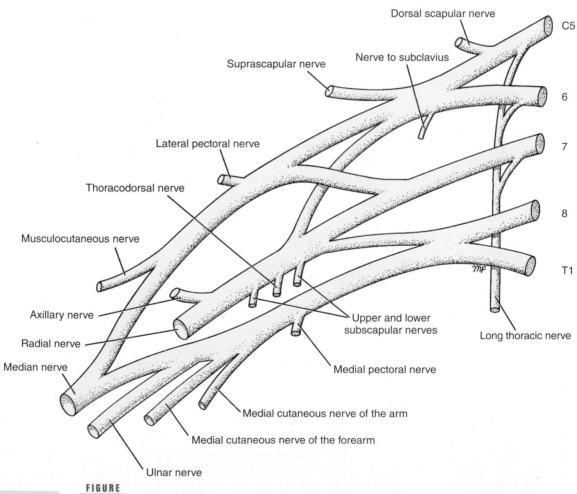

FIGURE 9-4 **Diagram of major neural branches of the brachial plexus.**

(From Snell, R. S. [2008]. *Clinical Anatomy By Regions* [8th ed., p. 772]. Philadelphia, PA: Lippincott Williams & Wilkins.)

TABLE 9-3	Common Brachial Plexus Disorders		
Condition	**Site of Injury**	**Cause of Injury**	**Clinical Features**
Erb-Duchenne palsy	Superior trunk	Hyperadduction of arm causing widening of the humeral-glenoid gap (e.g., **birth, shoulder dystocia**)	**Waiter's tip** (arm extended and adducted with pronated forearm)
Claw hand	Ulnar nerve	Epiphyseal separation of medial epicondyle of humerus	Weak finger adduction, poor fourth- or fifth-finger flexion, clawed fourth or fifth fingers from **lumbrical weakness**
Wrist drop	Posterior cord or radial nerve	Mid-humerus fracture causes nerve impingement or tear	Inability to extend wrist or fingers; loss of sensation from dorsal hand
Deltoid paralysis	Axillary nerve	**Anterior shoulder dislocation** causes axillary nerve impingement or stretching	Impaired shoulder abduction or elevation
Klumpke palsy	Posterior or medial cords	Hyperabduction of arm places excess tension on lower cords and nearby sympathetic chain	**Claw hand**, poor wrist and hand function, association with Horner syndrome

III. Metabolic Bone Diseases

A. Osteoporosis

1. Substantial osteopenia (i.e., decreased bone density) but normal mineralization in existing bone stock
2. Results from decreased bone formation or increased resorption of bone
3. Peak bone mass occurs at 20 to 25 years of age.
4. **Risk factors** = inadequate dietary calcium during young adulthood, smoking, excessive alcohol consumption, sedentary lifestyle, decreased estrogen or testosterone (e.g., postmenopausal), long-term steroid use, hyperparathyroidism, hyperthyroidism; typical patients are thin, white, postmenopausal women
5. **H/P** = usually asymptomatic until fractures (e.g., Colles, femoral neck, and vertebral) and neurovascular impingement occur
6. **Radiology** = decreased bone density evident on dual-energy X-ray absorptiometry (DEXA), X-ray, and CT
7. **Treatment**
   a. Prevention is key, with exercise and sufficient calcium and vitamin D in diet (especially before the peak bone density age of 35 years) important for maintaining bone stock.
   b. **Bisphosphonates** decrease osteoclast activity (less bone resorption), increase bone density, and decrease fracture risk.
   c. Selective estrogen receptor modulators (e.g., raloxifene) help increase bone density with fewer adverse effects than classic hormone replacement therapy.
   d. Pulsatile teriparatide (recombinant human parathyroid hormone) stimulates osteoblasts and bone remodeling; it may be used for up to 2 years.

B. Osteopetrosis

1. Increased bone density caused by impaired osteoclast activity
2. **H/P** = increased incidence of fractures, possible blindness or deafness, variable neurologic symptoms (from bony compression of nerves), impaired fracture healing
3. **Labs** = decreased hemoglobin (Hgb), decreased hematocrit (Hct) (via narrowing of marrow cavities), increased acid phosphatase, increased creatine kinase (CK)
4. **Radiology** = general increased bone density seen on X-ray, including thickening of cranium and vertebrae
5. **Treatment** = transfusion of marrow components necessary for osteoclast production, activity restriction

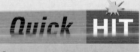

Quick HIT

Osteoporosis is **less** likely to occur in **obese** people, because the increased load placed on bones helps to prevent osteopenia.

Quick HIT

Hormone and electrolyte levels will be normal for age in osteoporosis unless an underlying **endocrine** disorder exists.

Quick HIT

X-rays will only show changes in osteoporotic bone after significant bone loss.

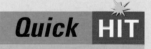

Quick HIT

Hormone replacement therapy is no longer considered acceptable for osteoporosis prevention because it carries increased risks for breast cancer, deep vein thrombosis (DVT), coronary artery disease (CAD), and stroke.

Musculoskeletal Disorders

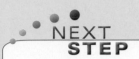

NEXT STEP

If a patient complains that "my hats no longer fit," consider a workup for Paget disease or osteopetrosis.

C. Paget disease of bone

1. Overactive osteoclasts and osteoblasts leading to excessive bone turnover and disorganized bony architecture
2. **H/P** = possibly, asymptomatic or deep bone pain, increased incidence of fractures; **tibial bowing**, kyphosis, **increased cranial diameter**, deafness (from changes in auditory ossicles)
3. **Labs** = increased alkaline phosphatase; increased urine hydroxyproline; normal calcium and phosphorus
4. **Radiology** = X-rays may demonstrate osteolytic lesions and expanded hyperdense bone; bone scan will detect diffuse "hot spots" in areas of active disease
5. **Treatment** = bisphosphonates, calcitonin

D. Osteogenesis imperfecta

1. Defective production of collagen from a genetic disorder
2. Diagnosis primarily made during childhood
3. **H/P** = frequent **fractures** from **minimal** trauma, **blue sclerae**, skin and teeth deformities, possible deafness, joint hypermobility (may resemble child abuse)
4. **Treatment** = activity restriction, surgical correction of bony misalignment, bisphosphonates decrease fracture risk

E. Gout

1. Peripheral monoarthritis caused by deposition of **sodium urate crystals** in joints
2. **Risk factors** = renal disease, male gender, obesity, excessive consumption of purine-rich foods, urate underexcretion, diuretic use, cyclosporine use, cancer, hemoglobinopathies
3. **H/P**
   a. **Sudden severe pain** and **swelling** in one joint that frequently starts at night
   b. First metatarsophalangeal joint most commonly affected (i.e., **podagra**); ankle, knee, and foot joints also common sites
   c. Possible concurrent fever, chills, or malaise
4. **Labs** = serum uric acid can be normal or increased; joint aspiration shows **needle-shaped**, **negatively birefringent crystals** and several white blood cells (WBCs) (see Figure 9-5)
5. **Radiology** = X-ray may rarely show bony erosions in chronic cases, and possibly tophi

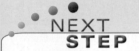

NEXT STEP

Allopurinol should **not** be administered in acute attacks of gout.

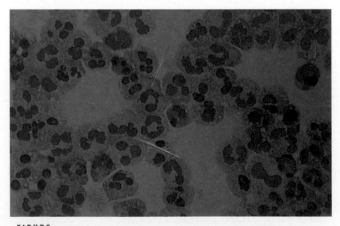

FIGURE 9-5 **Synovial aspirate from patient with gout.**

Note needle-shaped, negatively birefringent sodium urate crystals that are visible under polarized light microscopy. (From McClatchey, K. D. [2002]. *Clinical Laboratory Medicine* [2nd ed., Figure 27-17]. Philadelphia, PA: Lippincott Williams & Wilkins; with permission.)

6. **Treatment**
   a. NSAIDs (especially indomethacin), colchicine, corticosteroids
   b. Decreasing alcohol and diuretic use and avoiding foods high in purines (e.g., red meats, fish) may help prevent exacerbations.
   c. Allopurinol (inhibits uric acid formation) or probenecid (inhibits kidney uric acid resorption) used in cases of chronic gout to prevent flare-ups
7. **Complications** = long-standing disease leads to chronic tophaceous gout with formation of nodular tophi (large deposits of crystals in soft tissues), leading to permanent deformity

F. Pseudogout (calcium pyrophosphate dihydrate deposition disease or CPPD)

1. Calcium pyrophosphate dihydrate crystal deposition in joints
2. Familial condition associated with other endocrine diseases (e.g., DM, hyperparathyroidism)
3. **H/P** = similar presentation to gout but **less severe symptoms**; **knee** and **wrist** most commonly initially affected joints
4. **Labs** = joint aspiration shows **positively birefringent, rhomboid crystals** (see Figure 9-6)
5. **Radiology** = X-ray may show chondrocalcinosis (i.e., calcification of articular cartilage in joints)
6. **Treatment** = NSAIDs, colchicine

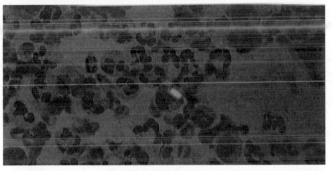

 FIGURE 9-6 Synovial aspirate from patient with calcium pyrophosphate dihydrate deposition disease; under polarized light microscopy, rhomboid-shaped calcium pyrophosphate dihydrate crystals appear positively birefringent.

(From McClatchey, K. D. [2002]. *Clinical Laboratory Medicine* [2nd ed., Figure 27-22]. Philadelphia, PA: Lippincott Williams & Wilkins; with permission.)

IV. Infection

A. Septic joint and septic arthritis

1. Most commonly occurs through **hematogenous spread** of bacteria, extension of local infection, or direct inoculation (e.g., open fracture)
2. Most commonly caused by *Staphylococcus aureus*; consider *Neisseria gonorrhoeae* in young, sexually active patients
3. Consider gram-negative rods in patients with DM, cancer, or other underlying illnesses.
4. Preexisting arthritis increases risk of progressive damage to cartilage.
5. **H/P** = sudden onset of joint pain (usually monoarticular); warm, red, tender, swollen joint, pain with any motion (i.e., micromotion tenderness), possible overlying skin lesions; children may show vague signs of pain and refusal to walk
6. **Labs** = increased WBCs, erythrocyte sedimentation rate (ESR), and C-reactive protein (CRP); joint aspiration shows **numerous WBCs** (lower for *N. gonorrhoeae* than *S. aureus*) with a high percentage of neutrophils and decreased glucose; positive cultures (frequent false-negative findings for *N. gonorrhoeae*) (see Table 9-4)

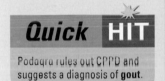

Quick HIT

Podagra rules out CPPD and suggests a diagnosis of **gout**.

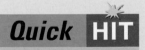

Quick HIT

The body's inflammatory response to bacteria in the joint is the cause of cartilage destruction in joint sepsis.

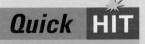

Quick HIT

Because the inflammatory response to *N. gonorrhoeae* is not as severe as that for other bacteria, I&D is not required for treatment.

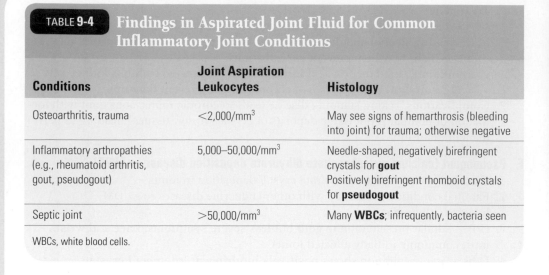

TABLE 9-4	Findings in Aspirated Joint Fluid for Common Inflammatory Joint Conditions	
Conditions	**Joint Aspiration Leukocytes**	**Histology**
Osteoarthritis, trauma	<2,000/mm³	May see signs of hemarthrosis (bleeding into joint) for trauma; otherwise negative
Inflammatory arthropathies (e.g., rheumatoid arthritis, gout, pseudogout)	5,000–50,000/mm³	Needle-shaped, negatively birefringent crystals for **gout** Positively birefringent rhomboid crystals for **pseudogout**
Septic joint	>50,000/mm³	Many **WBCs**; infrequently, bacteria seen

WBCs, white blood cells.

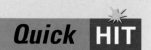
7. **Treatment = surgical irrigation and drainage** (I&D) required for any infection other than *N. gonorrhoeae*; for *N. gonorrhoeae*, use IV ceftriaxone and doxycycline for possible *Chlamydia* coinfection; for *S. aureus*, use penicillinase-resistant penicillin; for gram-negative bacteria, use aminoglycosides

B. Osteomyelitis

1. **Bone infection** via hematogenous spread or local extension
2. *S. aureus* and *Pseudomonas* most common causes; consider *Salmonella* in patients with **sickle cell disease**
3. **H/P** = bone pain, tenderness, fever, chills; possible skin involvement with a draining sinus
4. **Labs** = increased WBC, ESR, and CRP; cultures needed to define appropriate antibiotic therapy
5. **Radiology** = X-rays are not helpful initially and only show signs of infection after 10 days; MRI demonstrates bone edema early in disease; bone scan will show increased uptake after 72 hr; tagged-WBC scan is more sensitive than standard bone scan
6. **Treatment** = IV antibiotics for 4 to 6 weeks (empiric initially, pathogen specific following culture); I&D must be performed for an abscess inside the bone (i.e., sequestrum) or in surrounding tissue
7. **Complications** = inadequately treated infection can lead to chronic osteomyelitis that is difficult to cure or may require amputation

C. Lyme disease

1. Caused by *Borrelia burgdorferi*; the organism is delivered through the bite of the *Ixodes* tick
2. **H/P**
   a. Early localized stage: chills, fatigue, arthralgias, headache; **erythema chronicum migrans** (i.e., bull's eye rash), fever (see Figure 9-7)
   b. Early disseminated stage: **myocarditis weeks to months** after infection, cardiac arrhythmias, heart block, **Bell palsy**, sensory-motor neuropathies, aseptic meningitis, or meningoencephalitis
   c. Late disseminated stage: a **few months to years** later, chronic synovitis, **mono-arthritis or oligoarthritis**, subacute encephalopathy, or polyneuropathy may develop
3. **Labs** = positive enzyme-linked immunosorbent assay (ELISA) and western blot tests for antibodies; joint aspiration is not helpful
4. **Treatment = doxycycline**, amoxicillin, or cefuroxime (oral form can be used in early disease, but IV forms are required in disseminated disease)

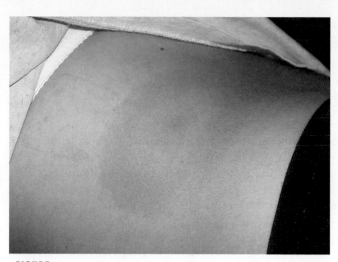

Patient with Lyme disease exhibiting erythema chronicum migrans (bull's eye rash).

(From Goodheart, H. P. [2003]. *Goodheart's Photoguide of Common Skin Disorders* [2nd ed., Figure 7-19]. Philadelphia, PA: Lippincott Williams & Wilkins; with permission.)

V. Osteoarthritis (OA)

A. Degenerative joint disease

1. Chronic, noninflammatory joint degeneration involving articular cartilage deterioration
2. Most commonly affects hips, knees, ankles, hands, wrists, and shoulders; can cause spinal stenosis in vertebral bodies
3. **Risk factors** — advanced age, family history, obesity, previous joint trauma, repetitive joint stress (heavy labor occupations)
4. **H/P** = joint crepitus, insidious onset of joint stiffness and pain that **worsens with activity and weight bearing** and is relieved by rest, no systemic symptoms; patients have decreased range of motion, bony protuberances in the distal interphalangeal (DIP) (i.e., **Heberden nodes**) and proximal interphalangeal (PIP) (i.e., **Bouchard nodes**) joints
5. **Labs** = normal ESR; <2,000 leukocytes on joint aspiration
6. **Radiology** = X-ray demonstrates osteophyte formation, joint space narrowing, subchondral bone sclerosis, and subchondral bone cyst formation (see Figure 9-8)

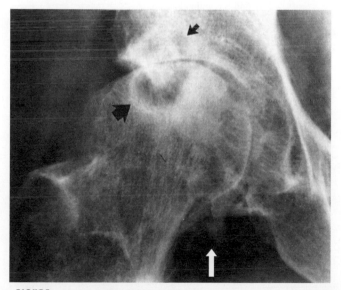

Osteoarthritis in a right hip joint; synovial cysts (*black arrows*) and osteophytes (*white arrow*) are evident.

(Modified from Daffner, R. H. & Hartman M. [2013]. *Clinical Radiology: The Essentials* [4th ed., p. 383]. Philadelphia, PA: Wolters Kluwer/Lippincott Williams & Wilkins.)

Quick HIT

- **Osteoarthritis**: typically **asymmetric** and may only affect one joint; DIP joints are frequently involved in hands.
- **RA**: affects joints on both sides of the body in a **symmetric** distribution; DIP joints are spared in hands.

Musculoskeletal Disorders

7. **Treatment** = activity modification, heat, analgesics (e.g., NSAIDs), weight loss, physical therapy, corticosteroid or hyaluronic acid injections, joint replacement in advanced cases

 # VI. Rheumatologic Diseases

A. Rheumatoid arthritis (RA)

1. Chronic inflammatory disorder with infiltration of synovial joints by inflammatory cells and progressive erosion of cartilage and bone
2. **Synovial hypertrophy** with granulation tissue formation on articular cartilage (i.e., **pannus formation**) caused by joint inflammation
3. Most commonly seen in middle-aged women; increased frequency in people with HLA-DR4 serotype
4. **PIP** and metacarpophalangeal (**MCP**) joints are usually first involved; **symmetric polyarthropathy** develops, involving ankles, knees, shoulders, hips, elbows, and spine.
5. **H/P**
   a. Malaise, weight loss, insidious onset of **morning stiffness with pain**, decreased mobility
   b. Warm joints, joint swelling, fevers, ulnar deviation of fingers; MCP hypertrophy, **swan-neck deformities** (i.e., flexed DIP plus hyperextended PIP), **boutonniere deformities** (i.e., flexed PIP), subcutaneous nodules, pleuritis, pericarditis, scleritis
6. **Labs**
   a. Rheumatoid factor (RF) positive in 75% of patients but not specific for the disease
   b. Positive anti-citrullinated peptide antibodies (ACPA) is >90% specific for RA
   c. Positive antinuclear antibodies (ANA) in 40% of patients (see Table 9-5)
   d. Joint aspiration shows 5,000 to 50,000 leukocytes.

TABLE 9-5	Immunologic Markers Found in Rheumatic Diseases
Disease	**Immunologic Markers**
Systemic lupus erythematosus (SLE)	ANA (95% of patients) Anti-dsDNA antibodies (60% of patients) Anti-Sm antibodies False-positive RPR or VDRL (syphilis test)
Drug-induced lupus	Antihistone antibodies ANA
Rheumatoid arthritis (RA)	RF (75% of patients) ACPA ANA (<50% of patients) HLA-DR4 common
Polymyositis or dermatomyositis	ANA Anti-Jo-1 antibodies
Ankylosing spondylitis	HLA-B27 (90% of patients)
Psoriatic arthritis	Possible HLA-B27
Scleroderma	Anti-scl-70 ANA
CREST syndrome	Anticentromere antibodies
Mixed connective tissue disease (MCTD)	Anti-RNP ANA
Sjögren syndrome	Anti-Ro (anti-SSA) ANA Anti-La (anti-SSB) ANA

ANA, antinuclear antibodies; CREST, calcinosis, Raynaud, esophageal dysmotility, sclerodactyly, and telangiectasias; dsDNA, double-stranded DNA; RF, rheumatoid factor; RPR, rapid plasma reagin.

7. **Radiology** = X-rays may demonstrate soft tissue swellings, joint space narrowing, marginal bony erosions, or subluxation; MRI is more sensitive than X-ray for detecting similar findings

8. Treatment = disease-modifying antirheumatic drugs (DMARDs)
   a. Hydroxychloroquine or sulfasalazine for mild disease
   b. Methotrexate or TNF-α inhibitors (e.g., etanercept, adalimumab) for moderate disease
   c. Leflunomide, anakinra, or combination therapy for severe or refractory disease
   d. Glucocorticoids and NSAIDs may be used for acute flares of arthritis

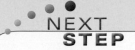

NEXT STEP

Check PPD to screen for latent tuberculosis before starting a TNF-α inhibitor.

B. Systemic lupus erythematosus (SLE)

1. Multisystem autoimmune disorder involving a variety of autoantibodies affecting several body systems
2. Antibody-mediated cellular attack occurs with deposition of antigen-antibody complexes in affected tissues.
3. **Risk factors** = young women, blacks, Asians, Hispanics
4. Sulfonamides, hydralazine, isoniazid, phenytoin, and procainamide can cause similar symptoms that **resolve** when the **drug is discontinued**.
5. H/P
   a. Common findings include malar and discoid rashes, serositis, oral ulcers, arthritis, photosensitivity, CNS symptoms, cardiac symptoms, and renal symptoms (see Figure 9-9).
   b. Can also experience fevers, malaise, weight loss, abdominal pain, vomiting, conjunctivitis, blindness
   c. Any combination of symptoms is possible and can change during the course of the disease.
6. Labs
   a. Positive ANA in 95% of patients (see Table 9-5)
   b. Anti–double-stranded DNA (dsDNA) antibodies found in 60% of patients but not found in other rheumatologic disorders
   c. Presence of anti-Sm antibodies is very specific for disease.
   d. Antihistone antibodies may be seen with drug-induced lupus-like symptoms.
   e. Patients frequently have a **false-positive test** for **syphilis**.
   f. Antiphospholipid (anticardiolipin) antibodies
   g. Decreased complement (C3 and C4)

Skin disorders

- **Malar (butterfly) rash**
- **Discoid rash**
- **Photosensitivity**
- **Oral ulcers**

Inflammatory disorders

- **Arthritis** (symmetric nonerosive arthritis in PIPs, MCPs, wrists, knees, feet)
- **Serositis** (pleuritis, pneumonitis, pericarditis)
- **Antinuclear antibodies (ANA)** increased

Organ system disorders

- **Renal disease** (immune complex glomerulonephritis, interstitial nephritis, proteinuria, increased BUN & creatinine)
- **Neurologic disorders** (psychosis, seizures, stroke, neuropathy)
- **Hematologic disorders** (autoimmune hemolytic anemia, leukopenia, thrombocytopenia)
- **Immunologic disorders** (anti-double-stranded DNA [dsDNA] antibodies, anti-Smith antibodies, antiphospholipid antibodies)

FIGURE 9-9 Diagnostic criteria for systemic lupus erythematosus.

BUN, blood urea nitrogen; MCPs, metacarpophalangeal joints; PIPs, proximal interphalangeal joints.

7. **Treatment** = avoidance of sun, NSAIDs given for pain, hydroxychloroquine improves skin and renal symptoms, corticosteroids given for immunosuppression and to decrease exacerbations, other immunosuppressant drugs given in cases resistant to corticosteroids, anticoagulation required if patient considered hypercoagulable

8. **Complications** = lupus anticoagulant and anticardiolipin antibodies increase the risks of miscarriage and fetal death; disease follows variable course, with some cases remaining benign and others progressing rapidly; patient death results from progressive impairment of lung, heart, brain, and kidney function

C. Polymyositis and dermatomyositis

1. Progressive systemic diseases with skeletal muscle inflammation; one-third of patients with polymyositis also have dermatomyositis (i.e., polymyositis with skin manifestations)
2. **Risk factors** = more common in women, blacks, elderly
3. **H/P**
   a. Symmetric progressive **proximal** muscle weakness (occurs in **legs first**) and myalgias, muscle atrophy in later stages of disease
   b. Cutaneous manifestations of dermatomyositis are a **red heliotropic rash** on the face, upper extremities, chest, or back; violet discoloration of eyelids or scaly patches over hand joints
   c. Patients with lung involvement have dyspnea and poor oxygenation saturation.
4. **Labs**
   a. Increased creatinine, aldolase, CK, aspartate aminotransferase (AST), alanine aminotransferase (ALT), and lactate dehydrogenase (LDH)
   b. ANA frequently positive
   c. Anti-Jo-1 antibodies in patients with interstitial lung disease (see Table 9-5)
   d. Muscle biopsy shows inflammatory cells and muscle degeneration, inflammatory cells **within** muscle fascicles in **polymyositis**, and **surrounding** muscle fascicles in **dermatomyositis**.
5. **EMG** = spontaneous fibrillations
6. **Treatment** = high-dose **glucocorticoids** for 4 to 6 weeks followed by a 6- to 12-month taper; azathioprine or methotrexate if unresponsive to glucocorticoids; IV immune globulin or rituximab can be added to regimen in resistant cases
7. **Complications** = possible interstitial lung disease, increased risk of several malignancies

D. Polymyalgia rheumatica (PMR)

1. Rheumatic disease with multiple sites of joint pain and frequently associated with **temporal arteritis**; most common in elderly women (see Chapter 1, **Cardiovascular Disorders**)
2. **H/P** = pain and stiffness in shoulder and pelvic girdle, difficulty raising arms and getting out of bed because of pain, malaise, unexplained weight loss; fever, minimal joint swelling, muscle strength maintained, although movement limited by pain
3. **Labs** = decreased Hct, **markedly increased ESR**, negative RF
4. **Radiology** = MRI demonstrates increased signal at tendon sheaths and synovial tissue outside of joints; positron emission tomographic (PET) scan shows increased uptake in large vessels
5. **Treatment** = low-dose corticosteroids, followed by tapered dosing

E. Fibromyalgia

1. Disease causing **chronic pain** in muscles and tendons in absence of apparent inflammation
2. Unknown etiology, but frequently associated with **depression**, anxiety, and irritable bowel disease
3. Possible predisposition with hypothyroidism, RA, sleep apnea; more common in women 20 to 50 years of age
4. **H/P** = myalgias and weakness without inflammation; "trigger points" on examination (i.e., specific locations that when stimulated reproduce pain symptoms),

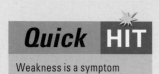

Quick HIT

Weakness is a symptom of **polymyositis** but not of polymyalgia rheumatica.

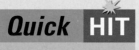

Quick HIT

Patients with PMR will frequently experience significant symptomatic improvement after just 1 day of corticosteroid administration.

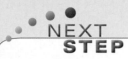

NEXT STEP

Once polymyalgia rheumatica has been diagnosed, the patient should automatically have a workup for **temporal arteritis**.

fatigue; possible depression, sleep disturbances, dizziness, headaches, and mood disturbances

5. **Treatment** = stretching, antidepressants (e.g., tricyclic antidepressants [TCAs], selective serotonin reuptake inhibitors [SSRIs]), patient education, physical therapy modalities

F. Ankylosing spondylitis

1. Chronic inflammatory disease of the **spine** and pelvis that results in eventual bone fusion
2. **Risk factors** = 20 to 40 years of age, male > female, white > black
3. **H/P**
   a. Hip and low back pain that is **worse in the morning** and **following inactivity; pain improves over course of day**
   b. Possible limited range of motion in spine, hip, or chest
   c. Painful kyphosis that is relieved by bending forward
   d. Possible self-limited anterior uveitis
4. **Labs** = positive HLA-B27 in 90% of patients, increased or normal ESR, negative RF, negative ANA (see Table 9-5)
5. **Radiology** = X-ray shows **bamboo spine** (multiple vertebral fusions); MRI shows increased signal in sacroiliac joints and vertebrae
6. **Treatment** = physical therapy, NSAIDs; exercise helps to prevent or delay permanent deformities; sulfasalazine, methotrexate, or anti-TNF drugs may be beneficial in more significant disease; joint replacement may be needed in extremities

G. Psoriatic arthritis

1. Arthritis that develops in 10% to 20% of patients with **psoriasis**; DIP joints and spine most commonly affected
2. **H/P** = asymmetric joint pain and stiffness, symptoms worse in morning and improve with activity, symptoms usually less severe than RA, possible anterior uveitis; joint line pain, pain with stress on joints, pitting of nails
3. **Labs** = negative RF and ANA, possible positive HLA-B27 (see Table 9-5)
4. **Radiology** = X-rays show findings similar to RA and highly destructive lesions of DIP and PIP joints (i.e., "pencil in cup" deformities); MRI is more sensitive in finding marrow edema
5. **Treatment** = NSAIDs, methotrexate, sulfasalazine, or anti-TNF drugs, depending on severity

H. Scleroderma

1. Chronic multisystem sclerosis with accumulation of connective tissue, skin thickening, and visceral involvement
2. **H/P** = arthralgias, myalgias, hand swelling, **Raynaud phenomenon** (i.e., blue distal extremities caused by arteriolar spasm), **skin thickening, esophageal dysmotility,** intestinal hypomotility, dyspnea, possible arrhythmias or heart failure
3. **Labs** = positive anti-scl-70 ANA (see Table 9-5)
4. **CREST syndrome** is a variant with Calcinosis, Raynaud phenomenon, Esophageal dysmotility, Sclerodactyly, and Telangiectasias
   a. Skin thickening limited to distal extremities and face
   b. Labs show anticentromere antibodies (see Table 9-5).
   c. Better prognosis than scleroderma
5. **Treatment** = supportive care; angiotensin-converting enzyme inhibitors (ACE-I) for malignant renal hypertension; calcium channel blockers and avoidance of caffeine, nicotine, and decongestants to relieve Raynaud symptoms; methotrexate or corticosteroids may improve skin thickening and pulmonary symptoms
6. **Complications** = pulmonary fibrosis, heart failure, acute renal failure caused by malignant renal hypertension

I. Mixed connective tissue disease (MCTD)

1. Overlapping features of SLE, scleroderma, and polymyositis
2. Can progress to a single diagnosis

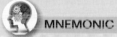

MNEMONIC

Remember the seronegative spondyloarthropathies (arthritic conditions involving the spine that are negative for rheumatoid factor) by the mnemonic **PAIR:**
Psoriatic arthritis
Ankylosing spondylitis
Inflammatory bowel disease-associated arthritis
Reactive arthritis

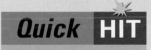

Quick HIT

Raynaud phenomenon may prohibit accurate measuring of pulse oximetry via a fingertip probe.

Musculoskeletal Disorders

3. **H/P** = **Raynaud phenomenon**, polyarthralgias, arthritis, swollen hands, proximal muscle weakness, esophageal hypomotility, pulmonary symptoms; absence of renal and neurologic symptoms
4. **Labs** = positive antiribonucleoprotein (RNP) ANA (see Table 9-5)
5. **Treatment** = NSAIDs, corticosteroids, ACE-I, supportive measures

J. Sjögren syndrome

1. Autoimmune disorder with lymphocytic infiltration of exocrine glands
2. Can be seen in association with RA, SLE, or primary biliary cirrhosis
3. **H/P** = **dry eyes, dry mouth**, enlarged parotid glands, purpura on legs, peripheral neuropathy, possible symmetric arthritis associated with other autoimmune conditions
4. **Labs** = positive anti-Ro (anti-SSA) and anti-La (anti-SSB) antibodies (see Table 9-5)
5. **Treatment** = supportive care, corticosteroids for significant symptoms

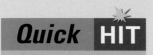

Quick HIT

Sicca syndrome is Sjögren syndrome **without** a secondary autoimmune association.

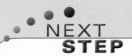

NEXT STEP

Because most bone tumors are metastases and not primary tumors, any patient with a new bone tumor should have a full workup to look for a tumor source.

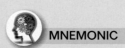

MNEMONIC

Remember the tumors that metastasize to bone by the mnemonic **P**ermanently **R**elocated **T**umors **L**ike **L**ong **B**ones: **P**rostate, **R**enal cell, **T**hyroid, **L**ung, **L**ymphoma, **B**reast.

VII. Neoplasms

A. Bone metastases

1. **Most common** bone tumors in adults
2. Can result from nearly any primary tumor (most commonly breast, renal cell, prostate, lung, thyroid, lymphoma)
3. **H/P** = presence of primary form of cancer; deep bone pain, possible palpable bone mass, **fractures following minor trauma**
4. **Labs** = biopsy is important to identifying source of metastasis
5. **Radiology** = X-ray identifies lesion in a bone; bone scan suggests extent of metastases in body; MRI useful to determine extent of a lesion
6. **Treatment** = chemotherapy as for primary tumor; bisphosphonates help slow bone loss; radiation therapy helps to decrease metastasis size; fixation of fractures required; prophylactic fixation may be performed for impending fractures

B. Osteosarcoma

1. Most common **primary** malignant bone tumor; more common in adolescents, male > female
2. Most frequently involves distal femur, proximal tibia, or proximal humerus
3. **Risk factors** = Paget disease of bone, p53 genetic mutations, familial retinoblastoma, radiation exposure, bone infarcts
4. **H/P** = deep bony pain, later development of palpable bony mass
5. **Labs** = increased alkaline phosphatase, increased ESR, increased LDH; biopsy provides definitive diagnosis
6. **Radiology** = X-ray shows bone lesion with a **sunburst** pattern and **Codman triangle** (i.e., periosteal new bone formation at the diaphyseal end of the lesion) (see Figure 9-10); MRI or PET scan useful for determining extent of lesion; chest CT routinely performed to look for metastases
7. **Treatment** = radical surgical excision, chemotherapy
8. **Complications** = 90% 5-year survival rate for low-grade disease, 50% 5-year survival for higher grade lesions

C. Ewing sarcoma

1. Highly malignant cartilage tumor occurring in diaphysis of long bones; most common in **children**, 5 to 15 years of age
2. **H/P** = bony pain, tissue swelling, fever, fatigue, weight loss, fractures with minor trauma; possible palpable mass
3. **Labs** = increased WBCs, decreased Hgb, increased ESR; biopsy important for making diagnosis
4. **Radiology** = X-ray may detect large destructive lesions with significant periosteal reaction (Codman triangle, or "onion-skin" bone lesion); MRI determines extent of lesion
5. **Treatment** = radiation, adjuvant chemotherapy, radical excision
6. **Complications** = 60% 5-year survival rate when both radiation and chemotherapy are used in nonmetastatic disease, 20% 5-year survival with metastases

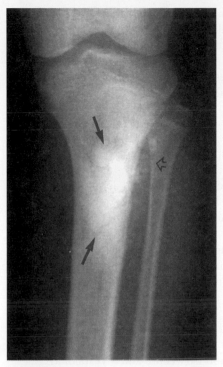

FIGURE
9-10 Osteosarcoma in left proximal tibia.

Note the dense sunburst pattern of the lesion (*solid black arrows*) and presence of Codman triangle (*open arrow*). (From Daffner, R. H. & Hartman, M. [2013]. *Clinical Radiology: The Essentials* [4th ed., p. 357]. Philadelphia, PA; Wolters Kluwer/Lippincott Williams & Wilkins.)

D. Osteochondroma
1. Most common **benign** bone tumor in metaphysis of long bones; more common in patients <25 years of age, male > female
2. Typically occurs in lower femur or upper tibia
3. H/P = irritated soft tissues overlying mass, mass itself frequently nontender; palpable hard mass
4. **Radiology** = X-ray shows bony growth off metaphysis of long bone; CT or MRI shows cancellous portion of long bone to be continuous with interior of lesion
5. **Treatment** = none necessary unless causing soft tissue irritation or neurovascular compromise or if continued growth occurs (surgical excision indicated)
6. **Complications** = rare (1%) transformation into chondrosarcoma

⬡ VIII. Pediatric Orthopedics

A. Developmental dysplasia of the hip (DDH)
1. Perinatal displacement of the femoral head from acetabulum disrupting normal development of the hip joint
2. Occurs because of poor development of acetabulum *in utero*
3. **Risk factors** = female > male, firstborn children, babies delivered in breech presentation, oligohydramnios
4. **H/P**
   a. Children have delayed walking or abnormal gait if diagnosis not made early.
   b. Positive **Barlow** and **Ortolani** maneuvers (provocation of hip dislocation or reduction)
   c. Knees at unequal heights when hips and knees flexed (i.e., **Galeazzi sign**)
   d. Trendelenburg gait (i.e., sagging of opposite hip)
   e. Asymmetric skin folds
5. **Radiology** = **ultrasound** is the most commonly used method of imaging hip congruity; X-rays are not helpful in making a diagnosis until after 4 months of age

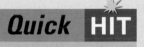

Quick **HIT**

A bony growth on a long bone that sits on top of cortical bone and is **not continuous** with the normal cancellous bone is concerning for a malignant lesion.

6. **Treatment** = **Pavlik harness** used in children <6 months of age; closed or open reduction and Spica casting performed in children 6 months to 2 years of age; open reduction performed after age 2 years; correction may not be performed after age 8 years because of reduced benefit
7. **Complications** = permanent hip dysplasia results from inadequately treated cases; likelihood of successful treatment and normal hip development improves with earlier treatment

B. Slipped capital femoral epiphysis (SCFE)

1. Separation through growth plate of femoral epiphysis from metaphysis
2. **Risk factors** = **adolescent, obese**, black race, hypothyroidism
3. **H/P** = thigh and knee pain; limp, limited internal rotation and abduction of the hip; hip flexion produces obligatory external hip rotation
4. **Radiology** = X-rays indicate posterior and medial displacement of the femoral head from the femoral metaphysis
5. **Treatment** = surgical pinning, weight-bearing restrictions following repair if unstable (unable to bear weight on presentation), prophylactic pinning of normal contralateral side performed in cases of hypothyroidism
6. **Complications** = increased risk of avascular necrosis (AVN) and premature osteoarthritis if treatment is not performed early

C. Legg-Calvé-Perthes disease

1. AVN of capital femoral epiphysis most common between 3 and 8 years of age
2. **H/P** = gradual progressive limp, insidious onset of pain, decreased range of motion
3. **Radiology** = X-ray shows asymmetric hips; affected femoral head appears small with sclerotic bone and widened joint space
4. **Treatment** = containment of hip within acetabulum via bracing or surgical means; **acetabular reconstruction performed in cases of permanent hip dysplasia**
5. **Complications** = 50% untreated cases recover fully; increased risk of hip complications in adulthood, including osteoarthritis, progressive AVN, and need for early arthroplasty in cases of permanent dysplasia

D. Osgood-Schlatter disease

1. Inflammation of the bone–cartilage interface of the tibial tubercle (i.e., osteochondritis)
2. Most common in young boys during pubertal growth spurt
3. **H/P** = pain at involved site that worsens with activity
4. **Treatment** = stretching exercises, NSAIDs

E. Club foot

1. Inversion of foot, plantar flexion of ankle, and adduction of forefoot
2. **H/P** = child who is slow to walk, limp; obvious defect on examination
3. **Treatment** = **serial casting** of foot in correct position; surgery required in long-standing cases to release contractures and modify bone alignment

F. Physeal fractures

1. Fractures involving the growth plate of growing bones; described by Salter-Harris classification system (see Table 9-6)
2. Most heal uneventfully, but some will result in impairment of bone growth at site of injury.
3. **H/P** = pain at site of injury; possible gross deformity, swelling, warmth at fracture site; growth disturbance with limb inequality seen in cases of permanent physeal damage
4. **Radiology** = X-ray demonstrates fracture at site of injury; premature closure of physis seen in cases of growth disturbance
5. **Treatment** = adequate reduction and immobilization, fixation for unstable fractures; growth disturbance may require limb-lengthening procedures, excision of closed portion of physis, or epiphysiodesis of contralateral physis (i.e., surgical disturbance of physis) to achieve equal limb size

TABLE 9-6	Salter-Harris Classification of Physeal Fractures	
Type	**Description**	**Prognosis**
I	Physeal separation without extension into adjacent bone	Good with adequate reduction, quick healing
II	Partial physeal separation with proximal extension into metaphysis	Good; rare growth disturbance
III	Partial physeal separation with distal extension into epiphysis	Poor unless accurate reduction; fixation usually required to maintain stability
IV	Fracture extends through metaphysis, physis, and epiphysis	Perfect reduction must be achieved; guarded prognosis even with good reduction
V	Crush injury of physis	High likelihood of partial growth arrest

G. Clavicular fracture

1. **Most common** fracture in children (e.g., birth trauma, falls)
2. H/P = pain overlying midshaft clavicle, most common fracture sustained during birth
3. Treatment = no treatment needed in neonates; figure-of-eight sling

H. Nursemaid's elbow

1. Radial head subluxation that occurs via pulling and lifting on the hand (e.g., yanking the child out of danger by his or her arm)
2. H/P = child with painful arm who will not bend elbow
3. Treatment = manual reduction via supination of the arm with flexion of the elbow from 0° to 90° of flexion

I. Rickets

1. **Impaired calcification** of bone in children caused by deficient vitamin D intake, absorption, or metabolism (i.e., hypocalcemic types) or impaired phosphate absorption (i.e., hypophosphatemic type)
2. Called **osteomalacia** in adults
3. Results from lack of sunlight and/or poor diet in absence of renal or metabolic defects
4. Epiphyseal cartilage becomes hypertrophic without calcification.
5. H/P = bone pain, delayed walking; **bowed legs**, kyphoscoliosis, proximal limb weakness, decreased height, softened skull bones; fractures that result from minimal trauma in adults
6. **Labs** = increased alkaline phosphatase (all types), decreased phosphorus (all types), decreased calcium (hypocalcemic), decreased (hypocalcemic) or increased (hypophosphatemic) 25-hydroxyvitamin D3 and 1,25-dihydroxycholecalciferol, increased parathyroid hormone (hypocalcemic)
7. **Radiology** = X-rays will demonstrate widening of physes, bowing of long bones, translucent lines in bones, flattening of skull, and enlarged costal cartilages
8. **Treatment** = phosphorus supplementation for all types, vitamin D supplementation for poor intake, 1,25-dihydroxycholecalciferol for impaired vitamin absorption or metabolism

J. Scoliosis

1. Resting lateral **curvature** of the spine with associated rotatory deformity
2. Curve is at risk of progressing during periods of rapid growth; risk of curve progression increases with size of curve.
3. Initially, mainly a **cosmetic** issue; progressive curvature interferes with activities
4. Severe cases result in decreased pulmonary function.

Musculoskeletal Disorders

TABLE 9-7	Variants of Juvenile Idiopathic Arthritis		
	Pauciarticular	**Polyarticular**	**Systemic**
Joints involved	Fewer than four joints; large joints **except hips**	Five or more joints; hips less common	Any number
Age of presentation	2–3 yr	2–5,10–14 yr	Any age <17 yr
Joint symptoms	Insidious swelling and decreased range of motion	Symmetric joint involvement, spine involvement, hand deformities, dactylitis	Acute significant pain, pain severity may follow fevers, neck stiffness common, occasional jaw involvement
Extraosseous symptoms	30% cases have **uveitis** or iridocyclitis	Growth retardation, fever, rare iridocyclitis	**Spiking fevers, maculopapular rash**, hepatosplenomegaly, **lymphadenopathy**, pericarditis, growth retardation
Labs	Weakly positive ANA	Mildly increased ESR, mildly decreased Hgb, weakly positive ANA in younger ages, positive RF in older ages	Increased WBC, anemia, increased ESR, negative ANA, rarely positive RF
Treatment	NSAIDs; methotrexate for chronic cases	NSAIDs, methotrexate, sulfasalazine, or etanercept	NSAIDs, methotrexate, corticosteroids, cytotoxic drugs
Prognosis	Most cases resolve in <6 months; uncommon chronic arthritis	60% patients enter remission within 15 yr; higher rate of severe chronic arthritis than pauciarticular; worse prognosis with older onset	Highly variable course; 50% patients will achieve eventual remission, significant minority have chronic disease
Complications	Blindness from iridocyclitis, leg length discrepancy, rare chronic disease with progressive arthritis	Chronic arthritis, leg length discrepancy	Leg length discrepancy, chronic arthritis, jaw arthritis, amyloidosis

ANA, antinuclear antibody; ESR, erythrocyte sedimentation rate; Hgb, hemoglobin; NSAIDs, nonsteroidal anti-inflammatory drugs; RF, rheumatoid factor; WBC, white blood cell.

5. **H/P** = asymmetry of back musculature and palpable curve of the spine that are augmented when patient bends at the waist; possible pulmonary compromise in severe cases
6. **Treatment** = observation for small curves; bracing for moderate curves in young patients; surgery for more severe curves or curves in older patients
7. **Complications** = severe curves can cause restrictive respiratory disease by limiting lung expansion

K. Juvenile idiopathic arthritis (JIA)
1. Nonmigratory arthropathy affecting one or more joints for >3 months
2. Classified as pauciarticular, polyarticular, or systemic, depending on the constellation of symptoms (see Table 9-7)
3. **H/P** = arthralgias of joints involved, morning stiffness; fever; additional findings depend on subtype
4. **Labs** = vary with subtype
5. **Radiology** = X-rays may demonstrate osteopenia and subchondral sclerosis around **involved joints**
6. **Treatment** = varies with subtype but usually consists of NSAIDs, methotrexate, or corticosteroids

L. Duchenne muscular dystrophy
1. X-linked disorder resulting from deficiency of **dystrophin** (subsarcolemmal cytoskeletal protein)
2. **Most common** lethal muscular dystrophy
3. Onset at 2 to 6 years of age

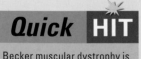

Quick HIT

Becker muscular dystrophy is similar to Duchenne muscular dystrophy, except symptoms are less severe and progression occurs more slowly.

4. **H/P** = progressive clumsiness, easy fatigability, **difficulty standing up and walking**, waddling gait, positive **Gower maneuver** (i.e., must push on thighs with hands to stand up); weakness occurs in proximal muscles before distal muscles; **pseudohypertrophy** occurs in calf muscles from fatty infiltration
5. **Labs** = increased CK; muscle biopsy shows muscle fiber degeneration and fibrosis and basophilic fibers; immunostaining for dystrophin (**absent** in disease) is diagnostic
6. **EMG** = polyphasic potentials and increased fiber recruitment
7. **Treatment** = physical therapy, corticosteroids, pulmonary support, ACE-I decrease cardiac afterload
8. **Complications** = progressive cardiac issues, scoliosis, and flexion contractures; death commonly occurs by 20 years of age because of respiratory issues

Dermatology

I. Infections

A. Cellulitis

1. Acute skin infection most frequently caused by *Staphylococcus aureus* or **group A streptococci**; methicillin-resistant *S. aureus* (**MRSA**) has increasingly evolved as a cause of cellulitis that is difficult to treat because of antibiotic resistance
2. **Risk factors** = **intravenous drug use, diabetes mellitus (DM)**, immunocompromise, penetration of skin (e.g., surgery, trauma), previous cellulitis, venous or lymphatic dysfunction
3. **History and physical (H/P)** = **erythema**, swollen and painful skin, myalgias, chills; warmth in involved area, fever, lymphadenopathy; skin findings may be near wound (see Figure 10-1)
4. **Labs** = increased white blood cell count (WBC), erythrocyte sedimentation rate (ESR), and C-reactive protein (CRP)
5. **Treatment** = oral cephalosporins or penicillinase-resistant β-lactams for 10 to 14 days; intravenous (IV) antibiotics for severe cases or bacteremia; linezolid or IV vancomycin used for MRSA or cases not responding to initial antibiotic therapy; diabetics should receive broad coverage antibiotics because of the increased risk for multiorganism infections
6. **Complications** = necrotizing fasciitis; 20% to 50% recurrence rate

B. Skin abscess

1. **Subcutaneous** collection of pus most commonly caused by staphylococcal bacteria
2. Can occur as collection of multiple infected hair follicles (i.e., carbuncle)

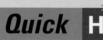

Skin and wound cultures are rarely useful in cellulitis because they frequently contain other normal skin flora or findings are false negative.

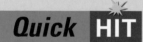

Anaerobic bacteria are more commonly a cause of abscesses in the lower back and perineal regions than in other parts of the body.

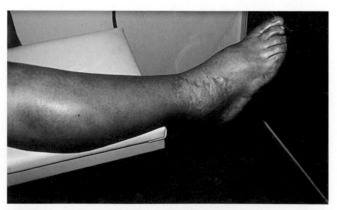

FIGURE

10-1 Cellulitis of the right pretibial region.

Note the erythematous, swollen skin with mild desquamation.
(From Goodheart, H. P. [2003]. *Photoguide of Common Disorders* [2nd ed., Figure 2-69]. Philadelphia, PA: Lippincott Williams & Wilkins; with permission.)

3. Hidradenitis suppurativa
   a. Chronic follicular occlusion and **apocrine gland** inflammation resulting in recurrent abscesses in the axilla, groin, and perineum
   b. Chronic infection leads to scarring.
   c. May require both antibiotics and surgical excision for treatment
4. **H/P** = erythematous, fluctuant, and localized swelling in skin; tender on palpation; pain frequently relieved by rupture of abscess
5. **Labs** = culture of abscess contents can determine pathogen but carries a high rate of false-positive findings if not performed under sterile conditions
6. **Treatment** = **incision and drainage** with healing by secondary intention; antibiotics (cephalosporins initially, then pathogen specific)
7. **Complications** = large, eroding facial abscess can cause cavernous sinus thrombosis

C. Necrotizing fasciitis

1. Quickly spreading group A *Streptococcus* or multipathogen infection of **fascial planes** leading to extensive soft tissue destruction and systemic infection
2. **H/P** = erythematous, warm, and swollen skin; **loss of sensation** in involved tissue, fever, crepitus in infected skin, purple discoloration, bullae over infected region
3. **Labs** = increased WBC, ESR, and CRP; operative culture useful for determining pathogen
4. **Radiology** = X-ray or computed tomography (CT) may detect subcutaneous collections of air
5. **Treatment** = prompt surgical debridement, incision, and drainage; IV antibiotics
6. **Complications** = sepsis, gangrene, high mortality (30% patients)

D. Gangrene

1. Tissue necrosis because of **poor vascular supply** or severe infection (occasionally, *Clostridium perfringens*); described as wet or dry, depending on appearance
2. **H/P** = prior skin infection or penetrating wound, severe pain in skin; fever, hypotension, skin crepitus, **rotten-smelling skin**
3. **Labs** = culture may be useful when caused by infection; ankle-brachial indices should demonstrate asymmetry between limbs
4. **Radiology** = subcutaneous air seen on X-ray or CT for wet gangrene; angiography or magnetic resonance angiography (MRA) demonstrates vascular insufficiency
5. **Treatment** = incision and drainage, debridement, antibiotics; amputation frequently required

E. Impetigo

1. **Contagious** skin infection most commonly found in **children**; caused by *S. aureus* or **group A streptococci**
2. **H/P** = facial pruritus; **yellow crusted lesions** around mucocutaneous surfaces; erythematous vesicles (blisters) seen in staphylococcal infection; erythematous pustules on face and extremities with streptococcal infections (see Figure 10-2)
3. **Treatment** = wash all affected areas; erythromycin, cephalosporins, or topical antibiotics; unaffected family members should not share towels or clothing to prevent spread until cure achieved

F. Acne vulgaris

1. Inflammation of hair follicles and sebaceous glands associated with *Propionibacterium acnes*, adolescence, androgens, and obstruction of pores by exfoliated skin or personal care products
2. **H/P**
   a. Most frequently occurs in **adolescents**
   b. Erythematous pustules predominantly on face, neck, chest, and back
   c. **Cystic lesions can form in severe cases.**
3. Treatment
   a. Topical **retinoids** decrease sebaceous gland activity and normalize follicular keratinization; they are the recommended first-line treatment.

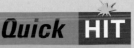

Dry gangrene, gradual necrosis of skin from vascular insufficiency, features hard and dry skin. **Wet gangrene,** necrosis caused by acute vascular obstruction or infection, features blistering and swelling of the involved area.

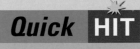

No proven association exists between acne vulgaris and certain types of food.

Quick **HIT**

Acne usually decreases in severity as adolescence ends. **Corticosteroid use** and **androgen** production disorders are common causes of outbreaks in adulthood.

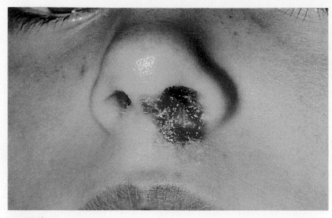

FIGURE
10-2 Impetigo involving left nostril caused by *Staphylococcus aureus* infection.

Note presence of greasy yellow scales within lesion.
(From Smeltzer S. C., Bare, B., Hinkle, J. L., & Cheever, K. H [2010]. *Brunner and Suddarth's Textbook of Medical-Surgical Nursing* [12th ed., p. 1687]. Philadelphia, PA: Lippincott Williams & Wilkins; with permission.)

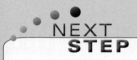

NEXT STEP

Women should have at least two **negative urine pregnancy tests** before an oral isotretinoin is prescribed.

Dermatology

    b. Antibiotics (oral or topical) may inhibit bacterial growth (second-line therapy, used in conjunction with a topical retinoid).

    c. Benzoyl peroxide has antimicrobial properties and also helps prevent follicular obstruction by comedolytic properties (second-line therapy, often used in conjunction with a topical retinoid and an antibiotic).

    d. Oral contraceptives may be useful in women with excess androgen production.

    e. Oral isotretinoin given for severe cases but requires close monitoring of liver enzymes (hepatotoxicity risk) and mandatory pharmacologic contraception (high teratogenic risks).

    f. Soaps and astringents have little effect on the condition.

  4. **Complications** = cystic acne can result in permanent scarring; oral vitamin A analogues can cause birth defects or hepatotoxicity

G. Herpes simplex virus (HSV)

  1. Recurrent viral infection of mucocutaneous surfaces caused by HSV-1 or HSV-2

  2. HSV transmitted through contact with **oral** or **genital fluids**

  3. **HSV-1** causes primarily **oral** disease; **HSV-2** causes primarily **genital** disease.

  4. After primary infection, viral genetic material remains in sensory ganglia; stress will cause reactivation of disease in distribution of involved nerves.

  5. **H/P** = small painful vesicles around mouth (HSV-1) or genitals (HSV-2) lasting several days (see Figure 10-3); primary infection usually presents with more severe symptoms and a flulike illness; disease affecting eyes causes impaired vision; disease affecting esophagus causes odynophagia and dysphagia

  6. **Labs** = Tzanck smear of lesions shows multinucleated giant cells; viral culture confirms diagnosis; Herpes antibodies

  7. **Treatment** = incurable, so treatment should be directed at minimizing symptoms and exacerbations; acyclovir, famciclovir, or valacyclovir shortens duration of recurrences and may decrease number of recurrences in patients with frequent eruptions; therapy can either be intermittent (episodic) or continuous (suppressive)

  8. **Complications**

    a. May be transmissible even when no vesicles are present

    b. Transmission from **infected mother to newborn** can cause disseminated disease with severe neurologic involvement.

    c. Rarely, mother-to-newborn transmission can occur in the absence of visible vesicles.

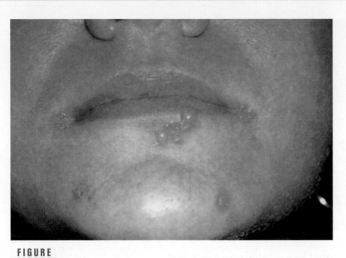

FIGURE
10-3 **Herpes simplex.**

These perioral vesicles are more indicative of infection with herpes simplex virus type 1 than type 2.
(From Weber, J., & Kelley, J. [2010]. *Health Assessment in Nursing* [4th ed., p. 294]. Philadelphia, PA: Lippincott Williams & Wilkins; with permission.)

H. Varicella

1. Infection by varicella-zoster virus (i.e., herpes zoster) that can present as primary disease (i.e., chickenpox) or recurrent disease (i.e., shingles) (see Figure 10-1)
2. Chickenpox and shingles have different presentations, despite being caused by the same viral infection (see Table 10-1).

TABLE **10-1**	Characteristics of Primary (Chickenpox) and Recurrent (Shingles) Varicella	
Varicella Condition	**Chickenpox (Primary)**	**Shingles (Recurrent)**
Patients affected	More common in **children**	Patient with prior history of varicella-zoster infection
Timing of presentation	Symptoms 2+ wk after infection occurs; symptoms of headache, malaise, myalgias, and fever precede development of lesions by <3 days	Myalgias, fever, malaise preceding lesions by approximately 3 days
Type of lesion	Small, red macules that evolve into papules and then vesicles that eventually become crusted	Small, red macules that evolve into papules and then vesicles that eventually become crusted
Distribution of lesions	**Wide** distribution	Limited to single or few distinct **dermatomes**; involvement of multiple dermatomes indicates **disseminated** disease
Course of disease	Lesions may develop up to 1 wk and resolve a few days after appearing; infective until lesions crust over	Lesions exist for a week and may be **painful**; infective until lesions crust over
Treatment	Antipruritics aid symptoms; acyclovir used in severe cases or in immunocompromised patients; **vaccination** has reduced disease incidence significantly	Analgesics, possible corticosteroids; acyclovir used in immunocompromised patients and trigeminal nerve distribution
Complications	More severe course in older and pregnant patients (increased risk of varicella pneumonia); can have severe consequences if passed from **infected mother to unborn fetus**	Postinfectious neuralgia (long-lasting pain at site of eruption), trigeminal neuropathy

NEXT STEP

Check varicella immunity status (received vaccine or had chickenpox as child) in all **pregnant** women; **varicella immune globulin** should be given to all nonimmune pregnant women who contract the disease.

Quick **HIT**

Immunocompromised patients are at an increased risk for developing **encephalopathy** or **retinitis** as complications from varicella infection.

Dermatology

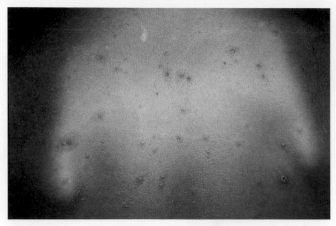

FIGURE
10-4 **Chicken pox in a child caused by varicella-zoster infection.**

While the small crusted vesicles are distributed across the body in the childhood form, reactivated infection in adults (shingles) occurs in a single dermatome.
(From Goodheart, H. P. [2003]. *Goodheart's Photoguide of Common Skin Disorders* [2nd ed., Figure 8-2]. Philadelphia, PA: Lippincott Willimas & Wilkins; with permission.)

I. Warts

1. Benign epithelial tumors caused by local infection by one of many types of **human papillomavirus** (HPV)
2. **H/P** = well-defined lesions of thickened epithelium, may appear flat (plantar warts) or raised; occasional tenderness to palpation
3. **Treatment** = occasionally self-limited; chemical, laser, or cryotherapy may be required for removal
4. **Complications** = some forms of HPV (types 6 and 11) that cause genital warts are associated with cervical cancer (see Chapter 11, **Gynecologic and Breast Disorders**)

J. Molluscum contagiosum

1. Viral skin infection most frequently seen in children and in patients positive for human immunodeficiency virus (HIV)
2. **H/P**
   a. Painless, **shiny papules** with **central umbilication** (<5 mm diameter)
   b. In children, found on face, back, chest, and extremities; in adults, found in perineal region
3. **Labs** = Giemsa and Wright stains on histology show large inclusion bodies
4. **Treatment** = frequently self-limited; chemical, laser, or cryotherapy for removal

K. Scabies

1. Cutaneous infestation by *Sarcoptes scabiei* mite
2. **Risk factors** = **crowded living conditions**, poor hygiene
3. **H/P** = severe pruritus at site of involvement (most commonly webs of fingers and toes) that worsens after a hot bath; **mite burrows** with nearby papules may be seen on close examination of skin
4. **Labs** = mites and eggs may be seen in skin scrapings under microscope
5. **Treatment**
   a. Permethrin cream or oral ivermectin; diphenhydramine to relieve pruritus
   b. All clothing, towels, and linens must be washed in hot water.
6. **Complications** = **infection of close contacts** common

L. Fungal infections

1. Cutaneous fungal infections typically characteristic for a specific body region (see Table 10-2 and Figure 10-5)
2. Frequently associated with **warm or moist environments**, obesity, DM, or recent antibiotic use

TABLE 10-2 Common Cutaneous Fungal Infections				
Condition	**Fungus**	**Lesions**	**Diagnosis**	**Treatment**
Tinea versicolor (pityriasis versicolor)	*Malassezia furfur*	Salmon-colored, light brown, or hypopigmented macules, most frequently on chest and back; lesions do not tan and may scale when scraped	KOH preparation shows short hyphae and spores ("spaghetti and meatballs"), Wood lamp examination shows extent of disease	Topical antifungal agent for several weeks or oral ketoconazole for 1–5 days
Tinea not caused by *M. furfur*. Described by location: corporis (body), cruris (groin), pedis (feet), unguium (nail beds), capitis (scalp)	• *Microsporum* • *Trichophyton* • *Epidermophyton*	Pruritic, erythematous, scaly plaques with central clearing	KOH preparation shows hyphae	• Topical antifungal agent for multiple weeks • Oral antifungal agent for resistant cases
Intertrigo	*Candida albicans*	Pruritic, painful, erythematous plaques with pustules most commonly in skin creases	KOH preparation shows pseudohyphae	• Topical antifungal agent • Topical corticosteroid

KOH, potassium hydroxide.

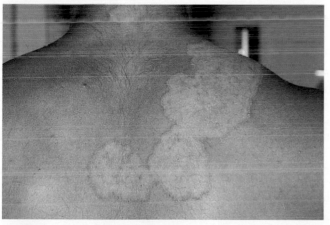

FIGURE 10-5 Tinea corporis; fungal infection of skin characterized by scaly rash on the body, with central clearing and a popular border.

(From Goodheart, H. P. [2009]. *Goodheart's Photoguide of Common Skin Disorders* [3rd ed., p. 121]. Philadelphia, PA: Lippincott Williams & Wilkins; with permission.)

II. Inflammatory Skin Conditions

A. Hypersensitivity reactions in skin

1. Allergic reaction seen in skin because of cutaneous **contact** or **ingestion** of a given allergen (e.g., drugs)
2. Mechanism of reaction
   a. **Type I**: caused by mast cell degranulation; light, diffuse rash (i.e., urticaria) appears soon after exposure and lasts only several hours
   b. **Type IV**: caused by lymphocyte activity; measles-like (i.e., morbilliform) rash appears several days after second exposure to allergen (mechanism for most allergic contact dermatitis)
3. H/P
   a. Pruritus, erythematous rash in distinct patterns (lines, shapes) in contact dermatitis
   b. Ingestion of an allergen (e.g., food, drug reaction) can cause rash in a characteristic location or in a poorly defined area.

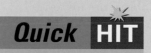

Quick HIT

Common causes of allergic contact dermatitis include plants (poison ivy, poison oak, etc.), nickel, soaps, and **latex**.

Dermatology

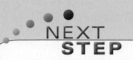

NEXT STEP

Use the pattern of a rash to distinguish an **external** cause (**defined** shape) from an **internal** cause (**nondefined** distribution) of rash.

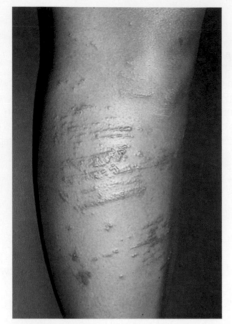

FIGURE 10-6 **Contact dermatitis.**

Contact dermatitis caused by exposure to poison ivy. Note the linearity of the rash consistent with an external cause. (From Goodheart, H. P. [2003]. *Goodheart's Photoguide of Common Skin Disorders* [2nd ed., Figure 2-48]. Philadelphia, PA: Lippincott Williams & Wilkins; with permission.)

   c. History of drug ingestion, contact with allergen, or previous reaction is helpful for diagnosis (see Figure 10-6).
 4. **Treatment**
   a. Stop offending agent or remove contact with allergen.
   b. Mild cases can be treated with topical corticosteroids and antihistamines.
   c. Oral corticosteroids may be required in worse cases.

B. Erythema multiforme

 1. More serious cutaneous hypersensitivity reaction caused by **drugs, infection**, or vaccination
 2. **H/P** = malaise, myalgias, pruritus; macules (i.e., small, nonpalpable lesions); plaques (i.e., large nonpalpable lesions) or vesicles on extremities (especially palms, soles); **target lesions** (i.e., erythematous center surrounded by pale inner ring and erythematous outer ring) may be evident
 3. **Labs** = increased eosinophils; skin biopsy shows increased lymphocytes and necrotic keratinocytes
 4. **Treatment** = may be self-limited; stop offending agent; corticosteroids, analgesics

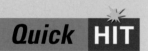

Quick HIT

Penicillins, sulfonamides, nonsteroidal anti-inflammatory drugs (NSAIDs), oral contraceptives, and anticonvulsant medications are agents most frequently associated with erythema multiforme.

C. Stevens-Johnson syndrome

 1. Severe form of erythema multiforme involving mucous membranes and severe plaque formation
 2. **Skin sloughing** may be evident; high risk of dehydration
 3. **H/P** = similar skin appearance to erythema multiforme but more severe; more likely to have myalgias, fever, nausea, vomiting, oral pain, and eye pain
 4. **Treatment** = **stop offending agent**; corticosteroids, analgesics, IV fluids; frequently treated in burn unit

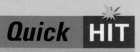

Quick HIT

HSV and *Mycoplasma pneumoniae* are common infectious causes of erythema multiforme.

D. Toxic epidermal necrolysis (TEN)

 1. Most severe form of hypersensitivity reaction with **significant skin sloughing** and **full-thickness epidermal necrosis** (see Figure 10-7)
 2. **Labs** = decreased WBC, decreased hemoglobin, decreased hematocrit, increased alanine aminotransferase (ALT), increased aspartate aminotransferase (AST)

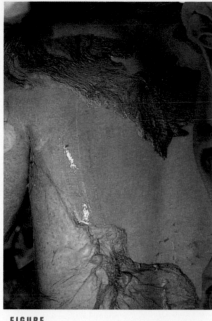

FIGURE
10-7 Toxic epidermal necrolysis (TEN).

This severe dermatologic condition begins as a generalized erythematous rash that progresses into widespread desquamation and erosion formation.
(From Elder, D. E., Elenitsas, R., Rubin, A. I., Ioffreda, M. Miller, J. & Miller, F. O. [2012]. *Atlas and Synopsis of Lever's Histopathology of the Skin* [3rd ed., p. 179]. Philadelphia, PA: Lippincott Williams & Wilkins; with permission.)

3. Treatment
   a. **Stop offending agent.**
   b. Treat patient in **burn center**, IV hydration, corticosteroids, intravenous immune globulin
   c. Acyclovir may be useful in cases caused by HSV.

E. Seborrheic dermatitis
1. Chronic hyperproliferation of epidermis most commonly on **scalp** or face
2. Most common in adolescents and infants
3. H/P = pruritus; erythematous **plaques with yellow, greasy scales**
4. **Treatment** = shampoo containing selenium, tar, or ketoconazole when scalp involved; topical corticosteroids and antifungals used for other regions
5. **Complications** = frequent recurrence

F. Atopic dermatitis (i.e., eczema)
1. Chronic inflammatory skin rash characterized by **dry skin patches** with papules
2. Both **infantile** (resolves with initial years of life) and **adult** (recurrent) forms exist.
3. **Risk factors** = asthma, allergic rhinitis, family history
4. H/P = pruritus; erythematous patches of dry skin with possible vesicles on flexor surfaces, dorsum of hands and feet, chest, back, or face; lesions more commonly on face and scalp in infants (see Figure 10-8)
5. **Treatment** = avoidance of precipitating factors, moisturizing creams, topical corticosteroids or tacrolimus; severe cases can be treated with oral corticosteroids and antihistamines

G. Psoriasis
1. Inflammatory skin disorder characterized by epidermal hyperproliferation
2. H/P = possible pruritus; well-defined **red plaques** with **silvery scales** on **extensor surfaces** (especially knees and elbows) that bleed easily with scale removal (i.e., Auspitz sign), possible small pustules, pitted nails, lifting of nails (see Figure 10-9)
3. **Labs** = negative for rheumatoid factor; skin biopsy shows thickened epidermis, absent granular cell layer, and nucleated cells in stratum corneum; possible increased uric acid, increased ESR

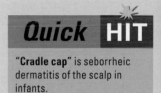

Quick **HIT**

"Cradle cap" is seborrheic dermatitis of the scalp in infants.

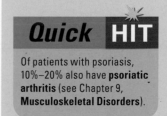

Quick **HIT**

Of patients with psoriasis, 10%–20% also have **psoriatic arthritis** (see Chapter 9, **Musculoskeletal Disorders**).

Dermatology

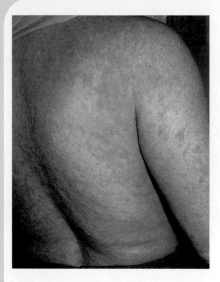

FIGURE
10-8 **Adult atopic dermatitis (eczema) characterized by erythematous patches of dry skin.**

(From Goodheart, H. P. [2003]. *Goodheart's Photoguide of Common Skin Disorders* [2nd ed., Figure 2-8]. Philadelphia, PA: Lippincott Williams & Wilkins; with permission.)

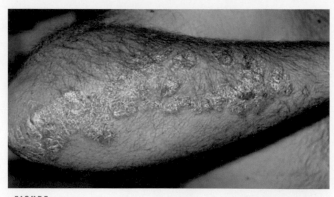

FIGURE
10-9 **Psoriasis**

Red plaques with silver scales on extensor forearm surface of a patient with psoriasis; similar lesions are also seen on the extensor surfaces of the knee.(From Goodheart, H. P. [2003]. *Goodheart's Photoguide of Common Skin Disorders* [2nd ed., Figure 2-23]. Philadelphia, PA: Lippincott Williams & Wilkins; with permission.)

4. **Treatment** = topical corticosteroids, tar, retinoids, tacrolimus, or antifungal agents; phototherapy, methotrexate, cyclosporine, or antitumor necrosis factor (anti-TNF) drugs can be used in severe disease

H. Pityriasis rosea

1. Mild inflammatory skin disorder in children and young adults with possible viral association characterized by papular lesions on the trunk and extremities
2. **H/P**
   a. Pruritus; oval erythematous papules covered with white scale located primarily on chest, back, and extremities
   b. Rash begins with appearance of **"herald patch"** (i.e., single round lesion up to 5 cm in diameter) a few days before generalized eruption (see Figure 10-10).

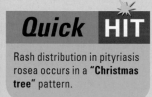

Quick HIT

Rash distribution in pityriasis rosea occurs in a **"Christmas tree"** pattern.

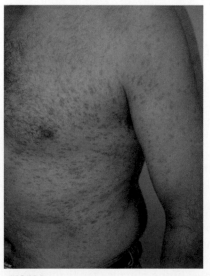

FIGURE
10-10 **Pityriasis rosea.**

These scaled papules fan out across the chest or back to give the overall appearance of a Christmas tree pattern. Image provided by Stedman's.

3. **Treatment** = self-limited; topical steroids, phototherapy, or erythromycin may decrease duration of exacerbation

I. Erythema nodosum

1. Inflammation of **subcutaneous fat septa** resulting in painful erythematous nodules; most commonly on anterior tibias but can also affect trunk and other extremities
2. Caused by delayed immunologic reaction to infection, collagen-vascular diseases, inflammatory bowel disease, or drugs
3. **H/P** = malaise, arthralgias; tender **erythematous nodules** (usually pretibial), fever
4. **Labs** = possible positive antistreptolysin 0 titer (when associated with streptococcal infection), increased ESR; skin biopsy may show fatty inflammation
5. **Treatment** = self-limited; NSAIDs, potassium iodide, corticosteroids

III. Bullous Diseases

A. Pemphigus vulgaris

1. Autoimmune disorder characterized by autoantibodies to adhesion molecules in epidermis
2. Patients usually middle aged or elderly
3. **H/P** = **painful, fragile blisters** in oropharynx and on chest, face, and perineal region; blisters rupture easily and erosions are common (see Figure 10-11)
4. **Labs** = skin biopsy shows separating of epidermal cells (i.e., **acantholysis**) with intact basement membrane; immunofluorescence demonstrates antiepidermal antibodies
5. **Treatment** = corticosteroids, azathioprine, or cyclophosphamide
6. **Complications** = sepsis, high mortality without treatment, osteoporosis (chronic corticosteroid use)

B. Bullous pemphigoid

1. Autoimmune disorder characterized by autoantibodies to epidermal basement membrane
2. Most patients >60 years of age
3. **H/P** = **widespread blistering** (especially on flexor surfaces and perineal region), pruritus; erosions can form with blister rupture (see Figure 10-12)
4. **Labs** = immunofluorescence shows antibasement membrane antibodies
5. **Treatment** = oral or topical corticosteroids or azathioprine

C. Porphyria cutanea tarda

1. Disease resulting from deficiency of hepatic uroporphyrinogen decarboxylase, an enzyme involved in heme metabolism

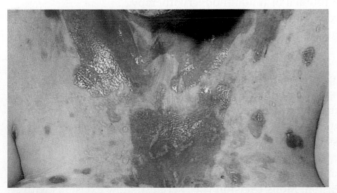

FIGURE

10-11 **Pemphigus vulgaris.**

Fragile bullae develop, which rupture, easily leading to widespread erosions and desquamation.
(From Elder, D. E., Elenitsas, R., Rubin, A. I., Ioffreda, M., Miller, J., & Miller, F. O. [2013]. *Atlas and Synopsis of Lever's Histopathology of the Skin* [3rd ed., p. 188]. Philadelphia, PA: Lippincott Williams & Wilkins; with permission.)

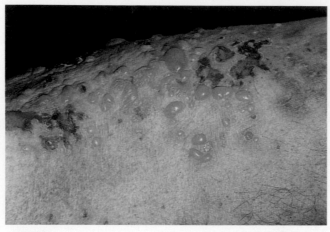

FIGURE 10-12 **Bullous pemphigoid.**

Multiple large bullae form on an erythematous base leading to severe erosions.
(From Elder, D. E., Elenitsas, R., Rubin, A. I., Ioffreda, M., Miller, J., & Miller, F. O. [2013]. *Atlas and Synopsis of Lever's Histopathology of the Skin* [3rd ed., p. 197]. Philadelphia, PA: Lippincott Williams & Wilkins; with permission.)

2. **Risk factors** = alcoholism, **hepatitis C**, iron overload, estrogen use, smoking
3. **H/P** = **chronic blistering lesions** on sun-exposed skin (especially the dorsa of hands, forearms, neck, face, ears, feet), **hyperpigmented skin, facial hypertrichosis**; ruptured blisters heal poorly and result in scarring
4. **Labs** = elevated AST and ALT, **increased total plasma porphyrin**, increased urine porphyrins, decreased uroporphyrinogen decarboxylase
5. **Treatment** = periodic phlebotomy, low-dose chloroquine or hydroxychloroquine, sunscreen use, avoidance of triggers such as alcohol, estrogens, tobacco, iron supplements

IV. Neoplasms

A. Actinic keratosis
1. **Precancerous** skin lesion that can progress to squamous cell cancer
2. **Risk factors** = **sun exposure**
3. **H/P** = erythematous **papule** with rough, **yellow-brown scales** <5 mm in diameter; lesions found in **sun-exposed** areas (see Figure 10-13)
4. **Labs** = biopsy shows dysplasia of epithelium (deeper epithelial cells show variations in shape and nuclei with increased staining)
5. **Treatment** = topical 5-flurouracil or imiquimod, cryotherapy
6. **Complications** = 0.1%/year risk of progression to **squamous cell carcinoma** (60% of squamous cell carcinomas arise from **actinic keratosis**)

B. Squamous cell carcinoma
1. Skin cancer involving **squamous** cells of epithelium
2. **Risk factors** = **sun exposure** (particularly UVB radiation), **actinic keratosis**, arsenic exposure, fair complexion, radiation
3. **H/P** = painless, erythematous papule with scaling or keratinized growths in sun-exposed area; progressive lesions may bleed, ulcerate, or be painful (see Figure 10-14)
4. **Labs** = biopsy shows anaplastic epidermal cells extending to dermis
5. **Treatment** = surgical excision; **Mohs excision** (i.e., serial shallow excisions with histologic analysis to minimize cosmetic damage) may be performed for lesions on face; radiation may be helpful in large lesions
6. **Complications** = progresses slowly but can be a large lesion by time of diagnosis if located in poorly visualized region (back, scalp); 5% to 10% of cases metastasize

Quick HIT

Seborrheic keratosis is a common, benign tumor of immature keratinocytes with a hyperpigmented, warty, "stuck on" appearance.

NEXT STEP

Even when actinic keratosis is the suggested diagnosis, biopsy a lesion to rule out squamous cell cancer.

Quick HIT

Use of a good **sunscreen** (≥SPF 15) is important in the prevention of skin cancer associated with sun exposure.

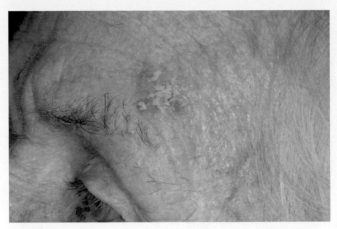

FIGURE
10-13 Actinic keratosis.

These lesions are superficial papules covered by dry scales and are a result of sun exposure. (From Elder, D. E. [2015]. *Lever's Histopathology of the Skin.* [11th ed., p. 987]. Philadelphia, PA: Lippincott Williams & Wilkins; with permission.)

C. Basal cell carcinoma

1. Skin cancer arising in **basal** epidermal cells
2. Risk factors = sun exposure
3. H/P = **pearly papule** with fine vascular markings (i.e., **telangiectasias**) (see Figure 10-15)
4. Labs = biopsy shows basophilic-staining basal epidermal cells arranged in palisades
5. **Treatment** = surgical excision, Mohs excision, radiation, or cryotherapy
6. **Complications** = lesions metastasize in <0.1% of cases

D. Melanoma

1. Malignant melanocyte tumor that spreads rapidly
2. Risk factors = sun exposure, fair complexion, family history, numerous nevi (i.e., moles)
3. Types
   a. **Superficial spreading**: most common type; grows laterally before invasive growth occurs
   b. **Nodular**: grows only vertically and becomes invasive rapidly; difficult to detect

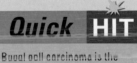

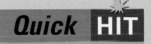

Quick HIT

Basal cell carcinoma is the **most common** type of skin cancer.

Quick HIT

Shave biopsy should **never** be used to study a suspicious melanotic lesion because it does not provide sufficient tissue for clear diagnosis and cannot be used to measure lesion depth.

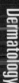

Dermatology

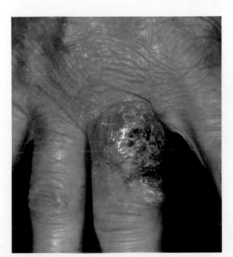

FIGURE
10-14 Squamous cell carcinoma with erythematous base and ulceration.

(From Rubin, R., & Strayer D. S. [2012]. *Rubin's. Pathology* [6th ed., p. 1163]. Philadelphia, PA: Wolters Kluwer/Lippincott Williams & Wilkins; with permission.)

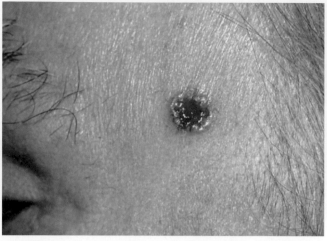

FIGURE
10-15 **Basal cell carcinoma.**

Note the pearly appearance of a papule with central ulceration.
(From Goodheart, H. P. [2003]. *Goodheart's Photoguide of Common Skin Disorders.* (2nd ed., Figure 22-17). Philadelphia, PA: Lippincott Williams & Wilkins; with permission.)

Quick HIT

Nevi should be followed to look for the ABCDEs of melanoma: **A**symmetry, **B**order (irregular), **C**olor (variable), **D**iameter (>6 mm), and **E**nlargement.

Dermatology

    c. **Acral lentiginous**: involves palms, soles, and nail beds
    d. **Lentigo maligna**: long-lasting in situ stage before vertical growth
4. H/P
    a. **Painless**, pigmented lesion with recent changes in appearance
    b. Lesions have irregular borders, multiple colors, and can be large or rapidly growing (see Figure 10-16).
    c. In contrast, melanocytic nevi are more symmetric, have more regular borders, are homogenously colored, and remain relatively the same size over time (see Figure 10-17).
5. **Labs** = excisional biopsy shows atypical melanocytes and possible invasion into dermis

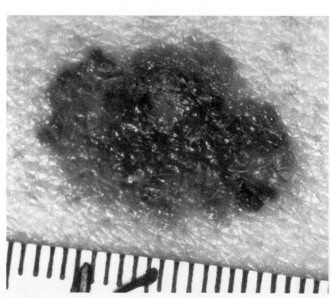

FIGURE
10-16 **Melanoma, superficial spreading type.**

Note the ABCDs of the lesion: asymmetry, irregular border, inconsistent color, and large diameter (>20 mm).
(From Rubin, R., & Strayer D. S. [2012]. *Rubin's Pathology* [6th ed., p. 1151]. Philadelphia, PA: Wolters Kluwer/Lippincott Williams & Wilkins; with permission.)

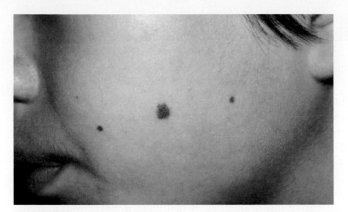

FIGURE
10-17 **Melanocytic nevus.**

Unlike melanoma, this lesion is nearly symmetric, has better border regularity, is a more consistent color, and is smaller in diameter.
(From Goodheart, H. P. [2008]. *Goodheart's Photoguide of Common Skin Disorders* [3rd ed., p. 364]. Philadelphia, PA: Lippincott Williams & Wilkins; with permission.)

6. **Treatment** = surgical excision (0.5 cm margin if in situ, 1 cm margin if <2 mm thick, 2 cm margin if >2 mm thick) with possible lymph node dissection; chemotherapy and radiation therapy if metastatic
7. **Complications** = aggressive cancer; lesions can have metastasized by time of discovery (most commonly, lung, brain, and gastrointestinal tract)

 ## V. Plastic Surgery

A. Grafts and flaps (*see* Table 10-3)
1. Transfer of skin and soft tissues from one location of body to another for use in wound repair
2. Skin grafts can be autografts (i.e., from healthy tissue on same patient), allografts (i.e., donor tissue from another individual), or xenografts (i.e., donor tissue from another species).
3. Flaps can be rotational or transpositional (i.e., left partially attached to donor site and rotated or stretched to cover wound) or free flaps (i.e., flap completely removed from donor site and transferred in whole to wound).

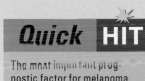

The most important prognostic factor for melanoma is **thickness of lesion** (>0.76 mm associated with increased risk of metastasis).

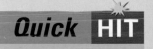

Periodic skin checks should be performed in anyone with a history of significant sun exposure and a positive family history for melanoma.

Dermatology

TABLE 10-3	Common Types of Skin Grafts and Tissue Flaps Used in Wound Repair		
Type	**Description**	**Common Donor Sites**	**Indications**
Split-thickness graft	Skin graft composed of epidermis and part of dermis	Abdomen, thighs, buttocks	Skin replacement in wounds; useful to cover extensive surface area (contracts over time)
Full-thickness graft	Skin graft composed of epidermis and full dermis	Above ears (for face), forearm, groin	Defects on face, hands
Composite graft	Skin grafts that also contain other tissues (cartilage, nail bed, fat)	Fingertip, ear, etc.	Site-specific anatomic reconstruction
Fasciocutaneous flap	Skin and subcutaneous tissue with attached vascular supply	Forehead, groin, deltopectoral region, thighs	Large defects with good vascular supply requiring padding
Muscle flap	Transferred muscle that either includes skin (myocutaneous flap) or requires additional skin graft	Tensor fascia lata, gluteal muscles, sartorius, rectus abdominus, latissimus dorsi	Areas requiring increased vascularized tissue, exposed deep tissues, severe radiation injury

B. Reconstructive surgery

1. Repair of soft tissue defects caused by surgery, congenital anomalies, or wounds
2. Multiple types of tissue are used to recreate normal anatomy (e.g., skin, muscle, bone, cartilage, vessels, nerves).
3. Examples
   a. Maxillofacial: cleft lip repair, cleft palate repair, facial trauma
   b. Breast: reconstruction with muscle flaps or implants following mastectomy
   c. Genitourinary: repair of epispadias, hypospadias, or genital agenesis
   d. Soft tissues: following sarcoma excision or for filling defects

C. Cosmetic surgery

1. Surgical alteration of appearance
2. Can be performed to remove anatomic anomalies or results of massive weight loss, surgery, or injury (e.g., gynecomastia, postmastectomy, excessive skin, difficulty breathing)
3. More often used to combat effects of **aging** or to **modify** physical appearance
4. Examples
   a. Facial: facelift, brow-lift, blepharoplasty (i.e., repair of baggy eyelids), rhinoplasty
   b. Skin: removal of scarring, spider veins, age wrinkles (dermabrasion, laser treatment, chemical peel)
   c. Breast: augmentation, reduction (may be helpful to reduce back strain)
   d. Fatty tissue reduction: abdominoplasty, liposuction
5. **Psychiatric** issues must be considered, especially in patients who repeatedly request "upgrades."

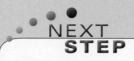

NEXT STEP

Genitourinary reconstruction or gender reassignment requires a careful preoperative evaluation to determine true gender of patient, genetic causes, realistic outcomes, expectations, and psychiatric issues.

Dermatology

GYNECOLOGIC AND BREAST DISORDERS

 I. Menstrual Physiology

A. Gynecologic development

1. Reproductive changes driven by follicle-stimulating hormone (FSH) and luteinizing hormone (LH) levels (see Table 11-1, Figure 11-1)
2. Secondary sexual characteristics are caused by androgens.
3. Tanner stages describe breast and pubic hair development during puberty (see Table 11-2).

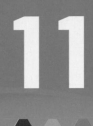

TABLE 11-1	Gynecologic Development by Age	
Age	**Hormone Levels**	**Characteristics**
Fetal to 4 yr	High intrauterine FSH and LH that peaks at 20 wk gestation and decreases until birth FSH and LH increase again from birth until 6 months of age then gradually decrease to low levels by age 4 yr	All oocytes formed and partially matured by 20 wk gestation Tanner stage 1 characteristics
4–8 yr	Low FSH, LH, and androgen levels caused by GnRH suppression	Tanner stage 1 characteristics Any sexual development considered precocious
8–11 yr	LH, FSH, and androgen levels begin to increase	Initial pubertal changes, including early breast development and pubic and axillary hair growth
11–17 yr	Further increase of LH, FSH, and androgens to baseline mature levels Hormones secreted in pulsatile fashion (higher at night) caused by sleep-associated increase in GnRH secretion	Puberty Progression through Tanner stages Development of secondary sexual characteristics and growth spurt Menarche in females (beginning of menstrual cycles) and further oocyte maturation
17–50 yr (females)	LH and FSH follow menstrual cycle Gradual increase in FSH and LH with ovarian insensitivity	Menstrual cycles Mature sexual characteristics
≥50 yr (females)	LH and FSH levels increase with onset of ovarian failure	Perimenopause: menstrual cycles become inconsistent (oligomenorrhea) Menopause: menstrual cycles cease (amenorrhea)

FSH, follicle-stimulating hormone; GnRH, gonadotropin-releasing hormone; LH, luteinizing hormone.

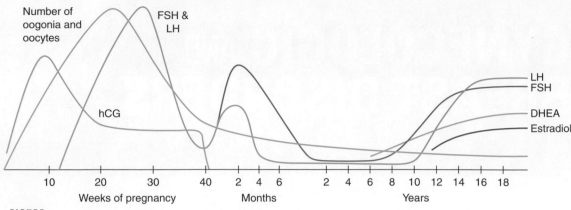

FIGURE 11-1 Changes in hormone and oogonia (egg) levels with gestation and age.

DHEA, dehydroepiandrosterone; FSH, follicle-stimulating hormone; hCG, human chorionic gonadotropin; LH, luteinizing hormone. (From Fritz, M. A. & Speroff, L. [2011]. *Clinical Gynecologic Endocrinology and Infertility* [8th ed., p. 939]. Philadelphia, PA: Lippincott Williams & Wilkins; with permission.)

TABLE 11-2	Tanner Stages for Female Breast and Hair Development	
Tanner Stage	**Breast Development**	**Pubic Hair Development**
1	Prepubertal: raised papilla (nipple) only	Prepubertal: no hair growth
2	Breast budding, areolar enlargement	Slight growth of fine labial hair
3	Further breast and areolar enlargement	Further growth of hair
4	Further breast enlargement: areola and papilla form secondary growth above level of breast	Hair becomes coarser and spreads over much of pubic region
5	Mature breast: areola recedes to level of breast while papilla remains extended	Coarse hair extends from pubic region to medial thighs

B. Precocious puberty

1. Development of pubertal changes in girls <8 years
2. Because of **early activation of the hypothalamic–pituitary–gonadal axis** (central precocious puberty) or autonomous excess secretion of sex steroids (pseudoprecocious puberty)
3. Types
   a. **Isosexual**
      (1) Premature sexual development appropriate for gender
      (2) Can be complete (i.e., all sexual characteristics develop prematurely) or incomplete (i.e., only one sexual characteristic develops prematurely)
   b. **Heterosexual**
      (1) Virilization/masculinization of girls or feminization of boys
      (2) In girls, most commonly results from congenital adrenal hyperplasia, exposure to exogenous androgens, or androgen-secreting neoplasm
4. **History and physical (H/P)**
   a. Complete isosexual: normal pubertal changes take place but at **earlier-than-normal age**
   b. Incomplete isosexual: premature breast budding (i.e., **thelarche**), axillary hair growth, or pubic hair growth (i.e., **pubarche**) may take place
5. **Labs**
   a. Increased LH and FSH with additional release following administration of gonadotropin-releasing hormone (GnRH) suggests central precocious puberty; low LH and FSH with no response to GnRH suggests pseudoprecocious puberty.
   b. Increased estrogen in the presence of low LH and FSH suggests ectopic hormone production (neoplasm) or consumption of exogenous estrogen; significantly high levels of adrenal steroids may be seen with neoplasm or congenital adrenal hyperplasia (CAH).

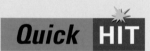

Quick HIT

Precocious puberty in boys occurs <9 years and is most commonly caused by adrenal hyperplasia.

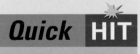

Quick HIT

Central nervous system lesions or **traumas** are causes of isosexual precocious puberty in approximately 10% of cases.

Gynecologic and Breast Disorders

    c. Increased thyroid-stimulating hormone (TSH) with low thyroxine (T_4) and triiodo-thyronine (T_3) suggest precocious puberty in response to chronic hypothyroidism.

6. **Radiology** = magnetic resonance imaging (MRI) or computed tomography (CT) with contrast may detect cerebral or adrenal lesions

7. **Treatment**
    a. **GnRH analogues** are useful for LH and FSH suppression in central precocious puberty.
    b. Precocious puberty secondary to ectopic hormone secretion should be treated by locating and removing the source of the hormone.
    c. Precocious puberty caused by CAH should be treated with cortisol replacement (see Chapter 5, **Endocrine Disorders**).
    d. Complete precocious puberty with an onset close to the expected start of puberty may not require treatment.
    e. Incomplete precocious puberty requires only observation to make sure that it does not become complete precocity.

8. **Complications** = short stature (bones fuse at early age); social and emotional adjustment issues

C. Normal menstrual cycle (see Figure 11-2)

1. LH, FSH, estrogen, progesterone, and human chorionic gonadotropin (hCG) all play roles in the menstrual cycle (see Table 11-3).

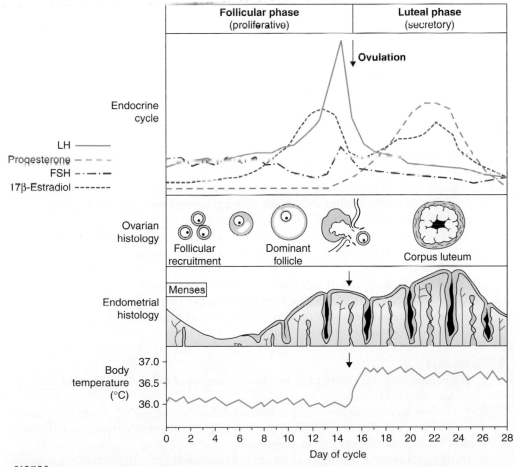

FIGURE 11-2 **Hormone levels during the menstrual cycle with appropriate ovarian, endometrial, and basal body temperature responses.**

FSH, follicle-stimulating hormone; LH, luteinizing hormone.
(Modified from Mehta, S., Milder, E. A., Mirachi, A. J., & Milder, E. [2006]. *Step-Up: A High-Yield, Systems-Based Review for the USMLE Step 1* [3rd ed., p. 196]. Philadelphia, PA: Lippincott Williams & Wilkins.)

Gynecologic and Breast Disorders

TABLE 11-3	**Roles of Hormones Involved in the Menstrual Cycle**
Hormone A	**Effects**
Luteinizing hormone (LH)	Midcycle **surge** induces **ovulation** Regulates cholesterol conversion to pregnenolone in ovarian theca cells as initial step in estrogen synthesis
Follicle-stimulating hormone (FSH)	Stimulates **development** of **ovarian follicle** Regulates ovarian granulosa cell activity to control estrogen synthesis
Estrogens (estradiol, estriol)	Stimulates **endometrial proliferation** Aids in follicle growth Induces LH surge High levels inhibit FSH secretion Principal role in sexual development
Progesterone	Stimulates **endometrial gland development** Inhibits uterine contraction Increases thickness of cervical mucus **Increases basal body temperature** Inhibits LH and FSH secretion; maintains pregnancy **Decrease** in levels leads to **menstruation**
Human chorionic gonadotropin (hCG)	Acts like LH after implantation of fertilized egg **Maintains corpus luteum viability** and progesterone secretion

2. **Follicular phase**
   a. Begins at first day of menses (i.e., menstruation)
   b. **FSH** stimulates **growth** of **ovarian follicle** (granulosa cells), which in turn secretes estradiol.
   c. **Estradiol** induces **endometrial proliferation** and further increases FSH and LH secretion from positive feedback of pituitary.
3. **Luteal phase**
   a. **LH surge** induces **ovulation**.
   b. Residual follicle (i.e., **corpus luteum**) secretes estradiol and progesterone to **maintain endometrium** and induce development of secretory ducts.
   c. High estradiol levels inhibit FSH and LH.
   d. If egg is **not** fertilized, corpus luteum degrades, progesterone and estradiol levels decrease, and the **endometrial lining degrades** (i.e., menses).
4. **Fertilization**
   a. If the egg is fertilized, it will implant in the endometrium.
   b. Endometrial tissue secretes **hCG to maintain the corpus luteum**.
   c. Corpus luteum continues to secrete progesterone until sufficient production is achieved by a developing placenta (~8 to 12 weeks).

D. Menopause
1. **Permanent** end of menstruation because of **ceasing of ovarian function** in later middle age (~51.5 years)
2. Premature menopause is defined as ovarian failure before age 40 years (more likely with history of tobacco use, radiation therapy, chemotherapy, autoimmune disorders, or abdominal or pelvic surgery).
3. During evolution of menopause (i.e., **perimenopausal** period), ovarian response to FSH and LH decreases, whereas FSH and LH levels increase and estrogen levels fluctuate.

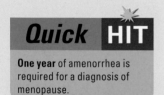

Quick HIT

One year of amenorrhea is required for a diagnosis of menopause.

4. **H/P** = **hot flashes** (secondary to thermoregulatory dysfunction), breast pain, sweating, **menstrual irregularity** with eventual **amenorrhea**, possible menorrhagia, fatigue, anxiety, irritability, depression, **dyspareunia** (caused by vaginal wall atrophy and decreased lubrication), urinary frequency, dysuria, change in bowel habits; examination detects vaginal atrophy
5. **Labs** = increased FSH, increased LH, decreased estradiol
6. **Treatment**
   a. Lubricating agents to treat dyspareunia (i.e., painful intercourse); short-term topical vaginal estrogen used in cases of significant vaginal symptoms
   b. Calcium, vitamin D, bisphosphonates, and exercise to prevent osteoporosis
   c. Selective estrogen receptor modulators, such as raloxifene and tamoxifen, may serve a role in reducing osteoporosis and cardiovascular risks.
   d. Regular cardiovascular follow-up
   e. Hormone replacement therapy was a mainstay of therapy for many years, but its benefits have more recently been shown to be less than previously believed, and it has been linked to increased risk for breast cancer and deep vein thrombosis.
7. **Complications** = osteoporosis, coronary artery disease, dementia

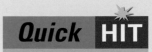

Quick HIT

Topical estrogen use is contraindicated in any patient with a history of breast cancer.

II. Contraception

A. Methods of contraception attempt to prevent pregnancy (see Table 11-4).

B. The various forms of contraception are each associated with certain side effects.

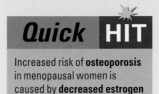

Quick HIT

Increased risk of **osteoporosis** in menopausal women is caused by **decreased estrogen** production by the ovaries.

TABLE 11-4	Methods of Contraception				
		Effectiveness[a]			
Method	Description	Ideal (%)	Typical (%)	Side Effects	
Hormonal methods					
Oral contraceptive pills (OCPs) (combined formulation)	• Estrogen–progestin combination of pills that inhibits follicle development and ovulation, changes endometrial quality, and increases cervical mucus viscosity to prevent fertilization and implantation	99	92	• Possible nausea, headache, bloating, mood changes • Increased risk of DVT • Contraindicated for heavy smokers or women with a history of DVT, estrogen-related cancer, liver disease, or hypertriglyceridemia	
Oral contraceptive pills (progestin formulation)	• Progestin-only pills that change endometrial quality and increase cervical mucus viscosity to prevent fertilization and implantation • May be option for women with contraindication for estrogen	98	88-91	• Increased breakthrough bleeding • Must be taken at same time every day to maximize efficacy	
Medroxyprogesterone acetate (Depo-Provera)	• Progestin analogue injected by health care provider every 3 months that inhibits ovulation and endometrial development	99	97	• Nausea, headache, weight gain, osteoporosis • Irregular bleeding	
Progestin implant	• Subcutaneous implant that slowly release progestin over ~3 yr (similar activity to progestin-only pill)	100[b]	100[b]	• Irregular bleeding, breast pain	

(continued)

Gynecologic and Breast Disorders

TABLE 11-4 **Methods of Contraception** (Continued)

Method	Description	Ideal (%)	Typical (%)	Side Effects
		Effectiveness[a]		
Transdermal contraceptive patch	• Transdermal delivery of estradiol and progestin analogue to act in similar manner to OCPs • Patch must be changed weekly	99	99	• Risk of patch detachment • Nausea, headache, weight gain • Irregular bleeding, breast pain • Less effective in heavier women because of diffusion into adipose tissue • Increased risk of DVT
Intravaginal ring	• Ring inserted intravaginally that releases ethinyl estradiol over 3 wk to prevent ovulation (less estrogen than OCPs) • Replaced each month	99	92	• Withdrawal bleeding, device-related discomfort, headache • Increased risk of DVT
Emergency contraception	• Regimen of estradiol and progestin taken within 72 hr of unprotected intercourse or intercourse with failed contraception method (e.g., broken condom) to prevent ovulation or inhibit fertilization • Levonorgestrel (Plan B) • Copper IUD inserted within 4–5 days of intercourse interferes with sperm function • Mifepristone (RU 486) interrupts new pregnancy	>90	>90	• Nausea, headache more severe than that seen with OCPs • Menstrual bleeding expected within 1 wk of administration
Barrier methods				
Condom	• Barrier (most frequently latex) placed over penis and left in place until withdrawal following ejaculation • Frequently used with spermicide • Polyurethane condoms are produced for those with latex allergy	98	85	• Risk of condom breakage • Latex significantly more effective than other materials (with possible exception of polyurethane) • Risk of latex allergy
Diaphragm or cervical cap	• Barrier inserted into vagina before intercourse to cover cervix • Used with spermicide and left in place for several hours after intercourse	94	84	• Inconvenient • Frequent poor compliance • Increased risk of UTI
Contraceptive sponge	• Polyurethane sponge implanted with spermicide that releases spermicide over 24 hr after insertion to inhibit fertilization	91[c]	80[c]	• Possible increased risk of toxic shock syndrome
Spermicide alone	• Insertion of spermicidal jelly or cream into vagina immediately before intercourse	82	71	• Correct usage and quantity difficult to achieve consistently
Sexual practice methods				
Abstinence	• Not engaging in intercourse	100	100	• None
Rhythm method	• Recording occurrence of menses, daily basal body temperature, and cervical mucus to determine timing of cycle, occurrence of ovulation, and period of fertility	95	83	• May be useful in diagnosing infertility
Withdrawal method	• Withdrawal of penis from vagina immediately before ejaculation	96	73	• Decreased pleasure • Difficult to conduct in effective manner
Lactation	• Unprotected intercourse during active postpartum lactation period	98	95	• Only able to be performed if actively breastfeeding, <6 months postpartum, and amenorrheic (pregnancy rate = no contraception rate otherwise)

(continued)

TABLE 11-4 Methods of Contraception (Continued)		Effectiveness[a]		
Method	**Description**	**Ideal (%)**	**Typical (%)**	**Side Effects**
Intrauterine devices				
Copper intrauterine device (IUD)	• Object inserted into uterus by physician with slow release of copper to prevent fertilization and interfere with sperm transportation • Left in place ~10 yr • May be placed soon after intercourse as emergency contraception (90% decrease in pregnancy rate)	99	99	• Small risk of spontaneous abortion and uterine perforation • Menorrhagia
Progestin-releasing IUD	• Object inserted into uterus by physician with slow release of progestin to prevent fertilization, interfere with sperm transportation, and inhibit ovulation • Left in place ~5 yr	99	99	• Small risk of spontaneous abortion and uterine perforation
Surgical methods				
Sterilization	• Cutting of vas deferens in men (vasectomy) or tubal ligation in women to prevent fertilization	~100	~100	• May be difficult to reverse • Increased risk of ectopic pregnancy in cases of failure or after voluntary ligation reversal

[a]As defined by pregnancy rate with 1 yr of use (6 months for lactation).
[b]Only one efficacy study performed; no pregnancies occurred in study.
[c]Effectiveness decreases to 80%/60% in women with prior vaginal birth history.
DVT, deep venous thrombosis; UTI, urinary tract infection.

C. Method choice

1. Should consider likelihood of patient compliance
2. Side effects must be tolerated by patient.
3. Certain methods may be contraindicated for comorbid medical conditions.

III. Menstrual Disorders and Issues

A. Amenorrhea

1. Absence of menstruation
   a. **Primary**: absence of menses (**never** has happened) with normal secondary sexual characteristics by a 16-year-old or absence of both menses and secondary sexual characteristics by a 13-year-old
   b. **Secondary**: absence of menses for 6 months in patient with **prior history of menses**
2. Causes
   a. Primary: hypothalamic or pituitary dysfunction, anatomic abnormalities (e.g., absent uterus, vaginal septa), **chromosome abnormalities** with gonadal dysgenesis
   b. Secondary: pregnancy, ovarian failure, hypothalamic or pituitary disease, uterine abnormalities (e.g., Asherman syndrome), polycystic ovary syndrome (PCOS), anorexia nervosa, malnutrition, thyroid disease
3. H/P
   a. History should address occurrence of any previous menstruation periods (e.g., primary or secondary amenorrhea), exercise and eating habits (e.g., substantial exercise or inadequate eating), family history, medications, androgenous symptoms (e.g., facial hair, voice deepening), and known comorbidity.
   b. Examination should note Tanner stages (see Table 11-2) and should check for normal sexual anatomy.

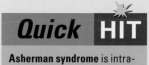

Asherman syndrome is intrauterine adhesions resulting from a surgical procedure or possibly infection.

Gynecologic and Breast Disorders

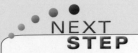

β-hCG **pregnancy test** is always the first step in the workup of any type of amenorrhea.

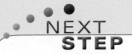

If testicles are present in an XY patient with androgen insensitivity syndrome, they should be **removed** at an early age because of increased risk of **testicular cancer**.

4. Labs
   a. **β-hCG test** used to rule out pregnancy (see Figure 11-3)
   b. TSH, T_4, and T_3-reuptake can diagnose thyroid dysfunction.
   c. Increased **prolactin** suggests prolactin-secreting tumor.
   d. FSH and LH levels measure hypothalamic-pituitary activity.
   e. Increased androgens (e.g., testosterone, dehydroepiandrosterone [DHEA]) suggest PCOS.
   f. **Progestin challenge** (i.e., patient is observed for bleeding after 5-day administration of progesterone) and **estrogen-progesterone challenge** (i.e., patient is observed for bleeding after administration of estrogen and progesterone) can help detect anatomic abnormalities (bleeding indicates normal outflow tract), hormonal abnormalities, or hypothalamic-pituitary activity.
5. Treatment
   a. Modify behaviors (e.g., eating disorders, exercise) to allow menstruation.
   b. Anatomic abnormalities require surgical correction.
   c. Hypothalamic-pituitary dysfunction may be treatable by GnRH or gonadotropin replacement.
   d. Prolactinoma may be treated with dopamine agonists.
   e. Hormone replacement therapy may be considered in ovarian failure.
   f. Lysis of adhesions and estrogen administration performed for Asherman syndrome
   g. Thyroid dysfunction and Cushing syndrome treated according to specific pathology
   h. In some untreatable patients with appropriate anatomy, pregnancy may be accomplished through egg donation, in vitro fertilization, and hormone modulation.

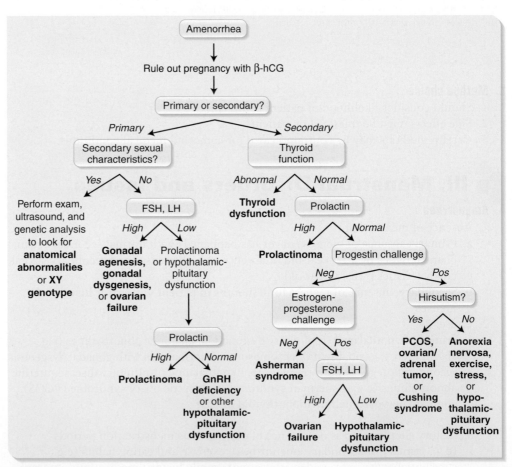

FIGURE
11-3 **Approach to the patient with amenorrhea.**

FSH, follicle-stimulating hormone; GnRH, gonadotropin-releasing hormone; β-hCG, human chorionic gonadotropin; LH, luteinizing hormone; Neg, negative; PCOS, polycystic ovary syndrome; Pos, positive.

6. **Complications** = patients with genetic disorders or ovarian failure may be **unable** to achieve normal menstrual cycles

B. Dysmenorrhea

1. Periodic pain associated with menses that may be primary (without pelvic pathology) or secondary (caused by endometriosis, pelvic inflammatory disease [PID], uterine fibroids, ovarian cysts, or adenomyosis)
2. **Risk factors** = menorrhagia, menarche <12 years, body mass index <20, PID, sexual assault, smoking, premenstrual syndrome
3. **H/P** = crampy lower abdominal pain associated with menstruation, nausea, vomiting, headache, diarrhea; mild abdominal tenderness
4. **Labs** = β-hCG and blood and vaginal cultures are helpful to rule out pregnancy and infection
5. **Radiology** = ultrasound (US) may be used to detect ovarian and uterine lesions; hysteroscopy or laparoscopy may be needed to detect intrauterine pathology, intra-abdominal pathology, or endometriosis
6. **Treatment** = nonsteroidal anti-inflammatory drugs (NSAIDs) or oral contraceptive pills (OCPs) for primary disorders; treat underlying infection or uterine disease

C. Premenstrual syndrome (PMS) and premenstrual dysphoric disorder (PMDD)

1. Syndromes seen in women with normal functioning ovaries that precede menses and are characterized by multiple pain, mood, and autonomic symptoms; mood symptoms are more severe in PMDD
2. Most women with menstrual cycles experience some symptoms, but 5% to 10% of women have severe symptoms that **interfere with daily life**.
3. **Risk factors** (for severe symptoms) = family history
4. **H/P**
   a. Weight gain, headache, abdominal or pelvic pain, abdominal bloating, change in bowel habits, food cravings, mood lability, depression, fatigue, irritability; breast tenderness, edema, abdominal tenderness, acne
   b. Findings precede menses and **occur at similar time points** in each cycle.
5. **Treatment** = exercise, vitamin B$_6$, NSAIDs, OCPs, progestins; selective serotonin reuptake inhibitors (SSRIs) ± alprazolam may improve mood symptoms in both PMS and PMDD

D. Endometriosis

1. Presence of **endometrial tissue outside the uterus** (e.g., ovaries, broad ligament); ectopic tissue follows same menstrual cycle as normal tissue
2. Retrograde menstruation, vascular/lymphatic spread of endometrial tissue from uterus to pelvic cavity, or iatrogenic spread of endometrial tissue (e.g., during caesarian section) are most plausible causes of condition.
3. **Risk factors** = family history, **infertility**, nulliparity (i.e., no history of childbirth), low body mass index
4. **H/P** = dysmenorrhea, dyspareunia, painful bowel movements (i.e., dyschezia), **pelvic pain**, possible infertility; uterine or adnexal tenderness; palpable adhesions on uterus or ovaries
5. **Labs** = biopsy of lesions shows **endometrial tissue**; β-hCG and urinalysis helpful to rule out pregnancy and urinary tract infection; CA-125 marker frequently increased but not a highly sensitive test
6. **Radiology** = **laparoscopy** will show "**powder-burn**" lesions and cysts on involved areas and is optimal diagnostic tool
7. **Treatment**
   a. Recording a journal of symptoms is useful for defining treatment.
   b. OCPs, progestins, danazol, or GnRH agonists may supply symptomatic relief.
   c. Laparoscopic ablation may successfully remove lesions while maintaining fertility potential.
   d. Hysterectomy, lysis of adhesions, or salpingo-oophorectomy may be required in severe cases.

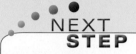

Quick HIT

Primary dysmenorrhea symptoms occur in the **beginning** of menstruation and resolve over several days; **secondary** dysmenorrhea symptoms often begin **midcycle** before the onset of menstruation and increase in severity until the conclusion of menstruation.

NEXT STEP

Any woman of childbearing age with abdominal pain must be given a β-hCG pregnancy test to rule out **ectopic pregnancy**.

NEXT STEP

If a patient suspected of having PMS or PMDD has mood symptoms **throughout** her menstrual cycle, initiate a psychiatric workup for a mood disorder. Menstrual-related symptoms should **only** occur in the **second half** of the cycle.

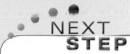

Quick HIT

Endometriosis is the most **common** cause of **female infertility** and may be responsible for up to 50% of cases.

Quick HIT

Adenomyosis is endometrial tissue that invades the myometrium, causing uterine enlargement and cyclical pain.

Gynecologic and Breast Disorders

8. **Complications** = fertility may not be achieved despite pharmacologic or laparoscopic intervention

E. Abnormal uterine bleeding

1. **Irregular** menstruation, excessive menses (i.e., menorrhagia), or **increased duration** of menses that may be the result of a variety of causes (e.g., uterine fibroids, cancer, hypothalamic-pituitary dysfunction, bleeding diatheses [e.g., von Willebrand disease], threatened abortion, molar pregnancy, ectopic pregnancy)
2. **H/P**
   a. Uterine bleeding that does not follow usual menstrual cycle or occurs in post-menopausal women
   b. Menses with **<24-day or >35-day intervals, lasting >7 days,** or blood loss **>80 mL** are considered abnormal.
   c. Associated symptoms (e.g., fever, abdominal pain, vaginal discharge, acne, changes in bowel or bladder function), family history, history of medical conditions useful to making diagnosis
   d. Visualization of bleeding site (e.g., cervix, vagina, anus, vulva), palpation of pelvic masses important
3. **Labs**
   a. β-hCG used to rule out pregnancy
   b. Complete blood count (CBC), coagulation studies, TSH, FSH, and LH are used to rule out anemia, coagulopathy, and endocrine abnormalities.
   c. Papanicolaou (Pap) smear and endometrial biopsy (possibly obtained during dilation and curettage [D&C]) used to rule out cancer
   d. Testing for STIs used to rule out infection
4. **Radiology** = US may detect uterine lesions; hysteroscopy frequently indicated to visualize lesions and perform D&C
5. **Treatment**
   a. Treat underlying disorder (e.g., coagulopathies, thyroid disease, infection).
   b. OCPs can be used for cycle irregularity.
   c. Endometrial ablation may be performed for severe or recurrent bleeding.

F. Polycystic ovary syndrome (PCOS)

1. Hypothalamic-pituitary disease characterized by **anovulation or oligoovulation** (manifested as amenorrhea/oligomenorrhea), **androgen excess**, and **polycystic ovaries**
2. **Excess LH secretion** induces overproduction of androgens by ovaries.
3. Some patients with PCOS may have hyperinsulinemia, which induces androgen production and increases risk of insulin resistance.
4. **Excess androgens** produced by ovaries and adrenals are converted to estrogen, which induces further ovarian androgen production.
5. Amenorrhea and infertility caused by abnormal LH levels and FSH inhibition by high estrogen level; hirsutism results from increased androgens
6. **H/P**
   a. **Obesity** (frequently initial sign)
   b. **Hirsutism:** excess growth of facial, chest, and abdominal hair
   c. **Acne**
   d. **Menstrual dysfunction:** amenorrhea, oligomenorrhea, breakthrough bleeding
   e. **Infertility**
   f. Bilateral ovarian enlargement on bimanual examination
7. **Labs** = increased LH, **LH:FSH ratio >2,** increased DHEA, increased total testosterone; positive progestin challenge
8. **Radiology** = US shows **enlarged ovaries** with **multiple cysts**
9. **Treatment**
   a. Exercise and weight loss
   b. OCPs can be used to suppress LH and FSH, regulate menstrual cycles, decrease circulating estrogen, and decrease endometrial cancer risk.

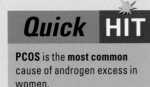

Quick **HIT**

PCOS is the **most common** cause of androgen excess in women.

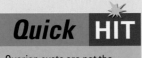

Quick **HIT**

Ovarian cysts are not the cause of disease in PCOS but are a result of androgen hypersecretion.

c. If OCPs are not an option, progestin alone for 7 days each month will induce bleeding and prevent endometrial hyperplasia.

d. Spironolactone has antiandrogen effects and may help treat hirsutism and acne, if response to OCPs is inadequate; it must be stopped in pregnancy due to risk of antiandrogen effects in male fetus.

e. Clomiphene (antiestrogen) induces follicle stimulation and maturation to allow pregnancy.

f. Metformin will facilitate weight loss, improve cholesterol profile, reduce blood pressure (BP), and reduce cardiovascular risk; some women may start ovulating solely with metformin therapy; management of glucose intolerance required to avoid complications of diabetes mellitus (DM)

g. Consider a statin to lower lipid and testosterone levels

h. Antibiotics as needed for acne

10. **Complications** = infertility; increased risk for DM, hypertension, ischemic heart disease, ovarian torsion, and endometrial cancer

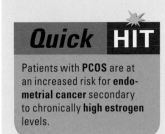

Patients with **PCOS** are at an increased risk for **endometrial cancer** secondary to chronically **high estrogen** levels.

 ## IV. Common Gynecologic Infections

A. Vaginitis

1. Vaginal infection caused by overgrowth of normal bacteria (*Gardnerella vaginalis*), protozoans (*Trichomonas*), or fungus (*Candida albicans*)

2. **Risk factors** = DM, human immunodeficiency virus (HIV), unprotected sex, multiple partners, young age at first intercourse, douching, intrauterine device (IUD) use, smoking

3. H/P = vaginal **irritation** or **pruritus**, vaginal discharge; examination detects vaginal inflammation with characteristic findings depending on cause (see Table 11-5, Figure 11-4)

4. **Labs** = **wet mount** (i.e., smear of vaginal fluid examined under microscope) with saline or potassium hydroxide (KOH) and **vaginal pH** testing useful to distinguish cause; smell a fishy odor when KOH is added to the vaginal discharge on a slide ("whiff test")

5. **Treatment** = metronidazole (*G. vaginalis* or *Trichomonas*), clindamycin (*G. vaginalis*), or fluconazole (*C. albicans*)

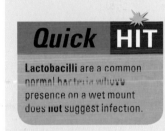

Lactobacilli are a common normal bacteria whose presence on a wet mount does **not** suggest infection.

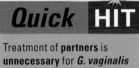

Treatment of **partners** is **unnecessary** for *G. vaginalis* or *C. albicans* but is required with *Trichomonas* infection (metronidazole).

B. Toxic shock syndrome

1. Severe systemic reaction to *Staphylococcus aureus* exotoxin associated with **prolonged tampon use**, prolonged intravaginal contraception use, or postpartum or postabortion infection

TABLE 11-5 Common Infections Causes of Vaginitis			
Characteristics	***Gardnerella vaginalis***	***Trichomonas vaginalis***	***Candida albicans***
Physical examination	Mild vaginal inflammation	Vaginal and cervical inflammation, **cervical petechiae**	Significant vaginal inflammation
Discharge	Thin, white, fishy odor	Malodorous, frothy, **greenish**	Thick, white, **"cottage cheese–like"**
Wet mount (saline)	**Clue cells** (epithelial cells with multiple attached bacteria)	**Motile trichomonads**	Normal
Wet mount (KOH)	Fishy odor (positive whiff test)	Possible fishy odor	**Pseudohyphae**
Vaginal pH	>4.5 (high)	>4.5 (high)	**3.5–4.5** (normal)
Treatment	Metronidazole	Metronidazole (also **treat partner**)	Topical clotrimazole, miconazole, or nystatin, or oral fluconazole (single dose)

KOH, potassium hydroxide.

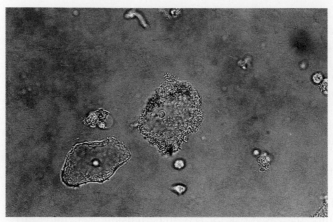

**FIGURE
11-4** **Vaginal wet mount (saline preparation) showing clue cell with multiple bacteria attached to the border.**

A normal epithelial cell is adjacent to the clue cell (1,000 × magnification).
(From Fleisher, G. R., Ludwig, S., Henretig, F. M., Ruddy, R. M., & Silverman, B. K. [2005]. *Textbook of Pediatric Emergency Medicine* [5th ed., Figure 94-8]. Philadelphia, PA: Lippincott Williams & Wilkins; with permission.)

2. **H/P** = vomiting, diarrhea, sore throat, headache; high fever, generalized macular rash; severe cases develop **hypotension**, shock, respiratory distress, and **desquamation of palms and soles**
3. **Labs** = vaginal fluid culture shows *S. aureus*; decreased platelets, increased alanine aminotransferase (ALT) and aspartate aminotransferase (AST), and increased blood urea nitrogen (BUN) and creatinine in progressing cases
4. **Treatment**
   a. Remove tampon or other intravaginal objects.
   b. Supportive care for hypotension; pressors may be required
   c. Clindamycin or penicillinase-resistant β-lactam antibiotics (e.g., oxacillin, nafcillin); vancomycin required for methicillin-resistant strains

V. Sexually Transmitted Infections (STIs)

A. Cervicitis
1. Infection of cervical columnar epithelium caused by *Neisseria gonorrhoeae* or *Chlamydia trachomatis*
2. Urethra, oral cavity, or rectal area can also become infected through sexual contact.
3. **H/P**
   a. Possibly asymptomatic (>50% of cases in chlamydial infection)
   b. Dyspareunia, bleeding after intercourse, **purulent vaginal discharge** (milder for *Chlamydia*)
   c. **Urethritis** associated with purulent discharge and dysuria
   d. Rectal and pharyngeal infections are frequently asymptomatic.
   e. Examination detects inflammation of cervix with associated purulent discharge.
4. **Labs**
   a. Gram stain of cervical scraping shows gram-negative diplococci with *N. gonorrhoeae* (usually nothing seen with *Chlamydia* infection).
   b. Culture on Thayer-Martin agar detects *N. gonorrhoeae*.
   c. **Enzyme immunoassays** are useful for detecting both pathogens.
   d. **DNA probes** and **DNA amplification** testing (i.e., polymerase chain reaction [PCR]) are highly sensitive means of detecting either pathogen on swabs of cervical fluid.
5. **Treatment** = ceftriaxone for *N. gonorrhoeae*, doxycycline (not in pregnancy) or azithromycin for *Chlamydia*; both antibiotics often given together because of **frequent dual infection**; sexual partners must be treated to reduce risk of reinfection
6. **Complication** = PID, septic arthritis

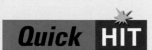

Chlamydia infection is **the most common reportable STD** because it can be **asymptomatic** (especially in men) and frequently goes unrecognized.

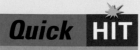

Clinical cervicitis with negative Gram stain and cultures is highly suggestive of *Chlamydia* infection.

Gynecologic and Breast Disorders

B. Pelvic inflammatory disease (PID)

1. Progressive *N. gonorrhoeae* or *Chlamydia* infection resulting in involvement of ovaries, uterus, fallopian tubes, or peritoneal cavity
2. Less frequently caused by *Bacteroides, Escherichia coli,* or streptococci
3. **Risk factors** = multiple sexual partners, unprotected intercourse, prior PID, douching, young age at first intercourse
4. **H/P** = lower abdominal pain starting within days of menses, nausea, vomiting, dysuria; purulent cervical discharge, abdominal tenderness, fever, **cervical motion tenderness**, adnexal tenderness, possible abdominal guarding
5. **Labs**
   a. Pregnancy test needed to rule out ectopic pregnancy
   b. Increased white blood cell count (WBC), increased erythrocyte sedimentation rate (ESR)
   c. Gram stain, culture, immunoassays useful for identifying agent
   d. **Culdocentesis** (i.e., aspiration of intraperitoneal fluid from cul-de-sac posterior to uterus) yields pus.
6. **Radiology** = transvaginal US may detect inflamed and enlarged uterus, abscess of fallopian tubes or ovaries, or free fluid (technique used for diagnosis less now than in the past); laparoscopy may visualize inflamed tissue
7. **Treatment** = empiric antibiotics until specific agent identified (doxycycline, ceftriaxone, cefoxitin); treat as inpatient if high fevers or young age; treat sexual partners
8. **Complications** = **infertility** because of adhesion formation, chronic pelvic pain, **tubo-ovarian abscess**, increased risk of ectopic pregnancy

C. Syphilis

1. Disease caused by the spirochete *Treponema pallidum* (only transmitted by sexual contact or from mother to child)
2. **H/P** — varies according to stage of disease
   a. **Primary**
      (1) One to 13 weeks after exposure (average **3 weeks**)
      (2) Solitary **chancre** (i.e., firm papule that evolves into **painless ulcer**) forms near area of contact and heals spontaneously within 9 weeks.
   b. **Secondary**
      (1) Begins as chancre heals and can last up to 12 weeks
      (2) Headache, malaise; fever, **maculopapular rash** on palms and soles, lymphadenopathy, papules in moist areas of body (i.e., condyloma lata)
      (3) Symptoms and lesions resolve spontaneously.
      (4) Brief relapses of secondary symptoms can occur for a few years after the initial presentation.
   c. **Latent**
      (1) Asymptomatic
      (2) Can last years
   d. **Tertiary**
      (1) One-third of untreated patients progress beyond latent stage in 1 to 30 years after infection.
      (2) Granulomatous lesions (i.e., **gummas**) of skin, bone, and liver
      (3) Loss of two-point discrimination and proprioception secondary to dorsal column degeneration (i.e., **tabes dorsalis**), Argyll-Robertson pupils
3. **Labs**
   a. VDRL and rapid plasma regain (RPR) are 80% sensitive screening tests.
   b. Fluorescent treponemal antibody absorption (FTA-ABS) or microhemagglutination assay for antibodies to treponemes (MHA-TP) used to confirm diagnosis
   c. Spirochetes may be seen with dark-field microscopy analysis of swabs of lesions.
   d. Examination of cerebrospinal fluid (CSF) should be performed to confirm tertiary syphilis in patients with neurologic findings.
4. **Treatment** = **penicillin G**, doxycycline, or tetracycline; IV penicillin G used in severe tertiary cases

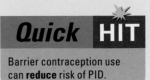

Quick HIT

Barrier contraception use can **reduce** risk of PID.

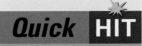

Quick HIT

Patients with PID may exhibit the **"chandelier sign"**: palpating the cervix during pelvic examination may be so painful that they almost jump off of the examination table.

NEXT STEP

Suspect **tubo-ovarian abscess** in a patient with PID who also has signs of sepsis or **peritonitis**. Inpatient treatment is required with intravenous (IV) hydration, IV antibiotics, and surgical drainage.

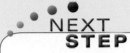

Quick HIT

RPR and VDRL may become negative following syphilis treatment, but FTA-ABS will remain positive for life.

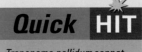

Quick HIT

Treponema pallidum cannot be cultured.

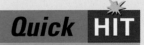

Gynecologic and Breast Disorders

    5. **Complications** = gummatous destruction of skin, bones, and liver; cardiovascular syphilis (aortic regurgitation, aortitis); neurosyphilis (cerebral atrophy, tabes dorsalis, meningitis)

D. Genital herpes: disease caused by herpes simplex virus type 2 (most cases) or type 1 (less common) (see Chapter 10, **Dermatology**)

E. Molluscum contagiosum (see Chapter 10, **Dermatology**)

F. Human papillomavirus (HPV)

1. Several types of papillomavirus (>100) that may be associated with **genital warts** (types 6 and 11) or **cervical cancer** (types 16 or 18 in 70% of cases)
2. **H/P** = frequent small pink papules at site of contact; infection caused by HPV types 6 or 11 can cause larger cauliflower-like warts on genital region
3. **Labs**
    a. An abnormal Pap smear should prompt HPV testing and colposcopy to look for lesions (see Figure 11-5).
    b. Application of acetic acid to lesions will turn them white during examination.
    c. Biopsy of lesions can be used to confirm infection and determine virus type through HPV DNA analysis.
4. **Treatment** = podophyllin, trichloroacetic acid, topical 5-fluorouracil, α-interferon injection of large lesions, cryotherapy, or laser therapy; a vaccine is now available for HPV types **6, 11, 16, and 18** that acts as prophylaxis against 90% of genital warts and 70% of cervical cancers
5. **Complications** = vaginal scarring for removal of large lesions, possible **increased risk** of **cervical cancer** depending on viral type

G. Chancroid

1. Highly contagious disease caused by *Haemophilus ducreyi* seen most commonly in tropical or subtropical regions or in immunocompromised patients
2. **H/P** = within 2 weeks of contact, small papule forms in area of contact and transforms into **painful ulcer** with grayish base and foul odor; possible inguinal lymphadenopathy that can cause **significant inguinal swelling** (i.e., bubo formation)
3. **Labs** = Gram stain of tissue at ulcer edge shows gram-negative rods
4. **Treatment** = ceftriaxone, erythromycin, or azithromycin

H. Lymphogranuloma venereum

1. Disease caused by L-1, L-2, or L-3 serotypes of *C. trachomatis* (differentiated from cervicitis); more common in developing nations
2. **H/P**
    a. Within 2 weeks of contact, malaise, headache, fever, and formation of papule at site of contact that becomes **painless ulcer** that heals after a few days

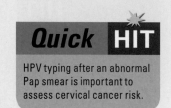

Quick HIT

HPV typing after an abnormal Pap smear is important to assess cervical cancer risk.

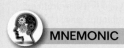

MNEMONIC

Remember the characterization of genital ulcers by the mnemonic **S**ome **G**irls **L**ove **L**icorice, but **F**ellows **H**ate **C**andy: **S**yphilis, **G**ranuloma inguinale, and **L**ymphogranuloma venereum = pain**L**ess. Pain**F**ul = **H**erpes simplex and **C**hancroid.

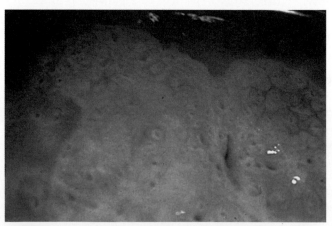

FIGURE

11-5 Colposcopy view of the cervix with multiple lesions consistent with human papillomavirus (HPV) infection.

Application of acetic acid to the cervix during the examination has made these lesions more apparent. (From Goodheart, H. P. [2008]. *Goodheart's Photoguide of Common Skin Disorders* [3rd ed., p. 323]. Philadelphia, PA: Lippincott Williams & Wilkins; with permission.)

b. After 1 month, **significant inguinal buboes** develop (more common in men than in women).
c. Can progress to bubo ulceration, elephantiasis (i.e., severe connective tissue swelling secondary to lymph vessel obstruction), fistula formation, and abscess formation
3. **Labs** = immunoassays for *Chlamydia* may be helpful for diagnosis
4. **Treatment** = tetracycline, erythromycin, or doxycycline

I. Granuloma inguinale
1. Disease caused by infection by *Klebsiella granulomatis*
2. **H/P**
   a. Papule on external genitalia forms several weeks after contact and rapidly becomes **painless ulcer** with **beefy red base** and **irregular borders**.
   b. Mild lymphadenopathy can occur.
   c. Infection of ulcers can lead to significant scarring, vaginal stenosis, or elephantiasis.
3. **Labs** = lesion biopsy on Giemsa stain shows **Donovan bodies** (i.e., red encapsulated intracellular bacteria)
4. **Treatment** = doxycycline or trimethoprim-sulfamethoxazole for 3 weeks

VI. Gynecologic Neoplasms

A. Uterine fibroids (uterine leiomyoma)
1. Benign uterine masses composed of smooth muscle; generally regress after menopause
2. **Risk factors** = nulliparity, African-American heritage, diet high in meats, alcohol consumption, family history
3. **H/P** = possibly asymptomatic; possible **menorrhagia**, pelvis pressure or pain, urinary frequency, or **infertility**; palpable mass on examination
4. **Radiology** = transvaginal US or hysteroscopy used to locate or visualize mass
5. **Treatment**
   a. Follow **asymptomatic** fibroids with US to detect **abnormal growth**.
   b. **GnRH agonists** reduce uterine bleeding and fibroid size but are only recommended as temporary therapy (reduce fibroid size before surgery or as temporizing measure before imminent menopause)
   c. **Myomectomy** (laparoscopic or hysteroscopic for isolated lesions, open for multiple lesions) indicated for resection of symptomatic fibroids in women wishing to maintain fertility
   d. **Hysterectomy** can be performed for symptomatic fibroids in patients for whom fertility is not a concern.
   e. **Uterine artery embolization** following a pelvic MRI to rule out other soft tissue pathology may be performed to selectively infarct small fibroids in women wishing to avoid surgery but carries a high likelihood of impaired fertility.

B. Endometrial cancer
1. Adenocarcinoma of uterine tissue most commonly related to **exposure to high estrogen levels**; most common in postmenopausal women
2. **Risk factors** = unopposed exogenous estrogen, PCOS, obesity, nulliparity, DM, hypertension, family history, increased age (postmenopausal), high-fat diet, colon cancer (hereditary nonpolyposis colon cancer [HNPCC])
3. **H/P** = heavy menses, midcycle bleeding, or **postmenopausal bleeding**, with possible abdominal pain; ovaries or uterus may feel fixed in position if tumor has local extension
4. **Labs** = endometrial biopsy (or examination of cells collected during D&C) shows hyperplastic abnormal glands with vascular invasion; **increased CA-125** tumor marker (not specific for endometrial cancer and not always increased) is useful in monitoring response to therapy
5. **Radiology** = chest X-ray (CXR) and CT can be used to detect metastases; transvaginal US may detect masses and can be used to measure endometrial wall thickness

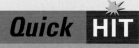
Quick HIT
Uterine fibroids do **not** continue to grow after menopause (because of estrogen sensitivity and decreased postmenopausal estrogen levels).

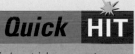
Quick HIT
Endometrial cancer **not related** to excess endogenous or exogenous estrogen exposure carries a **worse** prognosis than estrogen-related tumors.

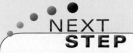
NEXT STEP
Although **atrophic vaginitis** is the **most common cause** of vaginal **bleeding** in postmenopausal women (80% cases), endometrial cancer must be ruled out for any postmenopausal woman presenting with this complaint (perform **endometrial biopsy**).

6. Treatment
   a. **Total abdominal hysterectomy** with **bilateral salpingo-oophorectomy** (TAH-BSO) and lymph node sampling
   b. Women who have cancer limited to the endometrial lining and who desire to maintain fertility can be treated temporarily with progestins to limit growth but should have TAH-BSO following childbearing years.
   c. Surgical debulking should be performed for large tumors unable to be completely resected.
   d. Any high-grade malignancy or tumors with spread beyond the endometrial lining should receive adjuvant radiation therapy in addition to surgery.
   e. Chemotherapy (in place of radiation) used for any cases with spread beyond the uterus
   f. Hormone therapy (e.g., progesterone, tamoxifen) may be beneficial for advanced tumors not cured by surgery and radiation.
7. **Complications**
   a. Local extension to fallopian tubes, ovaries, and cervix
   b. Metastases to peritoneum, aortic and pelvic lymph nodes, lungs, and vagina
   c. Ninety-six percent 5-year survival rate for localized disease; 25% 5-year survival rate with metastases

C. Cervical cancer

1. Squamous cell cancer (80% cases), adenocarcinoma (15% cases), or mixed adenosquamous carcinoma (5% cases) of the cervix that results from progression of **cervical dysplasia**
2. **Risk factors** = early first intercourse, tobacco, **HPV** (types 16, 18, 31, or 33), multiple sexual partners, high-risk sexual partners, history of STIs
3. Cervical dysplasia
   a. Precancerous squamous cell lesions of the cervix that progress to invasive cervical cancer in 1% to 22% of cases depending on cellular grade
   b. Usually detected by Pap smear or liquid-based cytology (abnormal cells seen on cytology)
   c. Cellular grading classified by Bethesda system (see Table 11-6)
4. **H/P** = usually asymptomatic in early stages; possible vaginal bleeding (postcoital or spontaneous), pelvic pain, or cervical discharge; cervical mass may be palpated; invasive cancer can be frequently seen on cervical examination
5. **Labs** = detected by **Pap smear**; punch biopsy of visible lesions; cone biopsy determines invasion extent
6. **Radiology** = CT, MRI, or US may be useful for determining extent of disease

Quick HIT

All women should receive **Pap smears** beginning at **21 years of age**, and most guidelines recommend stopping at age 65 years. Women 21–29 years of age should be screened **every 3 years.** Women ≥30 years may have HPV testing every 5 years in addition to the Pap smear cytology.

Gynecologic and Breast Disorders

TABLE 11-6	Bethesda Classification of Cervical Squamous Cell Dysplasia and Appropriate Therapy	
Grade	**Characteristics**	**Treatment**
Atypical squamous cells of undetermined significance (**ASCUS**)	Cellular abnormalities not explained by reactive changes; not suggestive of intraepithelial lesions	HPV screening; repeat Pap smear in 6 and 12 months; repeat HPV testing in 12 months
Atypical squamous cells, cannot exclude HSIL (**ASC-H**)	Cellular abnormalities not explained by reactive changes; HSIL cannot be excluded	HPV screening; endocervical biopsy; repeat Pap smear in 6 and 12 months; repeat HPV testing in 12 months
Low-grade squamous intraepithelial lesion (**LSIL**) (a.k.a. CIN 1)	Mild cellular dysplasia	Repeat Pap smear in 6 and 12 months; repeat HPV testing in 12 months; excision by loop electrocautery excision procedure (LEEP) or conization or laser ablation may be performed
High-grade squamous intraepithelial lesion (**HSIL**) (a.k.a. CIN 2 or 3)	Moderate or severe cellular dysplasia including carcinoma in situ	Excision by LEEP or conization or laser ablation; repeat cervical cytology every 6 months
Squamous cell carcinoma	Highly atypical cells with stromal invasion	Varies with degree of invasion and extent of involvement

CIN, cervical intraepithelial neoplasia; HPV, human papillomavirus.

7. **Treatment**
   a. Cervical dysplasia: treatment based on cellular grade (see Table 11-6)
   b. Invasive carcinoma
      (1) Lesions with microscopic invasion <5 mm treated with TAH or conization (i.e., cone-shaped endocervical resection) if patient desires to maintain fertility
      (2) For small lesions with close surgical margins, postoperative chemotherapy should be administered.
      (3) Visibly invasive lesions or those that involve the uterus but do not extend to the pelvic wall or lower third of the vagina should be treated by radical hysterectomy with lymphadenectomy or radiation therapy plus cisplatin-based chemotherapy.
      (4) Lesions with extension to parametrial tissue, pelvic wall, lower third of the vagina, or adjacent organs or any lesions with metastases should be treated with radiation therapy and chemotherapy.
8. **Complications** = 5-year survival is >90% for microscopic lesions, 65% to 85% for visible lesions limited to the uterus, 40% for lesions extending beyond the uterus, and 20% for metastatic lesions

D. Benign ovarian tumors

1. Benign ovarian lesions of functional ovarian cell, epithelial cell, or germ cell origin (see Table 11-7)

TABLE 11-7	Common Types of Benign Ovarian Masses			
Tumor	**Origin**	**Characteristics**	**History and Physical**	**Treatment**
Follicular cyst	Ovarian follicle	**Granulosa** cells, cystic (~3 cm diameter), occur in first 2 wk of cycle and **may regress** over menstrual period	Abdominal pain and fullness; palpable tender mass on bimanual examination Peritoneal signs if torsion or rupture occur	**Observation**; ovarian cystectomy if mass does not regress or for increased suspicion of cancer
Corpus luteum cyst	Corpus luteum	**Theca** cells, cystic or hemorrhagic corpus luteum, usually larger and firmer than follicular cyst, more common in later weeks of cycle	Abdominal pain; palpable tender mass on bimanual examination Greater risk of torsion or rupture with significant bleeding than follicular cyst	**Observation**; ovarian cystectomy if mass does not regress or for increased suspicion of cancer; rupture with significant hemorrhage requires surgical hemostasis and cystectomy
Mucinous or serous cystadenoma	Epithelial tissue	May resemble endometrial or tubal histology, cystic with serous or mucinous contents, may form calcifications **(psammoma bodies), may become extremely large**	Frequently asymptomatic until significant growth has occurred Palpable mass on bimanual examination that may be palpable during abdominal examination if large	Unilateral salpingo-oophorectomy; TAH/BSO if postmenopausal
Endometrioma	Endometrium	Spread of endometriosis to involve ovary, similar behavior to other sites of endometriosis	Frequently asymptomatic Abdominal pain, dyspareunia, infertility Tender palpable mass	OCPs, GnRH agonists, progestins, danazol may lessen symptoms; cystectomy or oophorectomy frequently required because of high recurrence rate
Benign cystic teratoma (i.e., dermoid cyst)	Germ cells	Composed of **multiple dermal tissues** including hair, teeth, and sebaceous glands	Frequently asymptomatic Oily contents released during rupture can cause peritonitis	Cystectomy with attempted preservation of ovary if benign; 1%–2% undergo malignant transformation and require salpingo-oophorectomy
Stromal cell tumor	Granulosa, theca, or Sertoli Leydig cells	Secrete hormones appropriate to cells of origin, malignant potential	**Precocious puberty** (granulosa theca cell tumors) or **virilization** (Sertoli-Leydig cell tumors)	Unilateral salpingo oophorectomy; TAH/BSO if postmenopausal

GnRH, gonadotropin-releasing hormone; OCPs, oral contraceptive pills; TAH/BSO, total abdominal hysterectomy with bilateral salpingo-oophorectomy.

2. H/P
   a. Frequently asymptomatic
   b. Lower abdominal pain (more common with functional tumors or tumor torsion), nausea, vomiting, abdominal fullness (only after significant growth)
   c. Palpable ovarian mass on bimanual examination, possible abdominal tenderness, fever
   d. In cases of ruptured mass, patient may have guarding, rebound tenderness, and abdominal rigidity.
3. **Labs** = frequently **increased CA-125**; biopsy of tumor used to determine benign or malignant nature
4. **Radiology** = US used to evaluate type of mass (cystic or solid) and quality of mass (irregular, multiple septa, smooth edges)
5. **Treatment** = observation common for functional cysts; oophorectomy performed for benign neoplasms; TAH-BSO considered for postmenopausal women
6. **Complications** = tumor torsion, tumor rupture with hemorrhage

E. Ovarian cancer

1. Cancer of ovaries most commonly of epithelial (65% cases) or germ cell (25% cases) origin; most cases are diagnosed only after considerable growth
2. **Risk factors** = **family history**, infertility, nulliparity, **BRCA1** or **BRCA2** gene mutations
3. H/P
   a. Usually **asymptomatic or minimally symptomatic until late in disease course**
   b. Abdominal pain, fatigue, weight loss, change in bowel habits, menstrual irregularity; ascites, mass may be palpated on bimanual examination
4. **Labs** = **increased CA-125** (80% of cases) in epithelial tumors; α-fetoprotein, hCG, and lactate dehydrogenase (LDH) may be increased in germ cell tumors
5. **Radiology** = US used to detect mass; MRI or CT useful to determine extent of involvement
6. **Treatment**
   a. Epithelial tumors
      (1) TAH/BSO, pelvic wall sampling, and appendectomy; adjuvant chemotherapy frequently prescribed
      (2) Tumor debulking with resection of involved bowel, liver, omentum, spleen, and lymph nodes performed for extensive disease with metastases
      (3) Single oophorectomy may be performed for tumors detected early in patients wanting to maintain fertility.
   b. Germ cell tumors
      (1) Unilateral salpingo-oophorectomy performed for limited disease
      (2) Surgical debulking performed for extensive tumors
      (3) Chemotherapy typically administered postoperatively
7. **Complications** = 5-year survival improves with early detection, but because tumor is frequently in advanced stages by time of detection, prognosis is often poor

VII. Disorders of the Breast

A. Breast abscess

1. Local infection of breast tissue caused by *S. aureus* or streptococcus (superficial infections) or anaerobic bacteria (subareolar infections)
2. Most are related to **breastfeeding**; more common in smokers
3. **H/P** = painful mass in breast; fever, palpable red and warm breast mass, breast tenderness, purulent drainage from mass or from nipple
4. **Labs** = increased WBCs; fine needle aspiration (FNA) of abscess confirms infection
5. **Radiology** = US helps to locate abscess within breast
6. **Treatment** = agent-appropriate oral or IV antibiotics; incision and drainage of fluctuant masses; continue breastfeeding
7. **Complications** = fistula formation with recurrent abscesses; high recurrence rate

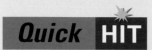

Quick HIT

CA-125 is useful only in **postmenopausal** women as an indicator for ovarian cancer.

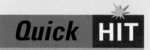

Quick HIT

US findings of cystic mass, smooth lesion edges, and few septa are more consistent with **benign** ovarian tumors.
• Findings of irregularity, nodularity, multiple septa, and pelvic extension are more suggestive of **malignancy**.

Quick HIT

Surgical resection is vital to establishing an accurate cytologic diagnosis of a suspected ovarian malignancy.

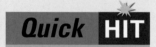

Quick HIT

Monthly **self-breast examinations** after each menstrual period are the best way to distinguish **developing lesions** from **monthly variations** in breast tissue make-up but have not been shown to decrease mortality.

B. Fibrocystic changes

1. Increased number of benign cysts and fibrous tissue found in women of childbearing age that varies in size during menstrual cycle
2. H/P = multiple bilateral small tender breast masses, possible mild breast pain preceding menses, symptoms improve after menses; breast examination detects mobile masses that **vary in size during menstrual cycle**
3. Labs = biopsy (performed when atypical lesions suspected) shows epithelial hyperplasia
4. **Radiology** = mammograms (yearly imaging starting by age 40 years) should be used to identify and follow lesions; US useful for detecting large cystic lesions
5. **Treatment** = caffeine and dietary fat reduction, OCPs, progesterone, or tamoxifen may improve symptoms in confirmed benign lesions

C. Fibroadenoma

1. Most common benign breast tumor (proliferative process in single duct); more common in **women <30 years of age**
2. H/P = **solitary**, solid, and **mobile mass** with **well-defined edges**; size may vary during menstrual cycle
3. Labs = biopsy (FNA or open) confirms benign nature
4. **Radiology** = US, mammogram, or MRI can determine location of mass and determine if solid or cystic
5. Treatment = surgical excision or US-guided cryotherapy
6. Complications = recurrence is common

D. Intraductal papilloma

1. Benign lesions of ductal tissue that may have malignant potential
2. H/P – **bloody or nonbloody discharge** from nipple on stimulation, breast pain; palpable mass behind areola
3. Labs = excisional biopsy used to rule out cancer; ductal lavage by microcatheter can be used to test for abnormal intraductal cells and is more accurate than examination of aspirated nipple fluid
4. Treatment = surgical excision

E. Breast cancer

1. Malignant neoplasms of the breast arising from either ductal (80% of cases, more aggressive) or lobular (20% of cases, less aggressive, more difficult to detect) tissue (see Table 11-8)
2. **Risk factors** = family history (first-degree relative), BRCA1 or BRCA2 gene mutations, ovarian cancer, endometrial cancer, prior breast cancer, increased estrogen exposure, early menarche, late menopause, nulliparity, late first pregnancy (35 years of age), increased age, obesity, alcohol, diethylstilbestrol (DES), industrial chemicals or pesticides, radiation exposure
3. H/P
   a. Possibly asymptomatic and undetected
   b. Painless breast lump, possible nipple discharge
   c. Palpable **solid** and **immobile** breast lump (when of sufficient size), peau d'orange (i.e., lymphatic obstruction causing lymphedema and skin thickening that makes breast look like an orange peel), possible nipple retraction
   d. Axillary lymphadenopathy in progressive cases
4. Labs
   a. **Biopsy** is indicated for any palpable breast mass or suspicious mammography findings.
      (1) FNA can be performed on palpable lesions or through US localization; it can be performed quickly with a high sensitivity and specificity by an experienced clinician but cannot differentiate between in situ and invasive carcinoma.
      (2) Core biopsy provides a better definitive histologic diagnosis and can determine if a lesion is invasive.
      (3) Needle localization under US guidance may be performed on nonpalpable lesions with calcifications to localize a mass for open biopsy.
   b. Testing for estrogen and progesterone receptors in tumor helps guide treatment.

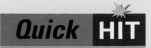
Quick HIT

Suspicious lesions on mammogram are those with **hyperdense regions** or **calcifications**.

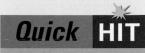
Quick HIT

Nonbloody nipple discharge is consistent with a **noncancerous** pathology and frequently does **not** require excision.

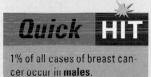
Quick HIT

1% of all cases of breast cancer occur in **males**.

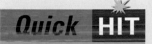
Quick HIT

Hormone replacement therapy has been linked to an **increased** incidence of breast cancer caused by exogenous estrogen administration.

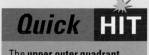
Quick HIT

The **upper outer quadrant** is the most common site of breast cancer.

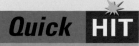
Quick HIT

Most breast cancers are detected through an **abnormal screening mammogram**, but **20%** of breast cancers are not detected on mammogram (typically in upper outer quadrant of breast).

TABLE 11-8	Features of Breast Cancer Variants	
Variant	**Characteristics**	**History and Physical**
Ductal carcinoma in situ (DCIS)	Malignant cells in ducts **without stromal invasion**; possible calcifications; unifocal; higher risk of subsequent invasive cancer than LCIS	Usually asymptomatic, possible nipple discharge or palpable lump
Lobular carcinoma in situ (LCIS)	Malignant cells in lobules **without stromal invasion**; no calcifications; can be multifocal; lower risk of invasion than DCIS, but **increased risk of contralateral malignancy**	Incidental finding, asymptomatic
Invasive ductal carcinoma	Malignant cells in ducts with stromal invasion and microcalcifications; **fibrotic response** in surrounding breast tissue; **most common** form of invasive breast cancer (80% of cases)	Firm palpable mass, skin dimpling, nipple retraction, peau d'orange, or nipple discharge
Invasive lobular carcinoma	Malignant cells in breast lobules with insidious infiltration and **less fibrous response**; more frequently **bilateral** or **multifocal** than ductal carcinoma; slower metastasis; greater association with hormone replacement therapy	Firm palpable mass, skin dimpling, nipple retraction, peau d'orange, or nipple discharge; may be more subtle than ductal carcinoma
Paget disease of the breast	Malignant adenocarcinoma cells infiltrate the epithelium of the nipple and areola; indicates carcinoma (usually ductal) in the deeper breast parenchyma	Scaly, eczematous, or ulcerated lesion on the nipple and areola; may be preceded by pain, burning, or itching
Inflammatory carcinoma	Subtype of ductal carcinoma characterized by **rapid progression** and **angioinvasive** behavior; **poor prognosis**	Breast pain, tender breast, erythema, warmth, peau d'orange, lymphadenopathy
Medullary carcinoma	Well-circumscribed mass; **rapid growth**; better prognosis than ductal carcinoma	**Soft**, well-circumscribed mass
Mucinous carcinoma	Well-circumscribed mass; **slow growth**; more common in older women; better prognosis than ductal carcinoma	**Gelatinous**, well-circumscribed mass
Tubular carcinoma	Slow-growing malignancy of well-formed **tubular** structures invading the stroma; patients typically in late 40s; excellent prognosis	Rarely detected before mammography

Gynecologic and Breast Disorders

5. **Radiology** = **mammography** is principal screening method; US can be used to differentiate cystic from solid lesions and to localize masses to guide intervention; MRI may be useful to determine extent of lesion; bone scan and CT can be used to identify metastases

6. **Treatment**
   a. Carcinoma in situ
      (1) **Ductal carcinoma in situ** (DCIS) treated with **lumpectomy** and possible radiation therapy; mastectomy considered in high-risk individuals
      (2) **Lobular carcinoma in situ** (LCIS) treated with **close observation** and tamoxifen or raloxifene
      (3) Prophylactic bilateral mastectomy can be performed in women with LCIS who do not desire lifelong observation.
   b. Invasive carcinoma
      (1) **Lumpectomy** with radiation therapy may be performed for **early** focal cancers.
      (2) **Mastectomy** should be performed for **multifocal** lesions or patients with prior breast radiation; radiation therapy is performed for tumors >5 cm.
      (3) **Sentinel lymph node biopsy** should be performed to look for spread to axillary nodes; positive sentinel node biopsy indicates need for axillary node dissection at time of tumor resection.
      (4) **Systemic therapy** (hormone or chemotherapy) is indicated for all **node-positive cancers**, tumors >1 cm, and tumors with aggressive histology; **hormone therapy** used for tumors with positive hormone

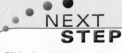

NEXT STEP

FNA of a solid breast mass carries a **20%** chance of a **false-negative** finding, so any negative FNA of a solid breast mass requires a more definitive biopsy.

receptors; **chemotherapy** can be used in patients with node-positive or negative tumor; **trastuzumab** (anti-HER-2/neu receptor antibody) used in patients with the appropriate receptors

c. Advanced cancer
   (1) Chemotherapy and hormone therapy used for locally advanced lesions with extension beyond breast
   (2) Surgical resection and/or radiation therapy can be performed after systemic therapy has decreased tumor size.
   (3) Metastases treated with systemic therapy; surgical resection or radiation therapy can be performed for solitary lesions
d. Inflammatory breast cancer
   (1) Best survival rates when mastectomy, radiation therapy, and chemotherapy are all utilized

7. **Complications**
   a. Tumors not responding to surgery and radiation are unlikely to be cured.
   b. Metastases to bone, thoracic cavity, brain, and liver
   c. Tumors with positive estrogen or progesterone hormone receptors or HER-2/neu protein receptors and those seen in older patients have a better prognosis.
   d. Lymphedema, a frequent sequela of lymph node dissection, can be complicated by cosmetic disfigurement, impaired wound healing, decreased range of motion, and increased risk of infection.

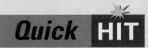

Quick HIT

Presence of **positive axillary lymph nodes** and **large tumor size** carries a **worse prognosis** in breast cancer.

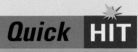

Quick HIT

Patients with BRCA1 or BRCA2 gene mutations should be followed very closely to look for breast or ovarian cancer and may want to consider prophylactic mastectomies and oophorectomies.

Gynecologic and Breast Disorders

OBSTETRICS

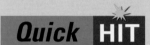

Quick HIT

Teratogens will either **kill** the fetus or will have **no effect** within the **initial 2 weeks** of gestation. They can cause **abnormal organ formation** between **2 and 12 weeks**.

I. Normal Pregnancy Physiology

A. Embryonic and fetal development begins with fertilization and takes approximately 38 weeks until fetal maturity occurs (see Figure 12-1).

    1. Gestational age is calculated from the mother's last menstrual period (LMP), which began roughly 14 days prior to fertilization. Therefore, **gestational age** is 2 weeks older than the **embryonic age**.

    2. Naegele's rule can be used to estimate delivery date by taking LMP, adding 7 days, subtracting 3 months, and adding 1 year (LMP + 7 days − 3 months + 1 year).

B. Normal changes in maternal physiology during pregnancy

    1. Several physiologic changes occur in the mother in response to the maintenance of fetal viability (see Table 12-1).

    2. Normal changes in maternal physiology affect every organ system.

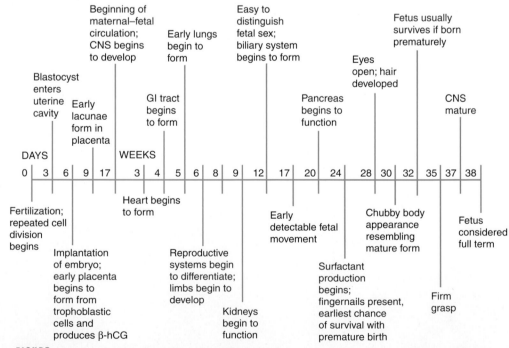

FIGURE

12-1 **Timeline of fetal development during gestation.**

β-hCG, β-human chorionic gonadotropin; CNS, central nervous system; GI, gastrointestinal. Dates are given using embryonic age, not gestational age.

TABLE 12-1	Normal Changes in Maternal Physiology during Pregnancy
Anatomy/System	**Changes**
Cardiovascular	• Cardiac output increases 40% with associated increases in SV (10%–30%) and HR (12–18 bpm) • Systolic murmur may be heard because of increased cardiac output • Myocardial O_2 demand increases • Systolic and diastolic blood pressures decrease slightly • Uterus displaces heart slightly superiorly
Respiratory	• Uterus displaces diaphragm superiorly and causes decrease of residual volume, functional residual capacity, and expiratory reserve volume • Total body O_2 consumption increases 20% • Tidal volume increases 40% with associated increase in minute ventilation because of stimulation by progesterone • Pco_2 decreases to ~30 mm Hg; dyspnea is frequent complaint despite increased minute ventilation and normal rate
Renal	• Renal plasma flow and glomerular filtration rate increase 40% • Decrease in BUN and creatinine • Increased renal loss of bicarbonate to compensate for respiratory alkalosis • Blood and interstitial fluid volumes increase
Endocrine	• Nondiabetic hyperinsulinemia with associated mild glucose intolerance • Production of human placental lactogen contributes to glucose intolerance by interfering with insulin activity • Fasting triglycerides increase • Cortisol increases • Thyroid-binding globulin (TBG) and total T_4 increase, but free T_4 is unchanged • TSH decreases slightly during early pregnancy (but still within normal limits)
Hematologic	• Hypercoagulable state • Increased RBC production • Hematocrit decreases because of increased blood volume
Gastrointestinal	• Increased salivation • Decreased gastric motility

bpm, beats per minute; BUN, blood urea nitrogen; HR, heart rate; RBC, red blood cell; SV, stroke volume; T_4, thyroxine

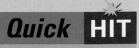

Quick HIT

Low-risk activity during pregnancy:
- **Exercise** is **encouraged** during pregnancy to improve maternal feelings of well-being, reduce symptoms caused by positional effects of the fetus, and promote healthy blood sugar levels.
- Sexual intercourse can be continued during pregnancy unless the mother is considered at high risk for spontaneous abortion, premature labor, or placenta previa.

II. Prenatal Care

A. Nutrition

1. Maternal nutritional demands alter during pregnancy to support both the mother and the developing fetus.
2. Some nutrients are specifically required to **reduce the risk of birth defects** (e.g., folate, iron) (see Table 12-2).
3. Ideal weight gain
   a. 28 to 40 lb in women with a body mass index (BMI) <19.8
   b. 25 to 35 lb for BMI 19.8 to 26 (~2 lb in first trimester, 0.75 to 1 lb/week in second and third trimesters)
   c. 15 to 25 lb for BMI >26
4. Fish (methylmercury contamination) and caffeine (increased risk of spontaneous abortion) consumption should be limited during pregnancy.

B. Prenatal visits

1. **Good prenatal care** is vital to healthy fetal development; its goals are to prevent or manage conditions that may be harmful to the mother or fetus.
2. Maternal weight (to monitor weight gain), urinalysis (to detect urinary tract infection [UTI] and gestational diabetes mellitus [DM]), blood pressure, fundal height

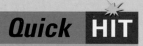

Quick HIT

Daily caloric intake during pregnancy should be approximately **2,500** kcal.

Quick HIT

Women at risk for poor nutrition during pregnancy include those who are teenagers, have a lower socioeconomic status, adhere to diets with certain food avoidances, are underweight, or who smoke, are alcoholics, or are drug abusers.

Obstetrics

TABLE 12-2	Important Increased Nutritional Demands during Pregnancy		
Substance	**Increased Need**	**Reason for Need**	**Effects of Insufficiency**
Folate	0.4–0.8 mg/day (should be started 4 wk before attempted conception)	Normal fetal neural tube development	Neural tube defects
Calcium	1,000–1,300 mg/day (50% increase)	Lactation reserves Increased utilization by fetus	Impaired maternal bone mineralization Hypertension Premature birth, low birth weight
Iron	30 mg/day (100% increase)	RBC production	Maternal anemia Premature birth, low birth weight, Maternal cardiac complications
Protein	60 g/day (30% increase)	Additional needs of maternal, fetal, and placental tissue	Impaired fetal and placental growth
Fluids	Adequate hydration important	Increased total maternal–fetal fluid volume	Relative dehydration

RBC, red blood cell.

(to estimate fetal growth), and fetal heart sounds (confirms fetal viability) are evaluated at each visit.
3. Initial visit includes detailed history, physical, and **risk assessment**.
4. Education should be provided to the patient concerning weight gain, nutrition, drug and substance abstinence, animal handling or avoidance, seat belt use, concerning symptoms and signs, scheduling of care and tests, childbirth and breastfeeding classes, and confidentiality issues.
5. Labs and ultrasound (US) are performed at certain time points during gestation to detect infection and fetal abnormalities (see Table 12-3).

TABLE 12-3	Common Screening Labs Performed during Pregnancy
Length of Gestation	**Labs or Study Performed**
Initial visit	CBC Blood antibody and Rh typing Pap smear Gonorrhea/chlamydia screening Urinalysis RPR or VDRL Rubella antibody titer Hepatitis B surface antigen HIV screening (with maternal consent)
16–18 wk	Quadruple screen[a] (maternal serum α-fetoprotein, hCG, unconjugated estriol, maternal serum inhibin A) to look for trisomies 21 and 18 and neural tube defects
18–20 wk	US dating of pregnancy and assessment for gross fetal abnormalities
24–28 wk	1-hr glucose challenge to screen for gestational DM
32–37 wk	Cervical culture for *Neisseria gonorrhoeae* and *Chlamydia trachomatis* (selected populations) Group B streptococcus screening

[a]See Table 12-4 for description of quadruple screen.
CBC, complete blood count; DM, diabetes mellitus; hCG, human chorionic gonadotropin; Rh, rhesus factor; RPR, rapid plasma reagin; US, ultrasound; VDRL, Venereal Disease Research Laboratories.

TABLE 12-4	Prenatal Assessment for Congenital Diseases in High-Risk Pregnancies	
Test	**Description**	**Indications**
Quadruple screen	Maternal serum α-fetoprotein, estriol, hCG, and maternal serum inhibin A levels measured to assess risk for neural tube defects and trisomies 18 and 21	• Performed in all pregnant women at 16–18 wk gestation • Frequently initial marker for fetal complications
Full integrated test	US measurement of nuchal translucency and serum measurement of pregnancy-associated plasma protein A (PAPP-A) in first trimester and quadruple screen in second trimester; lowest false-positive rate for noninvasive tests	• Women who present in first trimester who desire noninvasive testing with the lowest false-positive risk
Amniocentesis	Transabdominal needle aspiration of amniotic fluid from amniotic sac after 16 wk gestation to measure amniotic α-fetoprotein and determine karyotype (detects neural tube defects and chromosome disorders with greater sensitivity than triple screen alone)	• Abnormal quadruple screen, women >35 yr of age, risk of Rh sensitization • Carries an excess 0.5% risk of spontaneous abortion over normal risks for abortion
Chorionic villi sampling	Transabdominal or transcervical aspiration of chorionic villus tissue at 9–12 wk gestation to detect chromosomal abnormalities	• Early detection of chromosomal abnormalities in higher risk patients (advanced age, history of children with genetic defects)
Percutaneous umbilical blood sampling	Blood collection from umbilical vein after 18 wk gestation to identify chromosomal defects, fetal infection, Rh sensitization	• Late detection of genetic disorders, pregnancies with high risk for Rh sensitization

hCG, human chorionic gonadotropin; Rh, rhesus factor; US, ultrasound.

6. Screening lab tests that are not routinely performed at the first prenatal visit but should be considered in patients at risk: purified protein derivative (PPD) (for TB), red blood cell (RBC) indices, hemoglobin (Hgb) electrophoresis (anemias), hexosaminidase A (Tay Sachs), phenylalanine levels (phenylketonuria), hepatitis C serology, toxoplasmosis screening, and cystic fibrosis genetic screening.
7. **Leopold maneuvers** (i.e., external abdominal examination) can be performed in the third trimester to determine fetal presentation.
8. Specialized tests are performed in women with increased risk for congenital abnormalities (e.g., **>35 year of age**, history of spontaneous abortion, teratogen exposure, DM, history of fetal demise) (see Table 12-4, Table 12-5).

Quick HIT

Although the full integrated test is the most sensitive screening test for trisomies with the lowest rate of false-positive findings, it is not routinely performed because abnormal first trimester results frequently prompt the decision to abandon the second trimester tests and perform a more invasive test to find a definitive answer.

Quick HIT

Maternal serum α-fetoprotein levels:
• This screening test is **only valid** if performed during the correct gestational window (**16 to 18 weeks' gestation**).
• **High** levels are associated with an increased risk of **neural tube defects** or multiple gestations.
• **Low** levels are associated with increased risk of **trisomies 21** and **18**.

TABLE 12-5	Interpretation of Full Integrated Test and Quadruple Screen					
	Full Integrated Test (1st trimester)		**Quadruple Screen (2nd trimester)**			
Genetic disorder	**PAPP-A**	**NT**	**AFP**	**uE3**	**hCG**	**Inh A**
Trisomy 21 (Down syndrome)	↓	↑	↓	↓	↑	↑
Trisomy 18	↓↓	↑	↓	↓↓	↓↓	↔
Trisomy 13	↓↓	↑	↔	↔	↔	↔

AFP, α-fetoprotein; hCG, human chorionic gonadotropin; Inh A, Inhibin A; NT, nuchal translucency; PAPP-A, pregnancy-associated plasma protein A; uE3, estriol.

Obstetrics

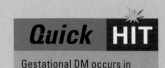

NEXT STEP

Gestational DM occurs most frequently in the **second** or **third trimesters**. If mother presents with signs of DM earlier in pregnancy, suspect nongestational (type I or II) DM.

III. Medical Complications of Pregnancy

A. Gestational diabetes mellitus (DM)

1. **New onset** glucose intolerance that begins during pregnancy (after 24 weeks)
2. **Risk factors** = family history of DM, >25 years of age, obesity, prior polyhydramnios, recurrent abortions, prior stillbirth, prior macrosomia, hypertension (HTN), African or Pacific Islander heritage, corticosteroid use, polycystic ovarian syndrome (PCOS)
3. **History and physical (H/P)** = usually asymptomatic
4. **Labs** = fasting glucose >126 mg/dL or **abnormal glucose tolerance test** performed at 24 to 28 weeks' gestation (see Figure 12-2)
5. **Treatment**
   a. Strict glucose control through **diet** and **exercise**
      (1) 40 kcal/kg/day in women with BMI <22
      (2) 30 kcal/kg/day in women with BMI 22 to 27
      (3) 24 kcal/kg/day in women with BMI 27 to 29
      (4) 12 to 15 kcal/kg/day in women with BMI >29
      (5) Self-monitoring of glucose performed to determine therapy efficacy
   b. Insulin should be used in patients failing nonpharmacologic therapy to keep fasting glucose <90 mg/dL and 1-hour postprandial glucose <120 mg/dL.
   c. Periodic fetal US and nonstress tests (discussed later) performed to assess fetal well-being
   d. Caesarean section may be indicated for macrosomic babies.

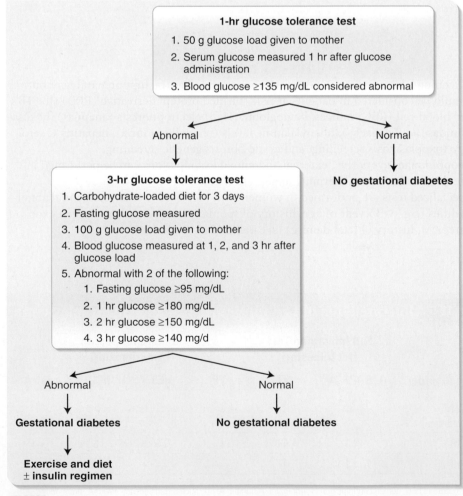

FIGURE
12-2 Screening for gestational diabetes mellitus performed at 24 to 28 weeks' gestation.

Obstetrics

6. Complications
   a. Fetal: macrosomia (i.e., baby of abnormally large size), polyhydramnios, delayed pulmonary maturity, uteroplacental insufficiency (resulting in intrauterine growth restriction [IUGR] or intrauterine fetal demise)
   b. Perinatal or postnatal: traumatic delivery, delayed neurologic maturity, fetal respiratory distress syndrome, hypoglycemia (secondary to therapy; can also occur after delivery), hypocalcemia

B. Pregestational diabetes mellitus (DM)

1. DM that exists **before** pregnancy; patient may or may not be aware of disease
2. H/P = consistent with typical presentation of DM (see Chapter 5, **Endocrine Disorders**); patients more likely to have significant hyperglycemia, postpartum hyperglycemia, and low BMI
3. **Labs** = increased serum glucose (prior to and during pregnancy), increased hemoglobin A1c with poor control; detection of anti-insulin and anti-islet cell antibodies is diagnostic for DM type I
4. **Treatment**
   a. Try to control glucose with diet and exercise.
   b. Insulin used for glucose control in type I and in type II DM not adequately controlled with lifestyle modification
   c. Fetal US and echocardiogram (especially third trimester) used to identify cardiac, neurologic, and growth abnormalities
   d. Early delivery after fetal lung assessment and corticosteroid administration recommended for poor glucose control or maternal complications
5. Complications
   a. Maternal: preeclampsia, renal insufficiency, retinopathy, diabetic ketoacidosis, hyperosmolar hyperglycemic state (HHS)
   b. Fetal: cardiac defects (especially transposition of the great vessels, tetralogy of Fallot), neural tube defects, sacral agenesis, renal agenesis, polyhydramnios, macrosomia, IUGR, intrauterine fetal demise

C. Preeclampsia

1. Pregnancy-induced **HTN** with **proteinuria** and **edema** that develops after 20 weeks' gestation in 5% of pregnancies owing to an unknown cause
2. **Risk factors** = HTN, **nulliparity, prior history of preeclampsia**, <15 or >35 years of age, multiple gestation (e.g., twins), vascular disease, chronic HTN or renal disease, DM, obesity, African-American ancestry
3. H/P
   a. Asymptomatic in mild cases
   b. **Edema** in **hands** and **face**, rapid weight gain, headache, epigastric abdominal pain, visual disturbances, hyperreflexia
   c. **Blood pressure ≥140/90** mm Hg during pregnancy in a patient who was formerly normotensive
4. **Labs**
   a. Urinalysis shows 2+ proteinuria on dipstick or >300 mg protein/24 hr.
   b. Decreased platelets, normal or mildly increased creatinine, increased alanine aminotransferase (ALT) and aspartate aminotransferase (AST), decreased glomerular filtration rate (GFR)
   c. Fetal nonstress test and amniocentesis (less commonly) can be useful to assess fetal well-being.
5. **Treatment**
   a. If near term, **induce delivery**.
   b. If mild and far from term, prescribe restricted activity, frequent maternal examinations for worsening symptoms, protein assessments, and fetal nonstress tests twice per week.
   c. If severe and far from term, closely monitor in inpatient setting and maintain blood pressure <155/105 with diastolic blood pressure >90 using antihypertensive medications (labetalol frequently used), give intravenous (IV) **MgSO₄**

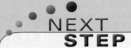

NEXT STEP

Continue glucose assessment after birth because maternal glucose needs will change suddenly for patients with gestational DM and because the mother has a low risk of remaining diabetic after pregnancy.

Obstetrics

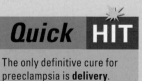

Quick HIT

The only definitive cure for preeclampsia is **delivery**.

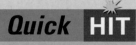

Quick HIT

Do not use angiotensin-converting enzyme inhibitors (**ACE-I**) or angiotensin receptor blockers (ARBs) to stabilize blood pressure in pregnancy because of risk of **teratogenic** effects.

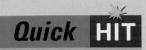

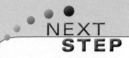

Do not confuse **eclampsia** with **epilepsy**. Know the patient's history before making a diagnosis because induced delivery **will not** cure the **epileptic** patient.

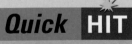

Anticonvulsant use in pregnancy:
- Patients with epilepsy should be kept on their regular anticonvulsant medication during pregnancy but should be given supplemental folate.
- Diazepam can be used to break active seizures (80% effective).

Obstetrics

Hyperemesis gravidarum is severe nausea and vomiting that affects 1% of pregnant women. It may be complicated by electrolyte abnormalities and treated with avoidance of large meals, adequate hydration, and pyridoxine and doxylamine.

for seizure prophylaxis, closely monitor maternal and fetal health, and induce delivery as soon as fetus is considered viable.

d. Continue antihypertensive medications and $MgSO_4$ postpartum and continue close observation for symptoms and lab abnormalities before discontinuing medications.

e. Mothers with preexistent HTN should be treated pharmacologically for HTN >140/95 mm Hg; labetalol or methyldopa is used initially, and a long-acting calcium channel blocker (e.g., nifedipine, amlodipine) may be added as a second agent.

6. **Complications** = eclampsia, seizures, stroke, IUGR, pulmonary edema, maternal organ dysfunction, oligohydramnios, preterm delivery; hemolysis, elevated liver enzymes, and low platelet counts (HELLP) syndrome can also cause abruptio placentae, renal insufficiency, encephalopathy, and disseminated intravascular coagulation (DIC)

D. Eclampsia

1. Progression of preeclampsia leading to **maternal seizures** that can be severe and fatal for both mother and child if untreated
2. H/P = headaches, visual disturbances (scotomata), and upper abdominal pain frequently precede onset of **seizures**
3. **Labs** = findings similar to preeclampsia
4. **Treatment**
   a. Treatment is similar to that for preeclampsia, with **delivery** being the definitive solution; labor should be induced as soon as stable.
   b. Use $MgSO_4$ and **IV diazepam** to control seizures.
   c. Stabilize patient with sufficient O_2 and blood pressure control (labetalol or hydralazine).
   d. **Continue** $MgSO_4$ and antihypertensive medications for **48 hr** following delivery because **25% of seizures** occur within 24 hr postpartum.
5. **Complications** = risk of maternal (<2%) and fetal (6% to 12%) death; 65% risk of preeclampsia and 2% risk of eclampsia in subsequent pregnancy

E. Maternal asthma (preexisting)

1. Severe maternal asthma is associated with preeclampsia, spontaneous abortion, intrauterine fetal demise, and IUGR.
2. H/P = course of disease frequently does not change during pregnancy from prior severity, but exacerbations may be less tolerated by the mother because of normal physiologic respiratory changes of pregnancy
3. **Treatment**
   a. Treat mild intermittent asthma with short-acting β-agonists (e.g., albuterol) as needed (also used as needed for all more severe variants)
   b. Treat mild persistent asthma with a short-acting β-agonist plus a low-dose inhaled corticosteroid.
   c. Treat moderate persistent asthma with either a medium-dose inhaled corticosteroid or combination of low-dose inhaled corticosteroid plus a long-acting β-agonist (e.g., salmeterol).
   d. Treat severe persistent asthma with a high-dose inhaled corticosteroid plus a long-acting β-agonist.
4. **Complications** = increased risk of preeclampsia, spontaneous abortion, intrauterine fetal death, and IUGR in untreated severe disease; oral corticosteroid use may be associated with IUGR and cleft palate (although unproved)

F. Maternal nausea and vomiting

1. Most pregnant women experience nausea and vomiting in the **first trimester** of pregnancy (i.e., morning sickness); most cases improve by the second trimester.
2. Most likely caused by increases in hCG or imbalance of progesterone and estrogen
3. H/P = nausea and vomiting that occurs frequently and may be daily; typically occurs in first trimester and improves after 16 weeks' gestation
4. **Treatment** = maintenance of hydration status, avoidance of large meals, elevating head in bed; antacids following meals may be helpful in worse cases

G. Maternal deep venous thrombosis (DVT)

1. Risk of DVT **increases** during pregnancy because of **venous stasis** and relative **increase** in **circulating clotting** factors.
2. H/P = similar presentation to that in nonpregnant patients (see Chapter 1, **Cardiovascular Disorders**); clinical diagnosis may be more difficult in pregnant patients because edema is also common in absence of DVT
3. **Radiology** = US and Doppler studies are safe means of finding thrombosis
4. **Treatment**
   a. At diagnosis, IV heparin dosed to maintain partial thromboplastin time (PTT) at two times normal, or low molecular weight heparin (LMWH) (e.g., enoxaparin) dosed to achieve consistent anti-factor Xa levels 0.5–1.2 U/mL at 4 hr after injection
   b. At discharge, patients should be switched to subcutaneous LMWH.
   c. If possible, discontinue anticoagulation 24 to 36 hours prior to delivery; patients at high risk may be switched to IV unfractionated heparin until 6 hours prior to delivery.
   d. Anticoagulants should be continued following delivery for 6 weeks (warfarin or enoxaparin can be used postpartum).
5. **Complications** = pulmonary embolus; heparin therapy can be complicated by hemorrhage or thrombocytopenia

H. Maternal UTIs

1. UTIs are **more common** during pregnancy because of maternal immunosuppression, outflow obstruction, and decreased ureteral peristalsis (secondary to increased progesterone).
2. H/P = similar symptoms to nonpregnant patients (e.g., dysuria, urinary frequency, urgency) or asymptomatic
3. **Labs** = urinalysis shows white blood cells (WBCs) and nitrites; urine culture shows bacteria
4. **Treatment** = amoxicillin, nitrofurantoin, or cephalexin × 3 to 7 days; recurrent cases or pyelonephritis may require longer therapy

I. Maternal drug use

1. Several prescribed and illicit drugs can have a negative effect on pregnancy (see Table 12-6, Table 12-7).

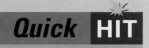

Quick HIT

Warfarin has teratogenic effects and should **not** be used during pregnancy but is safe to use during breastfeeding.

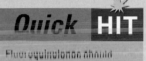

NEXT STEP

Stop all anticoagulation during active labor until 6 hours after delivery to prevent severe hemorrhage.

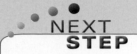

Quick HIT

Fluoroquinolones should not be used for treatment of UTI because of teratogenic effects.

TABLE 12-6	**Recreational Drug Use and Associated Risks to Mother and Fetus during Pregnancy**	
Drug	**Maternal Risks**	**Fetal Risks**
Marijuana	Minimal	IUGR, prematurity
Cocaine	**Arrhythmia**, myocardial infarction, subarachnoid hemorrhage, seizures, stroke, abruptio placentae	**Abruptio placentae**, IUGR, prematurity, facial abnormalities, delayed intellectual development, fetal demise
Ethanol	Minimal	**Fetal alcohol syndrome** (mental retardation, IUGR, sensory and motor neuropathy, facial abnormalities), spontaneous abortion, intrauterine fetal demise
Opioids	**Infection** (from needles), narcotic withdrawal, premature rupture of membranes	Prematurity, IUGR, meconium aspiration, neonatal infections, **narcotic withdrawal** (may be fatal)
Stimulants	Lack of appetite and **malnutrition**, arrhythmia, withdrawal depression, hypertension	IUGR, congenital heart defects, cleft palate
Tobacco	**Abruptio placentae, placenta previa**, premature rupture of membranes	Spontaneous abortion, prematurity, **IUGR**, intrauterine fetal demise, impaired intellectual development, higher risk of neonatal respiratory infections
Hallucinogens	Personal endangerment (poor decision making)	Possible developmental delays

IUGR, intrauterine growth restriction.

Obstetrics

TABLE 12-7	Common Medications That Carry Teratogenic Risks
Medication	**Teratogenic Risks**
ACE-I	Renal abnormalities, decreased skull ossification
Aminoglycosides	CN VIII damage, skeletal abnormalities, renal defects
Carbamazepine	Facial abnormalities, IUGR, mental retardation, cardiovascular abnormalities, neural tube defects
Chemotherapeutics (all drug classes)	Intrauterine fetal demise (~30% pregnancies), severe IUGR, multiple anatomic abnormalities (palate, bones, limbs, genitals, etc.), mental retardation, spontaneous abortion, secondary neoplasms
Diazepam	Cleft palate, renal defects, secondary neoplasms
DES	Vaginal and cervical cancer later in life (adenocarcinoma)
Fluoroquinolones	Cartilage abnormalities
Lithium	Ebstein anomaly
Phenobarbital	Neonatal withdrawal
Phenytoin	Facial abnormalities, IUGR, mental retardation, cardiovascular abnormalities
Retinoids	CNS abnormalities, cardiovascular abnormalities, facial abnormalities, spontaneous abortion
Sulfonamides	Kernicterus (bile infiltration of brain)
Tetracycline	Skeletal abnormalities, limb abnormalities, teeth discoloration
Thalidomide	Limb abnormalities
Valproic acid	Neural tube defects (~1% pregnancies), facial abnormalities, cardiovascular abnormalities, skeletal abnormalities
Warfarin	Spontaneous abortion, IUGR, CNS abnormalities, facial abnormalities, mental retardation, Dandy-Walker malformation

ACE-I, angiotensin-converting enzyme inhibitors; CN, cranial nerve; CNS, central nervous system; DES, diethylstilbestrol; IUGR, intrauterine growth restriction; OCPs, oral contraceptive pills.

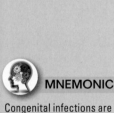

MNEMONIC

Congenital infections are frequently referred to as the TORCH infections:
Toxoplasmosis
Other (varicella-zoster, Parvovirus B19, group B streptococcus, chlamydia, gonorrhea)
Rubella/**R**ubeola/**R**PR (syphilis)
Cytomegalovirus
Herpes simplex/**H**epatitis B/**H**IV

2. **H/P** = a complete drug history should be taken to assess all potential fetal risks
3. **Treatment**
   a. Appropriate counseling and education for drug abuse
   b. Stop teratogenic drugs during pregnancy (unless stopping drug is more harmful than use) and select alternative medications or therapies to treat medical conditions.
   c. Careful screening for related domestic abuse

J. Congenital infections
1. Maternal infections during pregnancy that may have significant negative effects on fetal development or viability (see Table 12-8)
2. Prenatal screening is performed to detect certain infections that are of particular risk to the fetus.

TABLE 12-8	Congenital Infections and Effects upon the Fetus and Neonates		
Maternal Infection	**Possible Fetal/Neonatal Effects**	**Diagnosis**	**Treatment**
Toxoplasmosis	Hydrocephalus, intracranial calcifications, chorioretinitis, microcephaly, spontaneous abortion, seizures	• Possible mononucleosis-like illness • Amniotic fluid PCR for *Toxoplasma gondii* or serum antibody screening may be helpful for diagnosis	• Pyrimethamine, sulfadiazine, and folinic acid • Mother should avoid gardening, raw meat, cat litter boxes, and unpasteurized milk
Rubella	Increased risk of spontaneous abortion, skin lesions (**"blueberry muffin baby"**), **congenital rubella syndrome** (IUGR, deafness, cardiovascular abnormalities, vision abnormalities, CNS abnormalities, hepatitis) if disease transmission occurs	• Early prenatal IgG screening	• Mother should be immunized before attempting to become pregnant • No treatment if infection develops during pregnancy • No proved benefit from rubella immune globulin
Rubeola (measles)	Increased risk of prematurity, IUGR, and spontaneous abortion; **high risk** (20% if term birth, 55% if preterm) **of neonatal death** if disease transmission occurs	• Clinical diagnosis in mother confirmed by IgM or IgG antibodies after rash develops	• Mother should be immunized before attempting to become pregnant • Immune serum globulin given to mother if infection develops during pregnancy • Vaccine is contraindicated during pregnancy (live attenuated virus carries risk of fetal infection)
Syphilis	Neonatal anemia, deafness, hepatosplenomegaly, pneumonia, hepatitis, osteodystrophy, rash followed by hand/foot desquamation; 25% neonatal mortality	• Early prenatal RPR or VDRL • Confirm with FTA-ABS	• Maternal or neonatal penicillin
Cytomegalovirus	IUGR, chorioretinitis, **CNS abnormalities**, mental retardation, vision abnormalities, deafness, hydrocephalus, seizures, hepatosplenomegaly	• Possible mononucleosis-like illness • IgM antibody screening or PCR of viral DNA within first few weeks of life	• No treatment if infection develops during pregnancy • Ganciclovir may decrease effects in neonates • **Good hygiene** reduces risk of transmission
Herpes simplex	Increased risk of prematurity, IUGR, and spontaneous abortion; high risk of **neonatal death** or **CNS abnormalities** if disease transmission occurs	• Clinical diagnosis confirmed with viral culture or immunoassays	• Delivery by caesarean **section** to avoid disease transmission if active lesions present or if primary outbreak • Acyclovir may be beneficial in neonates
Hepatitis B	Increased risk of prematurity, IUGR; increased risk of neonatal death if acute disease develops	• Prenatal surface antigen screening	• Maternal **vaccination**; vaccination of neonate and administration of immune globulin shortly after birth
HIV	Viral transmission in utero (5% risk), **rapid progression** of disease to AIDS	• Early prenatal maternal blood screening (consent required)	• **AZT** significantly reduces vertical transmission risk • Continue prescribed antiviral regimen, but avoid efavirenz, didanosine, stavudine, and nevirapine
Gonorrhea/chlamydia	Increased risk of spontaneous abortion; neonatal sepsis, **conjunctivitis**	• Cervical culture and immunoassays	• Erythromycin given to mother or neonate
Varicella-zoster	Prematurity, **encephalitis, pneumonia**, IUGR, **CNS abnormalities**, limb abnormalities, blindness; high risk of neonatal death if birth occurs during active infection	• IgG titer screening in women with **no known history of disease** • IgM and IgG antibody titers can confirm diagnosis in neonates	• Varicella immune globulin given to nonimmune mother within 96 hr of exposure and to neonate if born during active infection • Vaccine is contraindicated during pregnancy (live-attenuated virus carries risk of fetal infection)
Group B streptococcus	Respiratory distress, pneumonia, **meningitis**, sepsis	• Antigen screening after 34 wk gestation	• IV β-lactams or clindamycin during labor or in infected neonates
Parvovirus B19	Decreased RBC production, hemolytic anemia, hydrops fetalis	• IgM antibody screening or PCR of viral DNA	• Monitor fetal hemoglobin by PUBS and give intrauterine transfusion for severe anemia

AIDS, acquired immunodeficiency syndrome; AZT, zidovudine; CNS, central nervous system; FTA-ABS, fluorescent treponemal antibody absorption test; HIV, human immunodeficiency virus; Ig, immunoglobulin; IUGR, intrauterine growth restriction; IV, intravenous; PCR, polymerase chain reaction; PUBS, percutaneous umbilical blood sampling; RBC, red blood cell; RPR, rapid plasma reagin; VDRL, Venereal Disease Research Laboratories.

Obstetrics

IV. Obstetric Complications of Pregnancy

A. Ectopic pregnancy

1. Implantation of zygote **outside of uterus**; most commonly occurs in **ampulla of fallopian tube** (95% of cases) but can also occur on ovary, cervix, or abdominal cavity
2. Risk factors = **pelvic inflammatory disease**, sexually transmitted diseases, gynecologic surgery, **prior ectopic pregnancy**, multiple sexual partners, smoking
3. H/P
   a. **Abdominal pain**, nausea, amenorrhea (due to pregnancy); **scant vaginal bleeding**, possible palpable pelvic mass
   b. In cases of rupture, abdominal pain becomes severe and can be accompanied by hypotension, tachycardia, and peritoneal signs.
4. **Labs** = elevated β-hCG (urine or serum) indicates pregnancy; β-hCG in intrauterine pregnancy will double every 48 hr; β-hCG that is **low for time of gestation** should raise suspicion for ectopic pregnancy)
5. Radiology
   a. Transabdominal and transvaginal US should be able to visualize pregnancy once β-hCG reaches **6,500 mIU/mL** and **1,500 mIU/mL**, respectively.
   b. **Absence of visible intrauterine pregnancy** should raise suspicion.
   c. US may show free abdominal fluid if rupture has occurred.
6. **Treatment** = unruptured ectopic pregnancy of <6 weeks' gestation is treated with methotrexate to abort pregnancy; longer term or ruptured ectopic pregnancy treated with IV hydration and **surgical excision** with attempt to preserve fallopian tube
7. **Complications** = unavoidable fetal death, severe maternal hemorrhage, increased risk of future ectopic pregnancy, infertility, Rh sensitization, **maternal death**

B. Spontaneous abortion (miscarriage) (see Table 12-9)

1. **Nonelective** termination of pregnancy **<20 weeks'** gestation (see Table 12-9)
   a. First-trimester spontaneous abortions are usually the result of **fetal chromosomal abnormalities** (especially trisomies).
   b. Second-trimester spontaneous abortions are usually caused by infection, **cervical incompetence, uterine abnormalities**, hypercoagulable state, poor maternal health, or **drug use** (prescription or recreational).
2. **Risk factors** = **increased maternal age**, multiple prior births, prior spontaneous abortion, uterine abnormalities, smoking, alcohol, nonsteroidal anti-inflammatory drugs (NSAIDs), cocaine, excessive caffeine use, certain maternal infections, low folate level, autoimmune disease

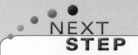

NEXT STEP

Any woman of childbearing age who presents with abdominal pain must be given a β-hCG **pregnancy test**.

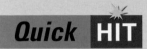

Quick HIT

The most common causes of vaginal bleeding in **early** pregnancy are **ectopic pregnancy**, threatened or inevitable **spontaneous abortion, physiologic** bleeding (related to implantation), and **uterine-cervical pathology**.

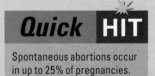

Quick HIT

Spontaneous abortions occur in up to 25% of pregnancies.

TABLE 12-9 Types of Spontaneous Abortions						
Abortion Type	**Threatened**	**Missed**	**Inevitable**	**Incomplete**	**Complete**
Sign/Symptoms					
Uterine bleeding	In initial 20 wk of gestation	Present or with pain	Initial 20 wk + pain	Initial 20 wk	Initial 20 wk
Cervical os	Closed	Closed	Open	Open	Open or closed
Uterine contents expelled	None	None	None	Some	All
Diagnosis	US detects **viable** fetus, **cervix is closed**	US detects **nonviable** intrauterine fetus	**Viable** fetus, **cervix is dilated**	Based on history of expelled products of conception	Based on history of expelled products of conception
Treatment	Bed rest, limited activity	Expectant management, misoprostol, or D&C; also give Rho(D) immune globulin	Same as missed abortion	Same as missed abortion	Rho(D) immune globulin

D&C, dilation and curettage; US, ultrasound.

3. **H/P** = history should focus on prior abortions, birth history, prior gynecologic infections, and family history of congenital diseases; vaginal bleeding, and possible open cervical os seen on examination
4. **Labs** = β-hCG used to assess gestational age and track progress of pregnancy
5. **Radiology** = US used to assess fetal viability
6. **Treatment** = depends on type of spontaneous abortion (see Table 12-9)

C. Intrauterine fetal demise

1. Intrauterine fetal death that occurs **after 20 weeks' gestation** and before the onset of labor
2. Caused by **placental** or **cord abnormalities** secondary to maternal cardiovascular or hematologic conditions, maternal HTN, **infection**, poor maternal health, or fetal congenital abnormalities
3. **H/P** = pregnant patient notes no fetal activity; uterus small for length of gestation, no fetal movement, no fetal heart tones
4. **Radiology** = US shows nonviable intrauterine fetus with no heart activity
5. **Treatment** = oxytocin, misoprostol (prostaglandin E_1), or prostaglandin E_2 can be used to induce labor and delivery; dilation and evacuation (D&E) might be used to remove fetus if <24 weeks' gestation
6. **Complications** = DIC if fetus is retained for prolonged amount of time

D. Intrauterine growth restriction (IUGR)

1. Fetal growth that lags behind gestational age (<10th percentile)
2. Types
   a. **Symmetric**
      (1) 20% of cases
      (2) Overall decrease in fetal size
      (3) Early in pregnancy
      (4) Most commonly caused by **congenital infection, chromosomal abnormalities**, or maternal drug use (illicit or therapeutic)
   b. **Asymmetric**
      (1) 80% of cases
      (2) Decreased abdominal size with preservation of head and extremities
      (3) Late in pregnancy
      (4) Caused by multiple gestation, **poor maternal health**, or placental insufficiency
3. **H/P** = fundal height is at least **3 cm smaller** than expected for gestational age (beginning at 20 weeks' gestation, distance in centimeters from pubis to top of fundus should equal gestational age in weeks)
4. **Radiology**
   a. US shows head circumference:abdominal circumference and femur length:abdominal circumference ratios **increased** in **asymmetric** IUGR and **normal** in **symmetric** IUGR.
   b. US can be used to estimate fetal weight.
   c. US frequently detects oligohydramnios.
   d. Doppler US studies may detect decreased fetal, umbilical, or maternal blood flow.
5. **Treatment**
   a. Fetal growth should be followed with US.
   b. Nutritional supplementation, maternal O_2 therapy, and maternal bed rest may aid fetal growth.
   c. Delivery should be induced if fetal growth slows further, maternal health worsens, or tests show fetal distress.
   d. Maternal antenatal corticosteroids help to speed fetal lung maturation in mothers expected to deliver early.

E. Oligohydramnios

1. **Deficiency** of **amniotic fluid** in gestational sac (amniotic fluid index <5 cm)
2. Associated with **IUGR**, fetal stress, fetal renal abnormalities, or poor fetal health
3. Significance of timing
   a. **First trimester**: frequently results in **spontaneous abortion**

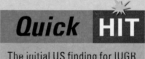

Quick HIT

The initial US finding for IUGR is frequently an **abdominal circumference <10th percentile** for gestational age.

Obstetrics

b. **Second trimester**: may be due to **fetal renal abnormalities**, maternal cause (e.g., preeclampsia, renal disease, HTN, collagen-vascular disease), or placental thrombosis

c. **Third trimester**: associated with **premature rupture of membranes** (PROM), preeclampsia, abruptio placentae, or idiopathic causes

4. **H/P** = possibly asymptomatic; fundal height may be small for gestational age

5. **Radiology** = US used to determine amniotic volume and perform fetal assessment; amniotic fluid index will be <5 cm, with no pockets at least 2 cm in size

6. **Treatment** = expectant management if fetus responds well to tests of well-being; induce delivery of viable fetus if risk of fetal demise is significant (poor response of fetus to tests of well-being); hydration, and bed rest may improve amniotic volume

7. **Complications** = spontaneous abortion, intrauterine fetal demise; abnormalities in limb, facial, lung, and abdominal development caused by **compression**

F. Polyhydramnios

1. **Excess** of amniotic fluid in gestational sac (amniotic fluid index >25 cm)

2. Can result from insufficient swallowing of amniotic fluid (e.g., esophageal atresia) by fetus or increased fetal urination related to **maternal diabetes**, multiple gestation, fetal anemia, or chromosomal abnormalities

3. **H/P** = fundal height may be larger than expected for gestational age

4. **Radiology** = US used to assess amniotic fluid volume; amniotic fluid index will be >25 cm or will show one pocket of at least 8 cm

5. **Treatment** = only administered if mother is uncomfortable or if a threat of preterm labor exists; pregnancies of <32 weeks' gestation treated with amnioreduction and indomethacin (tapered dosing); pregnancies >32 weeks' gestation treated with amnioreduction alone

6. **Complications** = preterm labor, PROM, fetal malpresentation, maternal respiratory compromise

G. Premature rupture of membranes (PROM)

1. Spontaneous **rupture of amniotic sac** with spillage of amniotic fluid **before** onset of labor

2. **Risk factors** = vaginal or cervical infection, cervical incompetence, poor maternal nutrition, prior PROM

3. **H/P** = loss of amniotic fluid from vagina; amniotic fluid may be seen pooling in vagina on visual examination

4. **Labs** = **microscopic examination** of vaginal fluid will show **"ferning"** if amniotic fluid is present; vaginal fluid will turn **nitrazine paper blue** in presence of amniotic fluid; vaginal fluid should be cultured to detect infection

5. **Radiology** = US should be used to confirm oligohydramnios and to assess volume of residual amniotic fluid and fetal position

6. **Treatment**

   a. If PROM occurs at <32 weeks' gestation, give corticosteroids (to hasten fetal lung maturation) and prophylactic antibiotics (for group B streptococcus); labor should be induced once amniotic fluid analysis indicates fetal lung maturity.

   b. If PROM occurs at 32 to 34 weeks' gestation, amniotic fluid analysis is performed to determine fetal lung maturity; labor is induced if lung maturity has occurred; corticosteroids and antibiotics are administered if lungs are immature until induction at 34 weeks.

   c. If PROM occurs after 34 weeks' gestation, antibiotics are administered and delivery is induced.

H. Preterm labor

1. Onset of labor <37 **weeks'** gestation

2. **Risk factors** = **multiple gestation, PROM**, infection, placenta previa, abruptio placentae, previous preterm labor, polyhydramnios, cervical incompetence, poor nutrition, stressful environment, **smoking**, substance abuse, or lower socioeconomic status

3. **H/P** = constant low back pain, cramping, signs of labor (painful contractions in the setting of cervical change) <37 **weeks'** gestation

4. **Labs** = urine, vaginal, and cervical cultures performed to detect infection

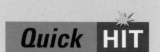

Quick **HIT**

Excessive amniotic fluid frequently **reaccumulates** following percutaneous drainage.

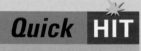

Quick **HIT**

Internal manual examination should **not** be performed by the physician in cases of PROM because of an **increased risk of introducing infection** into the vaginal canal.

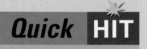

Quick **HIT**

Fetal lung maturity can be quantified by measuring lecithin (L) and sphingomyelin (S) levels in amniotic fluid and determining the **LS ratio** (**L: S >2** with the presence of phosphatidylglycerol [PG] in amniotic fluid **suggests lung maturity**).

5. **Radiology** = US used to assess amniotic fluid volume and fetal well-being and verify gestational age
6. **Treatment**
   a. At <34 weeks' gestation
      (1) Expectant management (even if PPROM)
      (2) Hospitalization, hydration, and activity restriction
      (3) **Tocolytic therapy** (with MgSO$_4$, **terbutaline**, indomethacin, or nifedipine) for 48 hours
      (4) Glucocorticoids (betamethasone or dexamethasone) for 48 hours to mature fetal lungs
      (5) Give empiric ampicillin for prophylaxis against group B streptococcus if delivery is imminent or if there is evidence of active infection.
   b. At >34 weeks' gestation
      (1) Expectant management if lung maturity is proven
      (2) Active management if there is an indication for delivery (e.g., nonreassuring fetal testing, infection, maternal threat)
      (3) Tocolysis and glucocorticoids are of no proven benefit beyond 34 weeks.
      (4) Give empiric ampicillin if delivery is imminent.
7. **Complications** = increased risk of neonatal complications and fetal respiratory distress syndrome with shorter gestational age

I. Placenta previa

1. **Implantation** of placenta **near cervical os** frequently associated with vaginal bleeding
2. **Types** (see Figure 12-3)
   a. **Low implantation**: placenta implanted in lower uterus but does not infringe on cervical os until dilation occurs
   b. **Partial** placenta previa: placenta partially covers os
   c. **Complete** placenta previa: placenta completely covers os
3. **Risk factors** = multiparity (i.e., prior pregnancy), increased maternal age, **prior placenta previa, prior caesarean section**, multiple gestation, uterine fibroids, history of abortion, smoking
4. **H/P** = **painless** vaginal bleeding in **third trimester** (30th week of gestation is most common time of onset)

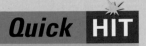

Quick HIT

Although not used to diagnose labor, ultrasound can measure cervical length. A cervical length >35 mm is associated with a very low risk of preterm birth; a cervical length <15 mm has high risk of preterm birth.

Obstetrics

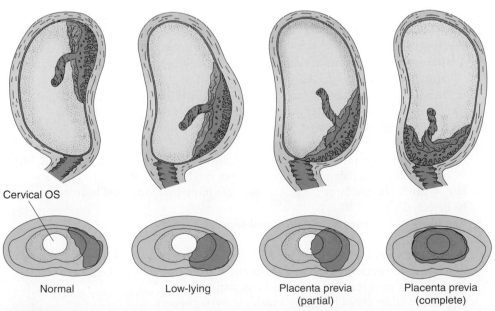

Cervical OS

Normal   Low-lying   Placenta previa (partial)   Placenta previa (complete)

FIGURE 12-3 Uterine profiles and cross sections demonstrating normal placental implantation and examples of low-lying placenta, partial placenta previa, and complete placenta previa.
(Modified from Simpson, K. R., & Creehan, P. A. [2014]. *Perinatal Nursing* [4th ed., p. 146]. Philadelphia, PA: Lippincott Williams & Wilkins; with permission.)

5. Radiology = US determines location of placenta (transvaginal or translabial US more sensitive)
6. Treatment
   a. Bed rest in cases of minor inconsistent bleeding; inpatient admission with maternal and fetal monitoring for active bleeding; give Rho(D) immune globulin to Rh-negative mothers for any bleeding in the third trimester
   b. **Tocolytics** can be used to delay delivery and reduce maternal bleeding risk in cases of a preterm fetus with **immature lungs** and **mild maternal bleeding**.
   c. When delivery is indicated, perform by **caesarean section**.
   d. Vaginal delivery can be performed with a low-lying placenta.
7. Complications = severe hemorrhage, IUGR, malpresentation, PROM, vasa previa (fetal vessels overlie the os and increase risk for fetal exsanguination); 1% of cases result in **maternal death**

J. Abruptio placentae
1. Premature separation of the placenta from uterine wall leading to **significant maternal hemorrhage**
2. **Risk factors** = HTN, prior abruptio placentae, trauma, **tobacco use**, cocaine use, PROM, multiple gestation, multiparity
3. **H/P** = **painful** vaginal bleeding in **third trimester**, back pain, abdominal pain; pelvic and abdominal tenderness, **increased uterine tone**; hypotension occurs with severe hemorrhage
4. **Radiology** = US **inconsistently** shows separation of placenta from uterus
5. Treatment
   a. Bed rest in inpatient setting for very mild cases
   b. Delivery typically occurs rapidly secondary to uterine irritation, but **caesarean section** should be performed in cases of **hemodynamic instability**.
   c. Transfusion is frequently required for significant hemorrhage.
6. **Complications** = DIC; **severe hemorrhage** that increases risk of maternal death; **fetal demise** occurs in 20% of cases; increased risk of abruption in future pregnancies

K. Multiple gestations
1. Any pregnancy in which **more than one fetus** develops at the same time
2. More likely to occur with fertility drug use
3. Types
   a. **Monozygotic**: division of zygote resulting in development of identical fetuses; fetuses may or may not share amnion or chorion
   b. **Dizygotic**: fertilization of more than one egg by different sperm resulting in development of dissimilar (i.e., fraternal) fetuses and separate amnions
4. Increased incidence of complications
   a. Maternal: HTN, DM, **preeclampsia**, **preterm labor**
   b. Fetal: **malpresentation**, placenta previa, abruptio placentae, PROM, **IUGR**, birth trauma, cerebral palsy, respiratory distress syndrome
5. **H/P** = fundal height large for gestational age; more than one fetal heart tone may be detected
6. **Radiology** = US detects 2+ gestational sacs
7. Treatment
   a. Close maternal follow-up (weekly or biweekly) starting at 24 weeks' gestation
   b. Activity restriction, frequent assessment of fetal growth with US, and weekly nonstress tests starting at 36 weeks' gestation
   c. Preterm labor should be halted with tocolytic therapy.
   d. Vertex-vertex (i.e., both heads downward) presentations may be delivered vaginally, but breech-vertex or breech-breech presentations require caesarean section; vertex-breech (first twin is head down, second is breech) presentation may often attempt vaginal delivery.

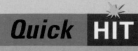

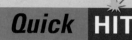
Placenta previa and **abruptio placentae** are the most common causes of vaginal bleeding **after 20 weeks'** gestation. Bleeding in **placenta previa** is **painless**, and bleeding in **placental abruption** is **painful**.

Do not perform a sterile vaginal examination in a patient with painless 3rd trimester bleeding until placenta previa is ruled out.

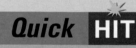
Conjoined twins only occur in cases of monozygotic twinning.

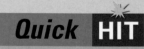
If the umbilical cords for multiple fetuses are fused, **twin–twin transfusion syndrome** can result, in which one twin is **inadequately** perfused, leading to an increased risk of fetal complications.

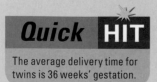
The average delivery time for twins is 36 weeks' gestation.

Obstetrics

V. Labor and Delivery

A. Assessment of fetal well-being

1. Tests of fetal activity, heart rate, and responses to stress used to confirm fetal wellbeing and to detect fetal distress
2. Nonstress test
   a. Used often during **prenatal assessment** and into labor
   b. Mother reclines in left lateral decubitus position.
   c. Fetal heart rate is monitored with external fetal heart rate and uterine contraction monitors.
   d. **Effects of fetal movement on heart rate** are noted.
   e. Normal ("reactive") test is considered to be two or more 15-bpm accelerations of fetal heart rate lasting at least 15 seconds, each within 20 minutes.
   f. An external sound device (vibroacoustic stimulator) can be attached to the mother's abdomen to encourage fetal activity and shorten the time of the test.
   g. Nonreactive test prompts the performance of a biophysical profile.
3. **Biophysical profile**
   a. Performed in follow-up to nonreactive nonstress test
   b. **Nonstress test repeated** and US assessment performed
   c. US used to measure **amniotic fluid index** (i.e., total linear measurement in centimeters of largest amniotic fluid pocket detected in each of four quadrants of amniotic sac), **fetal breathing rate, fetal movement, fetal tone** (i.e., extension of fetal spine or limb with return to flexion)
   d. Scoring system applied to nonstress test results and all US measurements; if test component satisfies criteria, it is given 2 points; if it does not meet criteria, it is assigned 0 points (no 1 point scores allowed).
      (1) Reactive nonstress test (2 points)
      (2) Amniotic fluid index = 5 to 23 cm (2 points)
      (3) 1+ episode of rhythmic breathing lasting 20 seconds within a 30-minute period (2 points)
      (4) 2+ episodes of discrete fetal movement within a 30-minute period (2 points)
      (5) 1+ episodes of spine and limb extension with return to flexion (2 points)
   e. **Reassuring** profile is a score of **8 or 10** and suggests minimal risk of fetal asphyxia; lower score suggests **fetal distress**.
4. **Contraction stress test**
   a. Used late in pregnancy or during labor to assess uteroplacental dysfunction
   b. Fetal heart rate is recorded with external fetal monitor or fetal scalp electrode.
   c. **Beat-to-beat variability** of ~5 bpm, **long-term heart rate variability**, and occasional **heart rate accelerations** (2+ accelerations of 15 bpm lasting at least 15 seconds within a 20-minute period) are **reassuring** signs.
   d. **Decelerations** of heart rate from baseline may indicate fetal head compression, umbilical cord compression, or fetal hypoxia (see Table 12-10, Figure 12-4).
5. **Fetal scalp blood sampling**
   a. Performed when a consistently abnormal fetal heart rate tracing seen
   b. Normal fetal blood pH is reassuring; **decreased pH** and **hypoxemia** and increased lactate indicate **fetal distress**.
6. **Fetal scalp monitoring**
   a. Monitor attached to fetal scalp to track pulse oximetry and perform continuous fetal heart rate monitoring and electrocardiogram (ECG)
   b. Should be used only in pregnancies >36 weeks' gestation with vertex presentation

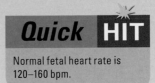

Quick HIT

Normal fetal heart rate is 120–160 bpm.

Quick HIT

A fetal **nonstress test** and **biophysical profile** are easy ways to assess fetal well-being and risk of fetal demise because of a stressful environment.

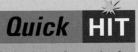

Quick HIT

During the last few weeks of gestation, a woman may experience multiple **false** (Braxton-Hicks) **contractions** not associated with true labor.

Obstetrics

TABLE 12-10	Types of Decelerations Seen on Fetal Heart Rate Tracings		
Deceleration	**Appearance**	**Cause**	**Treatment**
Early	Decelerations begin and end **with** uterine contractions	Head compression	• None required • **Not a sign of fetal distress**
Late	Begin **after** initiation of uterine contraction and end **after** contraction has finished	**Uteroplacental insufficiency**, maternal venous compression, maternal hypotension, or abruptio placentae; **may suggest fetal hypoxia**	• Test fetal blood from scalp sample to diagnose hypoxia or acidosis • Recurrent late decelerations or fetal hypoxia direct **prompt delivery**
Variable	**Inconsistent** onset, duration, and degree of decelerations	Umbilical cord compression	Change mother's position

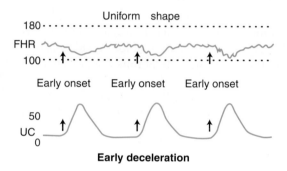

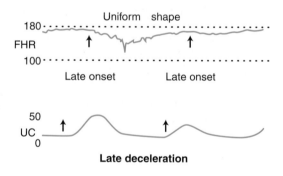

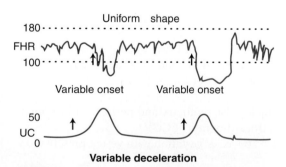

FIGURE 12-4 Examples of fetal heart and uterine tone tracings for early, late, and variable decelerations of fetal heart rate (*FHR*) following uterine contraction (*UC*).

(Modified from Hon, E. [1973]. *An Introduction to Fetal Heart Rate Monitoring.* Los Angeles, CA: University of Southern California. Also see Feibusch, K. C., Miroiu, M. Y., Breaden, R. S., Bader, C., & Gomperts, S. N. [2002]. *Prescription for the Boards: USMLE Step 2* (3rd ed.). Philadelphia, PA: Lippincott Williams & Wilkins.)

Obstetrics

B. Stages of labor

1. Labor (i.e., contractions with cervical change and effacement) typically begins at 37 to 42 weeks' gestation and involves four stages of progression (see Table 12-11).
2. Nulliparous and multiparous women proceed through labor at different rates.

TABLE 12-11 Stages of Labor					
				Duration	
Stage	Beginning/End	Activity	Management	Nulliparous	Multiparous
1	• Latent phase: start of uterine contractions until 6 cm cervical dilation and complete effacement • Active phase: 6 cm cervical dilation until near 10 cm cervical dilation with consistent progression • Deceleration phase: transition from active phase to second stage of labor	• Latent phase: cervical effacement and gradual dilation • Active phase: regular uterine contractions, quick progression of cervical dilation (1.2 cm/hr for nulliparous, 1.5 cm/hr for multiparous) and effacement • Deceleration phase: slowdown of dilation and effacement shortly before engagement of fetal head in pelvis	• Monitor fetal heart rate and uterine contractions, assess progression of cervical changes periodically during active phase	<20 hr (2/3 latent, 1/3 active)	<14 hr
2	Full (10 cm) cervical dilation until delivery	Fetal descent through birth canal driven by uterine contractions	Monitor fetal heart rate and movement through birth canal	<3 hr (<4 hr with epidural)	<2 hr (<3 hr with epidural)
3	Delivery of neonate until placental delivery	Placenta separates from uterine wall up to 30 min after delivery of neonate and emerges through birth canal, uterus contracts to expel placenta and prevent hemorrhage	Uterine massage, examination of placenta to confirm no intrauterine remnants	0–30 min	0–30 min
4	Initial postpartum hr	Hemodynamic stabilization of mother	Monitor maternal pulse and blood pressure, look for signs of hemorrhage	1 hr	1 hr

C. Induction of labor

1. Intervention (**oxytocin**, misoprostol, etc.) to initiate uterine contractions or speed progress of labor
2. Indications
   a. Maternal: preeclampsia, DM, stalled stage of labor, chorioamnionitis
   b. Fetal: prolonged pregnancy (i.e., >40 to 42 weeks), IUGR, PROM, some congenital defects
3. Contraindications to induction of labor are need for caesarean section, prior uterine surgery, fetal lung immaturity, malpresentation, acute fetal distress, active genital herpes, and placenta or vasa previa.
4. Likelihood of vaginal delivery following induction predicted by measuring fetal station and cervical dilation, effacement, consistency, and position (i.e., Bishop score) (see Table 12-12)
   a. Greater cervical dilation and effacement, softer cervix, more anterior cervical position, and greater station are associated with greater likelihood of vaginal delivery (i.e., higher Bishop score).
   b. Lower Bishop score is associated with higher likelihood of caesarean delivery (30% rate of caesarean delivery if Bishop score <3 after induction, 15% if >3).

TABLE 12-12	Bishop Scoring System[a]			
Score	**0**	**1**	**2**	**3**
Dilation (cm)	0	1–2	3–4	5–6
Effacement (%)	0–30	40–50	60–70	>70
Station (cm)[b]	−3	−2	−1, 0	+1, +2
Cervical consistency	Firm	Medium	Soft	
Cervical position	Posterior	Middle	Anterior	

[a]From Bishop, E. H. (1964). Pelvic scoring for elective induction. *Obstetrics and Gynecology, 24,* 266–268.
[b]Distance of presenting body part above (−) or below (+) ischial spines.

D. Malpresentation

1. **Normal** fetal presentation (i.e., cephalic or vertex) is with fetal head down, chin tucked, and occiput directed toward birth canal.
2. **Face** (i.e., full hyperextension of neck) presentation occurs rarely and usually undergoes normal vaginal delivery if chin is anterior.
3. **Brow** (i.e., partial hyperextension of neck) presentation occurs very rarely and requires caesarean delivery if the head does not spontaneously correct to a normal presentation.
4. **Breech presentation** is the most common **malpresentation** (Figure 12-5).
   a. **Frank breech**: 75% of cases; hips flexed and knees extended
   b. **Complete breech**: hips and knees flexed
   c. **Footling breech**: one or both legs extended
   d. **Risk factors** = prematurity, multiple gestation, polyhydramnios, uterine anomaly, placenta previa
   e. **H/P** = abdominal examination (i.e., Leopold maneuvers) detects fetal head in abdomen, vaginal examination may detect presenting part
   f. **Radiology** = US confirms fetal orientation
   g. **Treatment** = most cases will resolve before labor; **external cephalic version** may be applied to abdomen at 37 weeks' gestation to attempt repositioning of fetus (up to 75% effective); caesarean section performed in most cases
   h. **Complications** = cord prolapse, head entrapment, fetal hypoxia, abruptio placentae, birth trauma

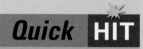

Quick HIT

Presentation at birth:
- Vertex presentation is position at time of delivery in >95% of pregnancies.
- Before 28 weeks' gestation, **25%** of pregnancies are in **breech** presentation, but **most** will assume **vertex** presentation by the time of birth.

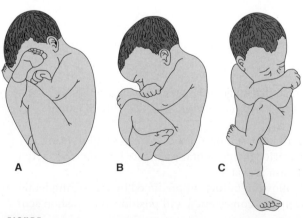

A B C

FIGURE 12-5 Examples of frank (A), complete (B), and incomplete (C) variations of breech presentation.

(Modified from Beckmann, C. R. B., Ling, F. W., Herbert, W. N. P., et al. [2014]. *Obstetrics and Gynecology* [7th ed., p. 104]. Baltimore, MD: Lippincott Williams & Wilkins; with permission.)

E. Caesarean section

1. Delivery of fetus through incision in uterine wall
2. Types
   a. **Vertical**: vertical incision in anterior muscular portion of the uterus (i.e., classic) or lower uterine segment (i.e., low vertical); chosen when fetus lies in transverse presentation, adhesions or fibroids prevent access to lower uterus, hysterectomy is scheduled to follow delivery, cervical cancer is present, or in postmortem delivery to remove living fetus from dead mother
   b. **Low transverse**: transverse incision in lower uterine segment; decreased risk of uterine rupture, bleeding, bowel adhesions, and infection (**preferred** to classic technique and performed more commonly)
3. Indications
   a. Maternal: **eclampsia, prior uterine surgery, prior classic caesarean section**, cardiac disease, birth canal obstruction, maternal death, cervical cancer, active genital herpes, HIV
   b. Fetal: **acute fetal distress, malpresentation**, cord prolapse, macrosomia
   c. Combined maternal and fetal: **failure to progress in labor**, placenta previa, abruptio placentae, cephalopelvic disproportion
4. In subsequent pregnancies, vaginal delivery can be attempted only if **transverse** caesarean section was performed.
5. If **vertical** incision has been used previously, repeat caesarean delivery must be performed because of risk of uterine rupture.
6. Complications = hemorrhage, infection and sepsis, thromboembolism, injury to surrounding structures; future pregnancies are at increased risk of placenta previa, placenta accreta, and miscarriage

F. Normal puerperium and postpartum activity

1. Care of the newborn
   a. Immediate suction of mouth and nose to aid in breathing and to prevent aspiration
   b. Neonate is dried and wrapped in clothes to prevent heat loss.
   c. Umbilical cord is clamped and cut; blood sample is taken from cord to measure blood gases and blood type.
   d. Onset of respiration within 30 seconds is confirmed; if spontaneous respiration does not begin, **resuscitation** must be initiated.
   e. Tracheal injection of synthetic or exogenous surfactant may be given in cases of lung immaturity.
   f. **Apgar score** is performed at 1 and 5 minutes after birth; a score of **7+ at 1 minute and 9+ at 5 minutes is reassuring** (see Table 12-13).

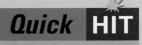

Quick HIT

Risk of maternal mortality is similar for elective caesarean section and vaginal delivery, but emergency caesarean section carries a higher risk of mortality.

Quick HIT

Breast milk is considered the ideal infant nutrient because it contains important **IgA antibodies** for the newborn, is in **sufficient supply**, is **cost-free**, and enhances mother–infant bonding.

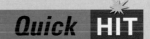

Quick HIT

Early breast milk (**colostrum**) is rich in proteins, fat, and minerals and contains IgA; after 1 week postpartum, breast milk contains proteins, fat, water, and lactose.

Obstetrics

TABLE 12-13	Apgar Scoring System for Determining Neonatal Well-Being

	Score		
Sign	**0**	**1**	**2**
Color	Blue, pale	Pink torso, blue extremities	Pink
Heart rate	None	<100 bpm	>100 bpm
Response to stimulation	None	Grimace	Strong cry
Muscle tone	Poor	Some movement	Active movement
Respirations	None	Poor, weak cry	Good, strong cry

Adapted from Apgar, V. (1953). A proposal of a new method of evaluation of the newborn infant. *Current Researches in Anesthesia and Analgesia*, 32, 261–267.

2. Maternal changes
   a. Uterus decreases in size and cervix becomes firm over 3 weeks.
   b. Uterine discharge (i.e., lochia) is red during initial days after birth but becomes paler and white by 10th day postpartum.
   c. Vaginal wall gradually becomes firmer.
   d. Total peripheral resistance increases rapidly because of elimination of utero-placental circulation; diuresis causes significant weight loss in first week postpartum; cardiac output gradually returns to normal.
   e. Mother may feel mild depression for few days after delivery (i.e., "postpartum blues"); most cases resolve without complications.
   f. Menstruation returns 6 to 8 weeks postpartum in non-nursing mothers.
   g. Ovulation and menstruation may not occur for several months in nursing mothers (98% effective in preventing pregnancy for 6 months after delivery if performed regularly).

G. Postpartum bleeding

1. Blood loss >500 mL/24 hr following vaginal delivery or >1,000 mL/24 hr after caesarean section is abnormal.
2. Because of **uterine atony** in most cases (more likely after multiple gestation, prolonged labor, and chorioamnionitis)
3. Can also result from **birth canal trauma**, **retained placental tissue**, or **coagulopathy** (e.g., DIC)
4. **H/P** = excessive postpartum bleeding from genital tract; soft, boggy uterus palpable with uterine atony; vaginal examination may detect lacerations; examination of placenta after birth should detect any missing segments
5. **Radiology** = US may show retained placental tissue
6. **Treatment**
   a. Uterine massage and oxytocin administration help increase uterine tone and decrease hemorrhage.
   b. Surgical repair of lacerations should be performed.
   c. Dilation and curettage (D&C) may successfully remove retained placental tissue.
   d. Hysterectomy may need to be performed in severe or refractory cases.

VI. Gestational Trophoblastic Disease

A. Hydatidiform mole

1. Benign neoplasms of trophoblastic cells (i.e., cells that make up placenta) that infrequently become malignant; **benign** trophoblastic neoplasms make up **80%** of trophoblastic disease
2. Types
   a. Complete: 46 XX or 46 XY genotype; completely derived from father (empty egg penetrated by two sperm)
   b. Incomplete: 69 XXY, 69 XXX, or 69 XYY genotype; fertilization of egg by two sperm; may be associated with abnormal fetus
3. **Risk factors** = low socioeconomic status, **extremes of age** (teen, >40 years), at time of pregnancy, history of prior molar pregnancy, **Asian heritage**, smoking
4. **H/P** = heavy or irregular painless vaginal bleeding during **first** or **second** trimester, hyperemesis gravidarum, dizziness, anxiety; large fundal height for gestational age, expulsion of "grape-like" vesicles from vagina, no fetal movement or heart tones detected
5. **Labs** = β-hCG is much **higher** than expected for gestational age
6. **Radiology** = US detects "**snowstorm**" pattern in uterus without presence of gestational sac
7. **Treatment** = D&C to remove neoplasm; follow β-hCG for 1 year (levels should gradually decrease); avoid pregnancy for 6 months to 1 year
8. **Complications** = malignant gestational trophoblastic neoplasm (20% of cases), choriocarcinoma (5% of cases, suggested by continued high β-hCG following D&C)

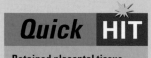

Quick HIT

Retained placental tissue causes the most substantial volume of postpartum bleeding.

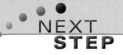

NEXT STEP

Highly suspect a molar pregnancy if **preeclampsia** occurs in the **first half** of pregnancy, and perform an US to confirm diagnosis.

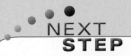

NEXT STEP

High β-hCG is seen in both **hydatidiform mole** and **multiple gestations**; differentiate the conditions with US.

Obstetrics

B. Choriocarcinoma

1. **Malignant** trophoblastic neoplasm that arises from hydatidiform moles (50% of cases) or following abortion, ectopic pregnancy, or normal pregnancy
2. **H/P** = vaginal bleeding and possible hemoptysis, dyspnea, headache, dizziness, or rectal bleeding; enlarged uterus on examination with bleeding seen from cervical os
3. **Labs** = increased β-hCG
4. **Radiology** = US detects uterine mass with mix of hemorrhagic and necrotic areas and possible parametrial invasion; computed tomography (CT) may detect metastases
5. **Treatment** = hysterectomy of disease limited to uterus; chemotherapy routinely administered; patient with early limited disease wishing to maintain fertility may choose chemotherapy alone; follow β-hCG to track cure; avoid pregnancy for 1 year after therapy
6. **Complications** = **metastases** to lungs, brain, liver, kidneys, or gastrointestinal tract; good prognosis unless presence of brain or liver metastases; frequently missed diagnosis if not caused by progression from molar pregnancy

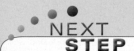

NEXT STEP

Be sure to collect a thorough **family history** while assessing growth or developmental delays to help distinguish a **hereditary** cause from an **environmental** one.

I. Development and Health Supervision

A. Physical growth

1. Characteristics of growth (i.e., weight, height, and head circumference) fall in a normal range; deviations from this range suggest abnormal growth, disease processes, or environmental concerns.

2. Pediatrician should keep a record of growth on a chart.

3. **Weight**

   a. Initial loss of weight in first few days after birth is normal; birth weight is regained by 2 weeks of age.

   b. Birth **weight doubles** by ~4 months, **triples** at ~12 months, and **quadruples at ~24 months**.

   c. From age 2 years to adolescence (age 13 years), annual weight gain is ~5 lb.

   d. Inadequate weight gain can result from **poor food intake** (including poor feeding and abuse), chronic vomiting or diarrhea, **malabsorption**, neoplasm, or congenital diseases (e.g., cardiac, endocrine).

   e. Weight <5th percentile on growth charts or a consistently low weight for a given height suggests **failure to thrive** (see Chapter 3, **Gastrointestinal Disorders**).

   f. The prevalence of **childhood obesity** (body mass index matched for age and gender >95th percentile) has steadily increased in the United States and is associated with rapid growth, sleep apnea, hypertension (HTN), slipped capital femoral epiphysis, precocious puberty, increased incidence of skin infections, social dysfunction, and earlier development of diabetes mellitus (DM).

4. **Height**

   a. **Height** (or birth length) is increased by 50% at ~1 year of age, **doubles** at **~4 years of age**, and **triples** at **~13 years of age**.

   b. Annual height gain from age 2 years to adolescence is ~2 in/year.

   c. Greater-than-normal height can be associated with familial tall stature, precocious puberty, gigantism, hyperthyroidism, Klinefelter syndrome, Marfan syndrome, or obesity.

   d. Lower-than-normal height can be associated with familial short stature, neglect, Turner syndrome, constitutional growth delay, chronic renal failure, asthma, cystic fibrosis, inflammatory bowel disease (IBD), immunologic disease, growth hormone deficiency, hypothyroidism, glucocorticoid excess, skeletal dysplasias, or neoplasm.

5. **Head circumference**

   a. Measured during first 1 to 3 years of life

   b. ~5 cm growth during age 0 to 3 months, ~4 cm in 3 to 6 months, 2 cm in 6 to 9 months, and 1 cm in 9 to 12 months

   c. Macrocephaly can be associated with cerebral metabolic diseases (e.g., Tay-Sachs, maple syrup urine disease), neurocutaneous syndromes (e.g., neurofibromatosis, tuberous sclerosis), hydrocephalus, increased intracranial pressure, skeletal dysplasia, acromegaly, or intracranial hemorrhage.

   d. Microcephaly can be associated with fetal toxin exposure (e.g., fetal alcohol syndrome), chromosomal trisomies, congenital infection, cranial anatomic abnormalities, metabolic disorders, or neural tube defects.

6. Trend of growth abnormalities helps suggest certain pathologies.
   a. Normal growth rate that declines **after birth** suggests **postnatal** onset.
   b. Growth that is **abnormal from the time of birth** suggests **prenatal** onset (e.g., genetic abnormalities, intrauterine pathology).
   c. Growth that is in low-normal range but eventually becomes closer to the mean suggests **constitutional growth delay**.
   d. Growth that is **consistently** low-normal suggests genetic short stature (i.e., compare with parents).

7. **History and physical (H/P)**
   a. Look for other symptoms and signs that suggest a particular disease.
     (1) Malabsorption: diarrhea
     (2) DM: hyperglycemia
     (3) Congenital heart disease: cyanosis, etc.
     (4) Signs of abuse: bruising, abnormal parent–child interaction
     (5) Psychosocial abnormalities: inattentiveness, apathy
   b. Growth should be assessed at **each health visit** to confirm normal patterns and catch abnormalities early.

8. Labs = should be directed at diagnosis of a specific disease when clinical suspicion exists (e.g., for DM, blood glucose; for congenital heart disease, arterial blood gas, etc.)

9. **Treatment**
   a. Treat underlying disorder.
   b. Seek intervention for cases of abuse.
   c. Provide parental education to help alleviate poor intake, poor-quality diets, or malnutrition and to help deal with psychosocial issues.

B. Developmental milestones

1. **Social, physical**, and **intellectual** achievements are reached by children at characteristic ages (see Table 13-1).
2. Absence or delay of milestones can suggest developmental delays.
3. Some delays are hereditary, but multiple or significant delays are a cause for concern.
4. Multiple or persistent delays can result from mental retardation, genetic disorders (e.g., fragile X syndrome, trisomy 21), language or hearing disorders, child abuse, or psychiatric conditions (e.g., attention deficit hyperactivity disorder [ADHD], autism).
5. Certain reflexes are prevalent during infancy but naturally disappear by **6 months** of age; absence or persistence of infantile reflexes beyond 6 months (especially with a history of perinatal complications or suspected congenital malformation) may suggest central nervous system (CNS) pathology (see Table 13-2).

C. Childhood health maintenance

1. Periodic physician visits are important during childhood to assess **growth**, detect growth and developmental **delays**, provide **vaccinations, screen** for certain disease processes, and provide **anticipatory guidance** (see Table 13-3).
   a. Visits 2 weeks after birth and at 1 month of age
   b. Visits at 2 months old, then every 2 months (2, 4, 6 months) until 6 months old
   c. Visits every 3 months from age 6–18 months (6, 9, 12, 15, 18 months)
   d. Visits at age 2 years and annually thereafter
2. Screening during visits should address common medical concerns (e.g., vision, hearing, dentition, diseases in high-risk populations).
3. Anticipatory guidance should address **nutrition, development, daily care, accident prevention**, and **behavioral issues**.
4. Vaccinations should be given at appropriate visits (see Table 13-4).

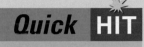

Quick HIT

It is **legally imperative** that **all suspected** cases of child abuse are **well documented** and **reported** to the appropriate authorities.

Quick HIT

Ages for developmental milestones are **guidelines.** It is normal for milestones to occur at an appropriate **range of ages**, and parents should be reassured that milestones occur within such a range and not at concrete ages.

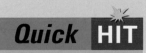

Quick HIT

Haemophilus influenzae type b (Hib) vaccine is **unnecessary** in previously unvaccinated children >**5 years** because of the low risk of severe infection at this age and older. **Asplenic** children should **always** receive Hib and pneumococcal vaccines regardless of their age.

Pediatrics

TABLE 13-1	Important Developmental Milestones during Childhood			
Age	**Social/Cognitive**	**Gross Motor**	**Fine Motor**	**Language**
2 months	Social smile	Lifts head 45°	Eyes follow object to midline	Coos
4 months	Laughs Aware of caregiver Localizes sound	Lifts head 90°	Eyes follow object past midline	
6 months	Differentiates parents from others Stranger anxiety	Rolls over Holds self up with hands Sits without support	Grasps/rakes Attempts to feed self	Babbles
9 months	Interactive games Separation anxiety (9–15 months)	Crawls Pulls to stand	Grasps with thumb	First words
12 months	Separation anxiety (9–15 months)	Walks with help	Pincer grasp Makes tower of two blocks	~5–10-word vocabulary
18 months	Parallel play	Walks well Walks backward	Makes tower of four blocks Uses cup or spoon	10–50-word vocabulary 2-word sentences
2 yr	Dresses self with help	Runs Climbs stairs (initially 2 feet/step, then 1 foot/step)	Makes tower of six blocks	50–75-word vocabulary 3-word sentences
3 yr	Magical thinking Gender identity (2–3 yr)	Climbs/descends stairs	Makes tower of nine blocks Able to draw circle	
4 yr	Plays with others	Hops on 1 foot	Able to draw line image (+); later able to draw closed line drawing (Δ)	250+ word vocabulary 4-word sentences
6 yr	Able to distinguish fantasy from reality	Skips	Draws a person	Fluent speech

TABLE 13-2	Childhood Reflexes and Their Relation to Central Nervous System Pathology			
Reflex	**Description**	**Time of Disappearance**	**Area of CNS Associated with Abnormal Persistence or Disappearance**
Moro	Extension of head causes extension and flexion of limbs; startle reflex	3 months	Medulla, vestibular nuclei
Grasp	Placing finger in palm causes grasping	3 months	Medulla, vestibular nuclei
Rooting	Rubbing cheek causes turning of mouth to stimuli	3 months	Medulla, trigeminal nuclei
Tonic neck	When head turned, arm on faced side extends and arm on opposite side flexes (fencer's position)	3 months	Medulla, vestibular nuclei
Placing	Rubbing foot dorsum causes foot to step up	2 months	Cortex

CNS, central nervous system.

| TABLE 13-3 | Screening Performed and Anticipatory Guidance Discussed during Regular Childhood Health Visits | | | | |

Visit	Screening	Nutrition	Daily Care	Accident Prevention	Behavioral Issues
Newborn/ 1 wk	Phenylketonuria, hypothyroidism, genetic metabolic disorders (maple syrup urine disease, cystic fibrosis, etc.) in high-risk patients; hearing; visual mobility and reflexes	Breast or bottle feeding	Crying, **sleep position** ("back to bed"), bathing	Smoke detectors, baby furniture, car seats	Parent–child interaction
1 month	Visual mobility and reflexes	Breast or bottle feeding, fluoride supplements	Sleep, bowel, and bladder habits	Sun exposure	Importance of close contact
2 months	Visual mobility and reflexes		Sleep, bowel habits	Close supervision, risks with ability to roll over	
4 months	Visual mobility and reflexes	**Solid foods** (iron-fortified cereal, pureed fruits, and vegetables) introduced at 4–6 months of age	Teething	Keeping small objects out of reach	Vocal interaction
6 months	Visual mobility and reflexes	Cup training, daily caloric needs, finger foods, avoidance of milk or juice at bedtime	Shoes	Preparation for increased mobility ("childproofing" the house), electrical socket covers, stair and door gates	Stranger anxiety, separation anxiety
9 months	Hgb/Hct; visual mobility and reflexes	Iron supplementation, self-feeding, spoon training	Tooth care, favorite toys	Aspiration risks	Communication, discipline
12 months	Visual mobility and reflexes, lead exposure; PPD in high-risk areas	Bottle weaning, eating at table, whole cow's milk		Poisoning risks, stair safety, burns	Speech, rules, positive reinforcement
15 months	Hgb/Hct; visual mobility and reflexes	Family meals			Toilet training, temper tantrums, punishment, listening to parent read
18 months	Visual mobility and reflexes	Reinforcement of utensil use	Nightmares, bedtime regimens	Supervised play, dangerous toys	Discipline, "terrible 2s," toilet training, games
2 yr	Lead exposure; visual mobility and reflexes	Avoiding unhealthy snacks, encouraging eating during meals	Transition from crib to bed, toothbrush training		Toddler independence, explanation of body parts, early play with other children
3 yr	Visual acuity; cholesterol (if family history of high cholesterol or CAD) Routine dental checkups begin at 2–3 yr	Healthy diet	Regular sleep schedule, **TV/media limitation**	Water safety, animal safety	Day care or babysitters (earlier if both parents work), play with other children, reinforce consistent toileting, conversation
4 yr	Hearing; lead exposure; visual acuity; PPD (if high-risk group); urinalysis	Meals as time for family bonding	Self-dental care	Pedestrian and bicycle safety, car seat or seat belt, dangers of strangers, guns, fires, poisons, teach phone number	Chores, interactions at day care or preschool, school preparation

Pediatrics

TABLE 13-3 Screening Performed and Anticipatory Guidance Discussed during Regular Childhood Health Visits (*Continued*)

Visit	Screening	Nutrition	Daily Care	Accident Prevention	Behavioral Issues
6 yr	Lead exposure; visual acuity	Avoidance of excess weight; obesity prevention counseling	Exercise, hygiene, school activities	Swimming	Allowance, encourage learning and development, reading
10 yr	Hearing. visual acuity			Hazardous activities, drug use (including alcohol and tobacco)	Friends, sexual education, puberty, responsibility
12 yr	Hearing; visual acuity; PPD (if high-risk group); Pap smear only if sexually active (girls)		Adequate sleep, school and extracurricular activities	Sexual responsibility	Body image, privacy issues
14 yr and older	Hearing; Hgb/Hct (girls); visual acuity; STD screening (if sexually active)	Weight maintenance	School and activities	Risk-taking behavior, driving, sexual responsibility	Dating, sexuality, goals, careers, independence issues

Note: anticipatory guidance from **prior** visits should be **reviewed**, when appropriate.

CAD, coronary artery disease; Hgb/Hct, hemoglobin and hematocrit; PPD, purified protein derivative of tuberculin (TB test); STD, sexually transmitted disease.

TABLE 13-4 Vaccination Schedule and Contraindications during Well-Child Health Visits (2015 Recommendations)

Vaccine	Birth	1 mo	2 mo	4 mo	6 mo	12 mo	15 mo	18 mo	24 mo	4–6 yr	11–12 yr	16–18 yr
HepB[a]	HepB	HepB				HepB						
Rota[b]			Rota	Rota	Rota							
DTaP[c]			DTaP	DTaP	DTaP		DTaP			DTaP	Tdap	
Hib[d]			Hib	Hib	Hib	Hib						
PCV[e]			PCV	PCV	PCV	PCV						
IPV[f]			IPV	IPV		IPV				IPV		
MMR[g]						MMR				MMR		
VZV[h]						VZV				VZV		
HepA[i]						HepA × 2						
MCV4[j]											MCV4	MCV4
HPV[k]											HPV × 3	

[a]Hepatitis B (HepB); contraindications: allergy to yeast or anaphylaxis following prior dose.

[b]Rotavirus (Rota); contraindications: anaphylaxis following prior dose.

[c]Diphtheria, tetanus, acellular pertussis (DTaP); tetanus booster (Td) given in adolescence; contraindications: encephalopathy or anaphylaxis following prior dose.

[d]*Haemophilus influenzae* type b (Hib); no contraindications.

[e]Pneumococcal vaccine (PCV); contraindications: anaphylaxis following prior dose.

[f]Inactivated polio vaccine (IPV); contraindications: pregnancy (or pregnant female at home) and anaphylaxis following prior dose.

[g]Measles, mumps, rubella (MMR); contraindications: pregnancy (or pregnant female at home), immunocompromise, thrombocytopenia, hematologic or solid neoplasm, anaphylaxis following prior dose.

[h]Varicella-zoster vaccine (VZV); contraindications: allergy to neomycin, anaphylaxis following prior dose, immunosuppression, pregnancy (or pregnant female at home), moderate or severe illness.

[i]Hepatitis A (HepA); given in two doses at least 6 months apart; contraindications: anaphylaxis following prior dose.

[j]Meningococcal vaccine (MCV4); possible rare association with Guillain-Barré syndrome.

[k]Human papilloma virus vaccine (HPV); given as three doses over 6-month period.

TABLE 13-5	Tanner Stages for Male Genital and Pubic Hair Development	
Tanner Stage	**Penile/Testicular Development**	**Pubic Hair Development**
1	Prepubertal; small genitals	Prepubertal; no hair growth
2	Testicular and scrotal enlargement with skin coarsening	Slight growth of fine genital and axillary hair
3	Penile enlargement and further testicular growth	Further growth of hair
4	Further penile glans enlargement and darkening of scrotal skin	Hair becomes coarser and spreads over much of pubic region
5	Adult genitalia	Coarse hair extends from pubic region to medial thighs

D. Adolescence

1. Period of **rapid physical**, **psychosocial**, and **sexual growth** and maturity leading into adulthood; encompasses time between 10 and 19 years of age
2. Puberty typically begins at age 9 to 10 years in girls and 9 to 11 years in boys; development of puberty before these ages is considered **precocious** puberty.
3. Physical changes are classified by Tanner stages (see Table 13-5; also refer to Chapter 11, Gynecologic and Breast Disorders).
4. Psychosocial issues
   a. Early adolescence (10 to 13 years) is typified by concrete thinking and early independent behavior.
   b. Middle adolescence (14 to 16 years) is typified by emergence of **sexuality** (e.g., sexual identity, sexual activity), an increased **desire for independence** (e.g., conflict with parents, need for guidance, self-absorption), and abstract thought.
   c. Late adolescence (17 to 21 years) is typified by increased self-awareness, increased confidence in own abilities, a more open relationship with parents, and cognitive maturity.
   d. Adolescents are at an increased risk for risk-taking behaviors (e.g., drug use, unprotected sexual activity, violence), **depression**, **suicidal ideation**, **homicide**, and **eating disorders**.
5. **H/P**
   a. History during visits should address **risk factors** (e.g., sexually transmitted diseases [STDs], violence, abuse), substance use, mood, physical changes, nutritional habits, menstrual issues (girls), and **concerns of patient**.
   b. Examination should focus on sexual maturation, dermatologic issues (e.g., acne, sun exposure, nevi), appropriate height and weight growth, and scrotal masses (i.e., detection of testicular cancer in boys).
   c. Additional medical screening should include that for HTN, obesity, DM, and hyperlipidemia.
6. **Treatment**
   a. Most teenagers proceed through adolescence without serious incidents even though accidents are the no. 1 cause of death in this age group.
   b. Risk-taking behavior can result in STDs and drug addiction that need to be treated appropriately.
   c. Emphasis should be placed on maintaining a good physician–patient relationship while addressing risk prevention.

II. Immune Disorders

A. Congenital immune deficiencies are uncommon and can result from defects in T cells and/or B cells, phagocytic cells, or complement (see Table 13-6).

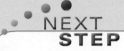

NEXT STEP

Because of adolescents' desire for independence and need for good self-esteem, adolescent patients should be approached in a **nonjudgmental** fashion to perform an accurate history and physical examination.

Pediatrics

Quick HIT

Confidentiality between a physician and patient must be maintained during adolescence **unless life-threatening** concerns are involved (e.g., suicidal ideation, homicidal ideation, life-threatening disease), and this right may need to be stressed to parents.

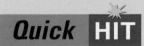

Quick HIT

Presentation of immune disorders does not occur immediately after birth because newborns retain **maternally derived antibodies** for ~3 months.

TABLE **13-6**	Types of Congenital Immunodeficiency Disorders		
Disease	**Description**	**Diagnosis**	**Treatment**
T-cell disorders			
DiGeorge syndrome	Chromosomal deletion in 22q11 resulting in **thymic and parathyroid hypoplasia, congenital heart disease**, tetany, and abnormal facial structure; recurrent viral and fungal infections occur because of insufficient T cells	**Tetany** and **facial abnormalities** on examination; decreased serum calcium; evidence of congenital heart disease; chest radiograph may show absence of thymic shadow; genetic screening can detect chromosomal abnormality	Calcium, vitamin D, thymic transplant, bone marrow transplant, surgical correction of heart abnormalities; IVIG or prophylactic antibiotics may be helpful
Chronic mucocutaneous candidiasis	Persistent infection of skin, mucous membranes, and nails by ***Candida albicans*** from T-cell deficiency; frequent associated adrenal pathology	Poor reaction to cutaneous *C. albicans* anergy test; possible decreased IgG	Antifungal agents (e.g., fluconazole)
B-cell disorders			
X-linked agammaglobulinemia	Abnormal B-cell differentiation resulting in low B-cell and antibody levels; X-linked disorder with **boys** experiencing recurrent bacterial infections after 6 months of age	**No B cells in peripheral smear**; low total immunoglobulin levels	IVIG, appropriate antibiotics, supportive pulmonary care
IgA deficiency	Specific IgA deficiency because of abnormal immune globulin production by B cells; patients have increased incidence of respiratory and gastrointestinal infections	**Decreased IgA** with **normal** levels of **other immune globulins**	Prophylactic antibiotics; IVIG with caution (small risk of anaphylaxis)
Hyper IgM disease	Defect in T-cell CD40 ligand resulting in poor interaction with B cells, low IgG, and excessive IgM; infection by **encapsulated bacteria** (pulmonary and gastrointestinal)	Decreased IgG and IgA, **increased IgM**; possible decreased Hgb, Hct, platelets, and neutrophils	IVIG, prophylactic antibiotics; bone marrow transplant
Common variable immunodeficiency	Autosomal disorder of B-cell differentiation resulting in low immune globulin levels; patients experience increased respiratory and gastrointestinal infections beginning in second decade of life; associated with increased risk of **malignant neoplasms** and **autoimmune disorders**	Low immune globulin levels; poor response to vaccines; decreased CD4:CD8 T-cell ratio; family history shows **both men and women affected**	IVIG, appropriate antibiotics
Combined B- and T-cell disorders			
Severe combined immunodeficiency syndrome (SCID)	Absent T cells and abnormal antibody function resulting in **severe immune compromise**; patients experience significant recurrent infections by all types of pathogens from an early age; **frequently fatal at an early age**	Significantly decreased WBCs, decreased immune globulins	IVIG, antibiotics, **bone marrow transplant; no live or attenuated vaccines** should be administered
Wiskott-Aldrich syndrome	X-linked disorder of immune development resulting in significant susceptibility to **encapsulated** bacteria and opportunistic pathogens; associated with **eczema** and **thrombocytopenia**	Recurrent infections in presence of **eczema** and **easy bleeding**; decreased platelets, decreased IgM with normal or high other immune globulins; genetic analysis detects abnormal WASP gene	**Splenectomy**, antibiotic prophylaxis, IVIG, bone marrow transplant
Ataxia-telangiectasia	Autosomal recessive disorder causing **cerebellar dysfunction, cutaneous telangiectasias**, increased risk of cancer, and impaired WBC and IgA development	**Telangiectasias** and **ataxia** develop after 3 yr of age; recurrent pulmonary infections begin a few years later; decreased WBCs, decreased IgA	IVIG and prophylactic antibiotics may be helpful, but treatment usually unable to limit disease progression

TABLE 13-6 Types of Congenital Immunodeficiency Disorders (*Continued*)			
Disease	**Description**	**Diagnosis**	**Treatment**
Phagocytic cell disorders			
Chronic granulomatous disease	Defect in which neutrophils **cannot digest** engulfed bacteria, resulting in recurrent bacterial and fungal infections	Cutaneous, pulmonary, and perirectal abscess formation; chronic lymphadenopathy; genetic analysis detects causative genetic mutations	Prophylactic antibiotics, γ-interferon, corticosteroids, bone marrow transplant
Hyper-IgE disease (Job syndrome)	Defect in neutrophil chemotaxis, T-cell signaling, and overproduction of IgE resulting in **chronic dermatitis, recurrent skin abscesses**, and pulmonary infections; patients commonly have coarse facial features and retained primary teeth	Increased IgE, increased eosinophils; defective chemotactic response of neutrophils on stimulation	Prophylactic antibiotics; skin hydration and emollient use
Chediak-Higashi syndrome	Autosomal recessive **dysfunction of neutrophils** resulting in recurrent *Staphylococcus aureus*, streptococcal, gram-negative bacteria, and fungal infections; associated with **abnormal platelets, albinism**, and **neurologic dysfunction**	Large granules seen in granulocytes on peripheral smear	Prophylactic antibiotics, bone marrow transplant
Leukocyte adhesion deficiency (types 1 and 2)	Inability of neutrophils to leave circulation because of abnormal leukocyte integrins (type 1) or E-selectin (type 2), recurrent bacterial infections of upper respiratory tract and skin, delayed separation of umbilical cord; short stature, abnormal facies, and cognitive impairment seen in type 2 disease	Increased serum neutrophils; defective chemotactic response of neutrophils upon stimulation	Prophylactic antibiotics; bone marrow transplant needed in type 1 disease; type 2 disease treated with fucose supplementation
Complement disorders			
Complement deficiencies	Multiple inherited deficiencies of one or more complement components, resulting in recurrent bacterial infections and **predisposition to autoimmune disorders (e.g., SLE)**	Hemolytic complement test results are abnormal and indicate problem in pathway; direct testing of components can detect exact deficiency	Appropriate antibiotics; treat autoimmune disorders, as needed

Hct, hematocrit; Hgb, hemoglobin; IVIG, intravenous immune globulin; SLE, systemic lupus erythematosus; WBC, white blood cell.

B. H/P = frequent and **recurrent infections** beginning after 3 months of age, including diseases caused by opportunistic pathogens; wound healing may be impaired

C. Labs = complete blood count (CBC) detects general white blood cell (WBC) abnormalities; determination of specific WBCs affected (T cells, B cells, neutrophils, etc.) and peripheral blood smear can help determine precise cell type abnormality

D. Treatment = antibiotics (both prophylactic and therapeutic) are required to treat infections; severe immune deficiencies may require immunotherapies or bone marrow transplant

E. Complications = recurrent infections, poor wound healing; death frequently occurs **before third decade of life** (younger for more severe deficiencies) because of body's inability to combat pathogens

III. Genetic Disorders (Chromosomal Pathology)

A. Sex chromosome disorders

1. Diseases caused by an abnormal number of sex chromosomes in the genetic karyotype (see Table 13-7)

Quick HIT

Most pregnancies with a 45XO karyotype end in spontaneous abortion.

Quick HIT

It was previously believed that males with an XYY genotype were at a higher risk for violent and antisocial behavior, but this trend has been disproved. They have the same rate of criminal activity as 46XY individuals with similar intelligence levels.

TABLE 13-7	Common Sex Chromosome Disorders	
Condition	**Karyotype**	**History and Physical**
Turner syndrome	45XO or mosaicism	Female with **short stature, infertility**, abnormal genital formation, increased incidence of renal and cardiac defects (**coarctation of aorta**), craniofacial abnormalities (protruding ears, **neck webbing**, low occipital hairline)
Klinefelter syndrome	47XXY	Male with **testicular atrophy**, tall and thin body, gynecomastia, infertility, mild mental retardation, and psychosocial adjustment abnormalities
XYY	47XYY	Male with tall body (>6 feet), significant acne, mild mental retardation
XXX	47XXX	Female with increased incidence of mental retardation, menstrual abnormalities

2. In females, sex chromosome abnormalities are usually less severe than autosomal disorders because **X chromosome inactivation** attempts to restore the normal number of active chromosomes and because Y chromosomes contain relatively **few** genes.
3. **Labs** = karyotyping will reveal an abnormal number of sex chromosomes
4. **Treatment**
   a. Turner syndrome requires regular cardiovascular assessments and estrogen and progestin replacement.
   b. Special education or behavior counseling may be needed for mental impairments.
   c. Generally, patients are able to live productive adult lives.

B. Trisomies
   1. Syndromes that occur because of **autosomal nondisjunction** or **genetic translocation** during sex cell production that result in extra copies of autosomal genetic material (see Table 13-8)

Quick HIT

Down syndrome is the most common cause of **congenital** mental retardation when both genders are considered.

Quick HIT

Nearly all trisomies result from nondisjunction during meiosis of **maternal** germ cells.

Quick HIT

The risk of trisomy increases exponentially in women after 35 years of age.

TABLE 13-8	Autosomal Trisomies	
Condition	**Incidence**	**History and Physical**
Trisomy 21 (Down syndrome)	~1/700 births (**increases with maternal age**)	**Mental retardation**, craniofacial abnormalities (protruding tongue, flat nose, small ears), vision and hearing loss, broad hands with simian crease, cervical spine instability, increased space between first and second toes; increased risk of **duodenal atresia** and other GI abnormalities, **Alzheimer disease**, ALL, and **cardiac defects**; usually survive into fourth decade of life or longer
Trisomy 18	1/6,000 births (**increases with maternal age**)	Severe mental retardation, small mouth, limb abnormalities (malposition, **rocker-bottom feet**, overlapping fingers on grasp), cardiac defects, GI abnormalities; frequently fatal within first year
Trisomy 13	1/5,000 births (**increases with maternal age**)	Cleft lip and palate, cardiac defects, CNS defects, severe mental retardation, rounded nose, **polydactyly**; frequently fatal within first year

ALL, acute lymphoblastic leukemia; CNS, central nervous system; GI, gastrointestinal.

2. **Labs**
   a. Karyotyping can detect extra chromosomes, and genetic screening can detect translocations.
   b. Prenatal quadruple screen can help detect potentially affected fetuses, and amniocentesis may be used to confirm the diagnosis.
3. **Treatment**
   a. Appropriate care for associated medical conditions
   b. Special education or selective environment used to handle mental retardation
   c. Surgical correction of anatomic defects, when appropriate
   d. Genetic counseling and prenatal preparation recommended for parents
   e. Degree of mental impairment determines ability to function in society or need for constant care.

C. Deletion syndromes

1. Diseases that result from deletion of all or part of an **autosomal** chromosome (see Table 13-9)
2. Usually severe disorders because of importance of missing genetic material
3. **Labs** = high-resolution chromosome banding and fluorescence in situ hybridization techniques are useful for detecting small defects; karyotyping may detect substantial defects
4. **Treatment** = supportive care; genetic counseling recommended for parents
5. **Complications** = early mortality can result from associated abnormalities or diseases and not from deletions directly

D. Fragile X syndrome

1. X-linked chromosomal disorder associated with mental retardation in males; females may be carriers and rarely show any effects of the abnormal gene
2. End of X chromosome appears fragile and does not condense normally because of a high number of terminal CGG codon repeats.
3. **H/P** = large face with **prominent jaw** and **large ears**; mild hand and foot abnormalities, large testicles (i.e., macroorchidism); **mental retardation**, hyperactivity, possible seizures

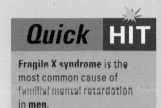

Quick HIT

Fragile X syndrome is the most common cause of familial mental retardation in **men**.

TABLE 13-9	Common Deletion Syndromes	
Syndrome	**Deletion**	**History and Physical**
Cri du chat	Entire 5p chromosome arm	**High-pitched, catlike cry**, small head, low birth weight, mental retardation; early mortality can result from failure to thrive
Wolf-Hirschhorn	4p16 to end of arm	Mental retardation, multiple **cranial abnormalities**, seizures
Prader-Willi	15q11-15q13 (deletion of **paternal** allele)	**Overeating, obesity**, decreased muscular tone in infancy, mental retardation, small hands and feet; obesity-related complications can decrease lifespan
Angelman	15q11-15q13 (deletion of **maternal** allele)	**Puppetlike movement, happy mood, unprovoked laughter**, mental retardation, seizures
Velocardiofacial	22q11	**Cleft palate**, cardiac defects, mild mental retardation, significant overbite, **speech disorders**, T-cell deficiency, hypocalcemia, association with DiGeorge syndrome; early mortality can result from associated cardiac complications or DiGeorge syndrome
Williams	7q11.23	**"Elfin facies"** (short, upturned nose; long philtrum, wide mouth), short stature, **mental retardation**, cheerful/friendly personality, **cardiac defects** (supravalvular stenosis)

MNEMONIC

Remember the differences between Prader-Willi syndrome and Angelman syndrome by the mnemonics **POP** and **MAMA**:
Prader-Willi
Overeating
Paternal
and
Maternal
Angelman
Mood (happy)
Animated movements

4. **Labs** = genetic screening detects hundreds of CGG repeats at end of X chromosome (number of repeats increases with each generation when inherited from a woman but not from a man); prenatal DNA analysis can be performed in mothers with a positive family history

5. **Treatment** = appropriate genetic counseling for parents; special education and monitoring will likely be needed by affected males

TABLE 13-10	Important Pediatric Pathologies to Remember	
Condition	**Brief Description**	**Cross-Reference Chapter**
Atrial/ventricular septal defect	Opening in septum of heart allowing shunting of blood	Chapter 1, Cardiovascular Disorders (p. 30)
Patent ductus arteriosus	Failure of ductus arteriosus to close after birth resulting in shunting of blood	Chapter 1, Cardiovascular Disorders (p. 30)
Tetralogy of Fallot	Ventricular septal defect, right ventricle hypertrophy, overriding aorta, and right ventricle outflow obstruction	Chapter 1, Cardiovascular Disorders (p. 32)
Croup	Inflammation of larynx	Chapter 2, Pulmonary Disorders (p. 53)
Epiglottitis	Infection of epiglottis, leading to airway obstruction	Chapter 2, Pulmonary Disorders (p. 53)
Respiratory distress of the newborn	Respiratory distress in premature infants caused by surfactant deficiency	Chapter 2, Pulmonary Disorders (p. 54)
Cystic fibrosis	Genetic exocrine gland disorder characterized by frequent respiratory infections and malabsorption	Chapter 2, Pulmonary Disorders (p. 55)
Pyloric stenosis	Pyloric hypertrophy causing gastric obstruction	Chapter 3, Gastrointestinal Disorders (p. 87)
Intussusception	Telescoping of bowel into adjacent bowel, resulting in obstruction	Chapter 3, Gastrointestinal Disorders (p. 88)
Wilms tumor	Malignant renal tumor in children	Chapter 4, Genitourinary Disorders (p. 108)
Cretinism	Congenital hypothyroidism, leading to poor physical and mental development	Chapter 5, Endocrine Disorders (p. 125)
Hemolytic disease of the newborn	Neonatal hemolysis caused by Rh sensitization of the mother before birth	Chapter 6, Hematology and Oncology (p. 151)
Childhood leukemias	Malignant transformation of myeloid or lymphoid cells in bloodstream and bone marrow	Chapter 6, Hematology and Oncology (p. 146)
Neural tube disorders	Failure of neural tube to close during fetal development, leading to spectrum of neurologic disorders	Chapter 8, Neurologic Disorders (p. 193)
Cerebral palsy	Neurologic injury during prenatal/perinatal insult, leading to motor deficits	Chapter 8, Neurologic Disorders (p. 194)
Retinoblastoma	Malignant tumor of retina in children	Chapter 8, Neurologic Disorders (p. 195)
Developmental dysplasia of the hip	Poor development of acetabulum in fetus, leading to congenital hip dislocation	Chapter 9, Musculoskeletal Disorders (p. 219)
Scoliosis	Noncorrecting curvature of the spine	Chapter 9, Musculoskeletal Disorders (p. 221)
Acne vulgaris	Inflammation of hair follicles and sebaceous glands common in adolescence	Chapter 10, Dermatology (p. 225)
Precocious puberty	Pubertal development beginning before anticipated age of sexual development	Chapter 11, Gynecologic and Breast Disorders (p. 240)
Primary amenorrhea	Absence of menses by time of anticipated initiation with normal secondary sexual characteristic development	Chapter 11, Gynecologic and Breast Disorders (p. 245)
Attention deficit hyperactivity disorder	Problematic inattention and hyperactivity in school-aged children	Chapter 14, Psychiatric Disorders (p. 301)

Rh, rhesus factor.

PSYCHIATRIC DISORDERS

 I. Psychotic Disorders

A. Schizophrenia

1. Severe psychosis that causes significant limitations in functional ability; typically begins in late adolescence or early adulthood
2. **Risk factors** = family history, maternal malnutrition, or illness during pregnancy; significantly higher rate in homeless and indigent patients likely secondary to their inability to function in society due to the disease
3. Diagnosis requires presence of two or more symptoms (see a–e below) for at least 1 month within a 6-month period and impaired social function for >6 months.
   a. **Delusions** (false beliefs about self or others which persist despite proof to the contrary)
   b. **Hallucinations** (sensory perception in the absence of external stimuli; e.g., hearing voices, "seeing things")
   c. **Disorganized thoughts or speech** (e.g., circumstantiality, tangentiality, loose associations, "word salad," neologisms)
   d. **Disorganized or catatonic behavior**
   e. **Negative symptoms** (e.g., social withdrawal, flat affect, avolition, apathy, anhedonia, poverty of speech, "thought blocking")
4. **Treatment**
   a. **Antipsychotics** (also known as neuroleptics) are the mainstay of therapy (see Table 14-1).
   b. Psychotic exacerbations may require hospitalization.
   c. Psychotherapy may be helpful in teaching the patient how to recognize symptoms.
5. Complications
   a. Generally poor prognosis, with gradual deterioration over several years in ability to function in society
   b. Patients with predominantly negative symptoms and/or poor support systems have a worse prognosis.

B. Other psychotic disorders

1. **Schizophreniform disorder**—psychosis characterized by at least two of the symptoms listed for schizophrenia, with a duration of at least 1 month but **fewer than 6 months**
2. **Brief psychotic disorder**—psychosis characterized by at least one of the symptoms listed for schizophrenia (except negative symptoms), with a duration of at least 1 day but **less than 1 month**
3. **Delusional disorder**—psychosis characterized by one or more delusions present for at least 1 month, but does not meet the criteria for schizophrenia; no impairment of functioning apart from the ramifications of the delusion(s)
4. **Schizoaffective disorder**—psychosis characterized by at least two of the symptoms listed for schizophrenia **concurrent with a major depressive or manic episode**; hallucinations or delusions must be present apart from the mood episode

Functional ability generally refers to a patient's ability to live independently, perform normal activities of daily living, and function as a contributing member of society.

High-potency antipsychotics have **more extrapyramidal** side effects and **fewer anticholinergic** side effects. Low-potency antipsychotics have **fewer extrapyramidal** side effects and **more anticholinergic** side effects.

Major depressive disorder (MDD) and mania may rarely cause psychosis, but the patient is never psychotic apart from the mood episode. In schizoaffective disorder, the psychosis **must** be present apart from the mood symptoms.

TABLE 14-1 Antipsychotic Medications			
Drug	**Mechanism**	**Indications**	**Adverse Effects**
Low-potency neuroleptics (chlorpromazine, thioridazine)	Block **D₂ dopamine** receptors	• Strong positive symptoms • Frequently second-line drugs for maintenance therapy	**Anticholinergic effects** (confusion, constipation, urinary retention, hypotension)
High-potency neuroleptics (fluphenazine, haloperidol, loxapine, thiothixene, trifluoperazine)	Block **D₂ dopamine** receptors	• Strong positive symptoms • **Emergency control** of psychosis or agitation • Frequently second-line drugs for maintenance therapy	**Extrapyramidal effects** (dystonia, parkinsonism, akinesia, akathisia), **tardive dyskinesia**, hyperprolactinemia, **neuroleptic malignant syndrome**, fewer anticholinergic effects
Atypical antipsychotics (aripiprazole, clozapine, olanzapine, quetiapine, risperidone, ziprasidone)	Block **dopamine** and **serotonin** receptors	• **First-line** drugs for maintenance therapy for psychotic disorders • Clozapine is the most effective antipsychotic but is reserved for refractory psychosis because of risk of agranulocytosis	Anticholinergic effects, weight gain; **clozapine** carries risk of **agranulocytosis**; fewer side effects than traditional neuroleptics

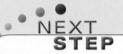

Tardive dyskinesia is a complication of antipsychotic medications characterized by **repetitive facial movements** (e.g., chewing, lip smacking) beginning **after several months** of therapy. It should be treated by stopping the offending drug if the patient's condition allows, but it may be **irreversible**.

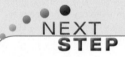

Neuroleptic malignant syndrome is:
• An uncommon complication of antipsychotic medications that starts within **days** of usage and carries a high mortality rate.
• Characterized by **high fever, muscle rigidity**, decreased consciousness, and increased blood pressure and heart rate.
• Treated by immediately **stopping** the drug and administering **dantrolene**.

Quick HIT

MDD with atypical features is the most common subtype of major depression.

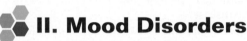

II. Mood Disorders

A. Major depressive disorder (MDD)

1. Experience of significant depression that:
   a. Lasts >2 weeks and impacts social and/or occupational function
   b. Is not attributable to drug use or medical conditions
      • Drugs that cause depressive symptoms include alcohol, benzodiazepines, antihistamines, traditional neuroleptics, glucocorticoids, and interferon-α.
      • Medical conditions that cause depressive symptoms include hypothyroidism, hyperparathyroidism, Parkinson disease, stroke, and brain tumors.
2. Following resolution, depressive episodes have a 50% chance of recurring.
3. Pathology may be due to low serotonin, norepinephrine, and dopamine activity in the central nervous system (CNS).
4. Diagnosis requires presence of **five of the following symptoms**, including either depressed mood or anhedonia (i.e., loss of interest in previously pleasurable activity) **lasting >2 weeks:**
   a. **Depressed mood**
   b. **Anhedonia**
   c. Change in sleep patterns (e.g., insomnia, hypersomnia)
   d. Feelings of guilt/worthlessness
   e. Fatigue
   f. Inability to concentrate
   g. Changes in appetite or weight
   h. Psychomotor retardation or agitation (i.e., impaired motor ability related to mental state)
   i. Thoughts about death (**suicidal ideation**)
5. Subtypes of MDD
   a. **MDD with atypical features** is major depression characterized by:
      • **Mood reactivity**
      • Hyperphagia (increased appetite and weight gain)
      • Hypersomnia
      • Psychomotor retardation ("leaden paralysis")
      • **Hypersensitivity to rejection** is common.
   b. **MDD with seasonal pattern** is depression that occurs in a regular pattern corresponding to certain seasons, usually fall and winter, due to decreased exposure to sunlight. Treat with phototherapy.

c. **MDD with peripartum onset** is depression that begins during pregnancy or within 4 weeks of delivery.

d. **MDD with psychotic features** is depression associated with delusions, hallucinations, or other psychotic symptoms.

6. **Treatment**

a. Psychotherapy (i.e., cognitive or behavioral counseling and instruction designed to provide insight into condition and modify behavior)

b. Pharmacologic therapy (may be combined with psychotherapy) (see Table 14-2)

c. Electroconvulsive therapy (ECT) can be used for refractory or severe cases to decrease frequency of major depressive episodes.

TABLE 14-2 Antidepressant Medications

Drug/Class	Mechanism	Indications	Adverse Effects
SSRIs (e.g., citalopram, escitalopram, fluoxetine, fluvoxamine, paroxetine, sertraline)	Inhibit presynaptic serotonin reuptake	**First-line** treatment for depression; anxiety	**Sexual dysfunction**, may increase risk of suicidal ideation in adolescents, risk of serotonin syndrome; require **3–4 weeks** of administration before they take effect
SNRIs (e.g., desvenlafaxine, duloxetine, venlafaxine)	Inhibit reuptake of both serotonin and norepinephrine	First-line treatment for depression with comorbid neurologic pain; second-line treatment for patients failing SSRIs	Nausea, dizziness, insomnia, sedation, sexual dysfunction, constipation, **HTN**, risk of serotonin syndrome
TCAs (e.g., amitriptyline, clomipramine, desipramine, doxepin, imipramine, nortriptyline)	Inhibit reuptake of norepinephrine	Second- or third-line treatment for depression; can be useful in patients with comorbid neurologic pain	Easy to overdose and may be **fatal at only five times therapeutic dose** (due to cardiac QT interval prolongation that causes arrhythmias), sedation, weight gain, sexual dysfunction, **anticholinergic symptoms**
MAOIs (e.g., isocarboxazid, phenelzine, selegiline, tranylcypromine)	Inhibit monoamine oxidase activity to inhibit deamination of serotonin, norepinephrine, and dopamine and increase levels of these substances	Infrequently used to treat depression due to side effect profile, dietary restrictions, and drug–drug interactions	Dry mouth, indigestion, fatigue, headache, **dizziness**; consumption of foods containing **tyramine** (cheese, aged meats, beer) can cause **hypertensive crisis**
Norepinephrine-dopamine reuptake inhibitor (bupropion)	Inhibit reuptake of dopamine and norepinephrine	Depression with **fatigue** and difficulty concentrating or comorbid ADHD; smoking cessation	Insomnia, weight loss, headache, **lowered seizure threshold**; **no sexual dysfunction**
Serotonin modulators (e.g., nefazodone, trazodone, vilazodone)	Inhibit reuptake of serotonin; and some direct actions on serotonin receptors	Depression with significant insomnia	Hypotension, nausea, **sedation**, **priapism**; seizure risk at high doses
Tetracyclic antidepressant (mirtazapine)	Block α_2-receptors and serotonin receptors to increase adrenergic neurotransmission	Depression with insomnia and/or anorexia	Dry mouth, sedation, **appetite stimulation**
St. John's wort (*Hypericum perforatum*)	Decrease reuptake of serotonin and, to a lesser extent, norepinephrine and dopamine	Used as first-line agent in Europe, but considered an **alternative therapy** in the United States	GI distress, dizziness, sedation; drug interactions common

SSRIs, selective serotonin–reuptake inhibitors; SNRIs, selective serotonin–norepinephrine reuptake inhibitors; MAOIs, monoamine oxidase inhibitors; ADHD, attention deficit hyperactivity disorder; GI, gastrointestinal; HTN, hypertension; TCAs, tricyclic antidepressants.

B. Persistent depressive disorder

1. Symptoms of **depression on more days than not** for >2 years. May include:

a. Chronic major depression

b. Chronic mild depression that does not meet the criteria for MDD

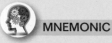

Psychiatric Disorders

2. H/P = diagnosis requires **dysphoria** (depressed mood) plus at least two other depressive symptoms for most days for >2 years
3. Treatment = pharmacotherapy with or without psychotherapy

C. Bipolar disorder

1. Cyclic episodes of **depression** and **mania** (or hypomania) that impair the patient's ability to function; patient is able to function normally between episodes

   a. **Manic episode**
   - Elevated, expansive, or irritable mood lasting at least 1 week
   - Three or more of the following symptoms: grandiosity, pressured speech, **decreased need for sleep**, flight of ideas, **easy distractibility, increased goal-oriented activity**, increased risky pleasurable activity
   - Episodes cause **significant impairment** of ability to function.

   b. **Hypomanic episode**
   - Elevated, expansive, or irritable mood lasting at least 4 days
   - Three or more of the symptoms of mania (see above)
   - Episode does not cause significant impairment of ability to function.

2. Types

   a. Bipolar I: at least **one manic episode**; episodes of major depressive are common but are not required for the diagnosis
   b. Bipolar II: at least **one hypomanic episode** and at least **one major depressive episode**

3. When present, depressive episodes are identical to those seen with MDD.

4. **Treatment**

   a. Patients should be hospitalized if psychotic or judged to be a risk to themselves or others until they can be stabilized.
   b. **Mood stabilizers** (e.g., lithium, valproate, lamotrigine, carbamazepine), which may be used alone or in combination with **atypical antipsychotics** (e.g., aripiprazole, quetiapine, risperidone), are used to control and prevent manic and hypomanic episodes and to treat depression.
   c. Lithium is frequently the first-line drug for long-term treatment of mania.
   - Mechanism is unknown but likely involves inositol triphosphate activity.
   - Adverse effects include tremor, nephrogenic diabetes insipidus, hypothyroidism, teratogenesis (Ebstein anomaly), renal insufficiency, weight gain.

D. Cyclothymic disorder

1. Rapid cycling of mild manic symptoms and mild depression lasting >2 years without a period of normal mood >2 months
2. Mood symptoms impair the ability to function, but criteria for major depression, mania, or hypomania are not met.
3. Treatment = psychotherapy or mood stabilizers

III. Anxiety Disorders

A. Panic disorder

1. Experience of recurrent, spontaneous panic attacks with associated fear that these episodes will occur; typically begins in late adolescence
2. H/P

   a. **Recurrent, unexpected panic attacks** that last up to 30 minutes and consist of extreme anxiety, feelings of impending danger, chest pain, shortness of breath, palpitations, diaphoresis, nausea, dizziness, paresthesias, chills or hot flashes, fear of losing control, or fear of dying.
   b. Diagnosis requires a history of recurrent episodes plus a **persistent fear that attacks will happen again**, or maladaptive change of behavior designed to avoid the attacks.

3. Treatment

   a. Cognitive behavioral therapy may help alleviate fear between attacks and decrease panic attack occurrence.

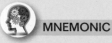
MNEMONIC

Remember the characteristics of manic episodes by the mnemonic **DIG FAST:**
- **D**istractibility
- **I**nsomnia
- **G**randiosity
- **F**light of ideas
- **A**ctivity (goal-oriented)
- **P**ressured **S**peech
- **T**aking risks/**T**houghtlessness

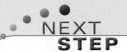
NEXT STEP

A history of **mania** must be ruled out by a thorough history in a patient suspected of having MDD before antidepressants are prescribed. **Antidepressants** given to a patient with **bipolar disorder** who is **not** taking mood stabilizers can induce a **manic episode.**

b. Selective serotonin–reuptake inhibitors (SSRIs) and serotonin–norepinephrine reuptake inhibitors (SNRIs) are used for long-term therapy in patients with frequent attacks.

c. Benzodiazepines can be used to break acute attacks (see Table 14-3).

TABLE 14-3	**Anxiolytic Medications**		
Drug	**Mechanism**	**Indications**	**Adverse Effects**
Benzodiazepines (e.g., alprazolam, clonazepam, diazepam, lorazepam)	Increase GABA inhibition of neuronal firing	Alprazolam has a rapid onset and short half-life and is particularly useful to break panic attacks; clonazepam and diazepam are more useful for prolonged therapy	Sedation, confusion; withdrawal symptoms may include restlessness, confusion, insomnia (especially with frequent use), and seizures
Buspirone	Unclear, but related to serotonin and dopamine receptors	Anxiety disorders in which abuse or sedation is a concern	Headaches, dizziness, nausea

GABA, γ-aminobutyric acid.

B. Generalized anxiety disorder

1. Excessive, **persistent** anxiety and worry that occur more days than not for >6 months and impairs ability to function

2. **Epidemiology** = women twice as likely affected than men. Typically begins in early adulthood.

3. **H/P**

   a. Diagnosis requires excessive anxiety for most days, impairment of ability to function, and three of the symptoms listed below for >6 months.

   b. Symptoms include restlessness or feeling "on edge," fatigue, inability to concentrate, irritability, muscle tension, sleep disturbance.

4. **Treatment** = cognitive behavioral therapy; SSRIs or SNRIs; buspirone is considered safer for long-term therapy than benzodiazepines (see Table 14-3) because of the chronic nature of the anxiety

C. Social anxiety disorder

1. Excessive fear or anxiety about **social situations** in which the individual is exposed to scrutiny by others, which is out of proportion to the actual threat that the social situation poses

2. **H/P** = social situations (e.g., performances, conversations) cause anxiety that can be mild or severe (i.e., panic attacks); patients avoid these situations and have a persistent fear of being embarrassed

3. **Treatment**

   a. Cognitive behavioral therapy

   b. β-Blockers can be used in mild cases to prevent tachycardia when engaging in an anxiety-provoking situation.

   c. SSRIs frequently are effective at reducing anxiety and permitting social interactions.

   d. Benzodiazepines are an alternative option for reducing acute anxiety.

D. Specific phobia

1. Fear of a **particular object, activity**, or **situation** that causes the patient to avoid feared subject; typically begins in childhood

2. **H/P** = encountering feared subject incites panic attack, the patient makes great effort to avoid feared subject and realizes that behavior is irrational; some patients may experience vasovagal response (i.e., fainting) during episodes

3. **Treatment** = psychotherapy involving systematic desensitization through repeated exposure, relaxation techniques, hypnosis, or insight modification

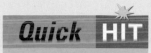

Quick HIT

It is **very difficult** to commit suicide using an overdose of benzodiazepines because their lethal dose is >1,000 times the therapeutic dose. **Flumazenil** is a benzodiazepine antagonist that can reverse the effects of an overdose.

Psychiatric Disorders

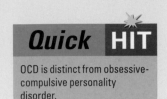

 IV. Obsessive-Compulsive and Related Disorders

A. Obsessive-compulsive disorder (OCD)

1. Presence of obsessions and/or compulsions which cause impairment in function and affect daily life
   a. **Obsessions** are recurrent, persistent thoughts or urges that are intrusive and unwanted and that cause anxiety or distress.
   b. **Compulsions** are repetitive, ritualized behaviors (e.g., hand-washing) or mental acts (e.g., reciting specific words, counting) that are aimed at reducing or preventing the anxiety or distress caused by obsessive thoughts.
2. H/P
   a. Diagnosis requires presence of obsessions or compulsions that significantly affect daily life.
   b. Stressful events can exacerbate compulsive behaviors.
   c. Patients are aware of compulsive behaviors but feel unable to control them.
3. **Treatment** = cognitive behavioral therapy and pharmacologic therapy (SSRIs, SNRIs) help limit and control behavior

B. Body dysmorphic disorder

1. Preoccupation with a perceived defect in physical appearance that limits ability to function; typically begins in adolescence
2. Patient performs repetitive behaviors (e.g., mirror checking, excessive grooming) related to the concerns about his or her appearance.
3. H/P = patient imagines physical defect in distinct body region, frequently presents to dermatologist or plastic surgeon to "improve" defect, and continues to imagine defect following treatment
4. **Treatment**
   a. Psychotherapy addressing self-perception
   b. Antidepressants may help in refractory cases.
   c. Avoid performing needless surgery.

C. Hoarding disorder

1. Patient has difficulty discarding or parting with possessions, even if they have no real value; discarding possessions results in significant distress.
2. Accumulation of possessions results in excessive clutter and potentially dangerous/unhealthy living conditions.
3. **Treatment** = cognitive behavioral therapy, SSRIs

 V. Stress- and Trauma-Related Disorders

A. Adjustment disorder

1. Behavioral and emotional symptoms in response to a specific **stressful event or situation** (e.g., death in family, assault, divorce), occurring within 3 months of the event and causing **significant impairment** of ability to function
2. H/P
   a. **Distress out of proportion** of what is expected following a stressful event, inability to concentrate, **self-isolation**, change in sleep patterns, change in appetite
   b. May be characterized as adjustment disorder with depressed mood, with anxiety, with mixed anxiety and depressed mood, with disturbance of conduct, etc.
   c. Symptoms **begin within 3 months** of stressful event and **end 6 months after** end of stressor.
3. **Treatment** = cognitive behavioral therapy; antidepressants or anxiolytics can be used if psychotherapy alone is unable to effect normal daily functioning

B. Posttraumatic stress disorder (PTSD)

1. Complex syndrome of symptoms that occurs following **psychological trauma** (exposure to actual or threatened death, serious injury, or sexual violation)
   a. The event can be directly experienced by the patient, witnessed in person, or experienced by a close family member or friend.
   b. Symptoms typically begin within a few months of the event, and must last **at least 1 month.**
2. **H/P**
   a. Intrusion symptoms in which the individual reexperiences the traumatic event (e.g., **intrusive memories; recurrent, distressing dreams; flashbacks;** psychological distress; or physiological reactions to internal or external cues that resemble the event)
   b. **Avoidance** of activities or settings associated with the event
   c. **Persistent negative alterations in cognition or mood** associated with the event (e.g., amnesia of certain aspects of the event, exaggerated negative beliefs about self or others, blaming self for the event, anhedonia, feelings of **detachment**, increased state of arousal, survivor guilt, social withdrawal)
3. **Treatment** = cognitive behavioral therapy, alone or in combination with SSRI or SNRI; atypical antipsychotics may be beneficial for symptoms refractory to SSRIs or SNRIs.

VI. Somatic Symptom and Related Disorders

A. Conversion disorder

1. Development of **sensory** or **voluntary motor deficits** without a recognized medical or neurologic condition to cause the deficits
2. **H/P** = symptoms may include weakness/paralysis, tremor, dystonia, gait disturbance, dysphagia, dysphonia/dysarthria, seizures, numbness/paresthesias, visual or hearing disturbance, or any combination thereof.
3. **Treatment** = Simply presenting the diagnosis and educating the patient about the psychogenic nature of the deficit may lead to spontaneous resolution of symptoms in 40% to 50% of cases; second-line treatments include cognitive behavioral therapy and physical therapy; SSRIs and SNRIs are sometimes helpful

B. Somatic symptom disorder

1. One or more somatic symptoms which may or may not be due to a recognized medical condition, but which are distressing or disruptively to daily life; accompanied by **anxiety about health** and persistent worry about the seriousness of the symptoms
2. While the specific symptoms may change over time, the worry and impaired psychosocial functioning are persistent, generally lasts >6 months.
3. **H/P** = somatic symptoms may include:
   a. Pain symptoms
   b. Sexual symptoms (e.g., erectile dysfunction, decreased libido)
   c. Neurologic symptoms
   d. Gastrointestinal symptoms (e.g., vomiting, diarrhea)
4. **Treatment** = tricyclic antidepressants (TCAs) and SSRIs are beneficial, as is cognitive behavioral therapy

C. Illness anxiety disorder

1. **Preoccupation with having or acquiring a serious illness** in the **absence of significant somatic symptoms,** accompanied by:
   a. A high level of anxiety about health
   b. Performance of excessive health-related behaviors (such as repeatedly checking for evidence of a serious illness)
2. Treatment
   a. Regular physician visits help to alleviate fears.
   b. Cognitive behavioral therapy and SSRIs are beneficial.

D. Factitious disorder (Münchausen syndrome)

1. Falsification of physical or psychological signs or symptoms of a disease or injury in the absence of obvious reward or clear benefit to the patient

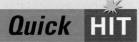

Malingering is the falsification of disease in order to obtain some benefit or reward, such as being excused from work or school, obtaining narcotics, etc.

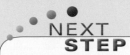

NEXT
STEP

Münchausen syndrome *by proxy* is a disorder in which **parents** try to make their **children** appear to have a certain disease. It is considered **child abuse** and must be reported to the appropriate authorities.

2. H/P
   a. Patient reports symptoms or signs of a given disease and attempts to induce disease process (e.g., self-injections of insulin or excrement, attempts to become infected by a pathogen, induction of vomiting/diarrhea, etc.).
   b. Patient may deny intentional production of symptoms; may wander from one physician to another
3. Treatment
   a. Patient denial makes treatment difficult.
   b. No unnecessary therapies should be administered.
   c. Attempt to limit medical care to one physician and one hospital.
   d. If patient is willing, psychotherapy may be beneficial.

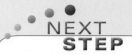

NEXT STEP

Patients with anorexia nervosa should be screened for **depression**, and SSRIs should be included in treatment if depression is diagnosed.

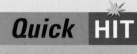

Anorexia nervosa carries a 6% 10-year mortality rate caused by disease complications or suicide.

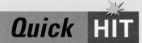

Refeeding syndrome results from the sudden shift from fat to carbohydrate metabolism in severe anorexics who resume eating and is characterized by **hypophosphatemia, cardiovascular collapse, rhabdomyolysis, confusion,** and **seizures**.

VII. Eating Disorders

A. Anorexia nervosa
1. Eating disorder characterized by:
   a. **Distorted body image** (patients believe that they are overweight)
   b. Intense **fear of gaining weight**
   c. **Reduced caloric intake** relative to energy requirements and **refusal to maintain a normal body weight**; may involve fasting, excessive exercise, purging, etc.
2. **Risk factors** = adolescence, high socioeconomic status; 90% of cases are women
3. H/P = low body weight (generally <85% ideal body weight), fixation on prevention of weight gain, severe body image disturbance, amenorrhea, cold intolerance, hypothermia, dry skin, lanugo hair growth (i.e., fine, short hair similar to that in the newborn), bradycardia. Osteoporosis may be present. Patients often have co-morbid depression.
4. **Treatment**
   a. Inpatient treatment is frequently required to aid in weight gain.
   b. Psychotherapy that focuses on body image, weight gain; sufficient caloric intake is needed to maintain long-term control.
   c. Pharmacologic therapy has not been proved beneficial.
5. **Complications** = electrolyte abnormalities, arrhythmias (especially ventricular types), refeeding syndrome

B. Bulimia nervosa
1. Eating disorder characterized by:
   a. **Binge eating** (inappropriate high caloric intake within a short period of time, which the patient often perceives as uncontrollable)
   b. **Inappropriate compensatory behaviors** (e.g., purging, strict caloric restriction, excessive exercise) following binges, to prevent weight gain
   c. **Unhealthy preoccupation with weight and body shape**; these patients generally maintain a normal (not low) body weight
2. H/P
   a. Bingeing–compensation episodes occur at least once a week for >3 months.
   b. Physical examination may reveal dental enamel erosion (from repeated vomiting), scars on hands (from inducing vomiting), parotid enlargement/inflammation (which may elevate serum amylase), and oligomenorrhea.
3. **Treatment** = nutritional counseling; psychotherapy (cognitive behavioral therapy) directed at body image and reduction of bingeing–compensation cycles; SSRIs or TCAs help in behavior modification

C. Binge eating disorder
1. Eating disorder characterized by uncontrollable **episodes of binge eating** without inappropriate compensatory behaviors
   a. On average, binges occur at least once a week for >3 months.
   b. Patients are often overweight or obese due to excessive caloric intake.
2. **Treatment** = psychotherapy (cognitive behavioral therapy and intrapersonal therapy) is first line and is generally more effective than pharmacotherapy; SSRIs may be used.

VIII. Personality Disorders

A. Persistent pattern of inner experience and behavior that **deviates significantly from cultural norms**

1. Manifested through perception of others, affect, interpersonal relationships, and impulse control
2. Is **persistent** and **inflexible** despite situation
3. Leads to impaired ability to function
4. Typically begins in late adolescence
5. Is not attributable to drug use, medical condition, or other psychiatric disorder

B. Clusters (see Table 14-4)

1. Classification system of personality disorders
   a. Cluster A: odd or eccentric ("weird")
   b. Cluster B: dramatic or emotional ("wild")
   c. Cluster C: anxious or fearful ("wimpy or worried")
2. Personality disorders not meeting criteria for any of the defined variants are classified as "personality disorder not otherwise specified (NOS)."

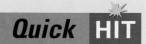

Quick HIT

A patient who exhibits mild signs of a personality disorder but is able to function normally in society is said to have a **personality trait** and may not require treatment.

TABLE 14-4 Personality Disorders

Disorder	Characteristics	Treatment
Cluster A		
Paranoid	Persistent distrust and suspicion of others, others' actions consistently interpreted as harmful or deceptive, reluctant to share information, frequent misinterpretation of comments, frequent angry reactions, common suspicions of partner fidelity	Supportive, nonjudgmental psychotherapy, low-dose antipsychotics
Schizoid	Inability to form close relationships, social detachment, emotionally restricted, anhedonia, flat affect, lack of sexual interests	Antipsychotics initially to resolve behavior, supportive psychotherapy focusing on achieving comfortable interactions with others
Schizotypal	Paranoia, ideas of reference, eccentric and inappropriate behavior, social anxiety, disorganized speech, odd beliefs	Supportive psychotherapy focusing on recognition of reality, low-dose antipsychotics or anxiolytics
Cluster B		
Antisocial	Aggressive behavior toward people and animals, destruction of property, illegal activity, pathologic lying, irritability, risk-taking behavior, lack of responsibility, lack of remorse for actions; patient >18 yr of age, history of conduct disorder prior to 15 yr of age; more common in men	Structured environment, psychotherapy with defined limit-setting may be helpful in controlling behavior
Borderline	Unstable relationships, feelings of emptiness, fear of abandonment, poor self-esteem, impulsivity, mood lability, suicidal ideation, inappropriate irritability, paranoia, splitting (seeing others as either all good or all bad); much more common in women	Extensive psychotherapy using multiple techniques combined with low-dose antipsychotics, SSRIs, or mood stabilizers
Histrionic	Attention-seeking, inappropriate seductive or theatrical behavior, emotional lability, shallow relationships, dramatic speech, uses appearance to draw attention to self, easily influenced by others, believes relationships more intimate than they are	Long-term psychotherapy focusing on relationship development and limit-setting
Narcissistic	Grandiosity, fantasies of success, manipulation of others, expectation of admiration, arrogance, sense of entitlement, believes self to be "special," lacks empathy, envious of others	Psychotherapy focusing on acceptance of shortcomings
Cluster C		
Avoidant	Fear of criticism and embarrassment, social withdrawal, fear of intimacy, poor self-esteem, reluctance to try new activities, preoccupied by fear of rejection, inhibited by feelings of inadequacy	Psychotherapy (initially individualized, then group therapy later) focusing on self-confidence combined with antidepressants or anxiolytics
Dependent	Difficulty making decisions, fear of responsibility, difficulty expressing disagreement, lack of confidence in judgment, need for others' support, fear of being alone, requires constant close relationships	Psychotherapy focusing on developing social skills and development of decisive behavior
Obsessive-compulsive	Preoccupied with details, perfectionistic, excessively devoted to work, inflexible in beliefs, miserly, difficulty working with others, hoarding of worthless objects, stubbornness	Psychotherapy focusing on accepting alternative ideas and working with others

SSRIs, selective serotonin–reuptake inhibitors.

Psychiatric Disorders

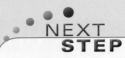

NEXT STEP

Use the **CAGE** questionnaire to screen for alcohol abuse. More than one "yes" response to any of these conditions should raise suspicion for excessive use:
- Desire to **Cut down** on usage
- **Annoyance** over others' suggestions to stop usage
- **Guilt** over usage
- Drug use on waking (i.e., **Eye-opener**)

 # IX. Substance Abuse

A. **Substance use disorder:** problematic substance (e.g., alcohol, drug) use that results in significant functional impairment or stress; formerly labeled "substance abuse" or "substance dependence"; symptoms may include:
1. Consumption of larger amounts of the substance than intended
2. Significant energy spent obtaining, using, or recovering from the substance
3. Tolerance
4. Cravings
5. Persistent desire or unsuccessful attempts to quit or cut down on substance use

B. **Intoxication:** reversible CNS effect of a substance following usage (see Table 14-5)

C. **Physical dependence:** physical adaptation to repetitive substance use in which abrupt cessation or antagonist use causes a withdrawal syndrome (see Table 14-5)

D. **Psychological dependence:** perceived need for a given substance because of its associated positive effects or because of fear of effects from lack of use

E. Patients who successfully change habits or behaviors frequently progress through the following **stages of change:**
1. **Precontemplation**—no acknowledgment that a problem exists or that a change needs to be made (i.e., denial)
2. **Contemplation**—admitting the need to change at some unspecified point in the future, but no immediate plans for change
3. **Preparation**—making concrete plans to deal with problem
4. **Action**—implementing changes
5. **Maintenance**—making sure changes are continued

 # X. Pediatric Psychiatric Disorders

A. Autism spectrum disorder
1. Severe, persistent impairment in **social communication and interpersonal interactions** as well as restricted, **repetitive patterns of behavior and interests**; generally presents in early childhood
2. H/P
   a. **Impaired social interactions:** impaired use of nonverbal behaviors, failure to develop peer relationships, failure to seek social interaction, lack of social reciprocity
   b. **Impaired communication:** developmental language delays, poor initiation or sustenance of conversation, repetitive language, poor eye contact, lack of imaginative or imitative play for age
   c. **Restricted behavior:** inflexible routines, preoccupation with a restricted pattern of interest, repetitive motor mannerisms, preoccupation with parts of objects
3. **Treatment**
   a. Behavior, speech, and social psychotherapy with peers and family may help improve social interaction.
   b. Aggressive, irritable behavior can be treated with atypical antipsychotics.
   c. Supervised environment may be required long term.

TABLE 14-5	Characteristics of Substance Abuse

Substance	Intoxication	Withdrawal	Complications of Chronic Use	Treatment
Alcohol	**Decreased inhibition**, slurred speech, **impaired coordination**, inattentiveness, decreased consciousness, retrograde amnesia	Diaphoresis, **tachycardia**, anxiety, nausea, vomiting, tremor, **delirium tremens** (seizures, delirium), tactile hallucinations	**Malnutrition** (vitamin B$_{12}$, thiamine), encephalopathy (Wernicke-Korsakoff), **accidents**, suicide, **cirrhosis**, GI bleeding, aspiration pneumonia; higher incidence of abuse in patients with other psychiatric disorders	Supplemental nutrition; supportive psychotherapy or **group counseling**; naltrexone decreases cravings; disulfiram causes unpleasant nausea and vomiting if taken before alcohol consumption; benzodiazepines prevent delirium tremens during withdrawal
Amphetamines (methamphetamine, methylphenidate, etc.)	**Hyperactivity**, psychomotor agitation, **pupillary dilation**, tachycardia, HTN, psychosis	Anxiety, depression, increased appetite, fatigue	Psychosis, depression, fatigue, Parkinsonian symptoms	Rehabilitative counseling, antipsychotics, benzodiazepines
Benzodiazepines (alprazolam, etc.)	Sedation, amnesia, slurred speech, decreased coordination	Anxiety, insomnia, tremor, **seizures**	Memory loss	Rehabilitative counseling, anticonvulsants
Caffeine	**Insomnia**, restlessness, tremor, anxiety, tachycardia	Headaches, fatigue, inattentiveness	GI irritation, fatigue, inattentiveness	Gradual reduction in usage
Cocaine	**Euphoria**, tachycardia, psychomotor agitation, pupillary dilation, hypertension, paranoia, **grandiosity**	Sedation, **depression**, psychomotor retardation, fatigue, anhedonia	Arrhythmias, **sudden cardiac death**, stroke, suicidal ideation, inattentiveness	Reduction of hypertension, antipsychotics, benzodiazepines, rehabilitative counseling
Hallucinogens (LSD, mescaline, ketamine)	**Hallucinations**, delusions, anxiety, paranoia, tachycardia, pupillary dilation, tremors	Minimal	Psychosis, "flashbacks"	Remove patient from dangerous environment until intoxication resolves, antipsychotics
Marijuana	**Euphoria**, paranoia, psychomotor retardation, impaired judgment, increased appetite, **conjunctival injection**, dry mouth	Irritability, depression, insomnia, nausea, tremor	**Amotivational syndrome**, infertility, depression, psychosis	Rehabilitative counseling, antipsychotics
Nicotine (and other substances found in tobacco and cigarettes)	Restlessness, nausea, vomiting, abdominal pain	Insomnia, weight gain, irritability, inability to concentrate, nervousness, headaches	Smoking (but not necessarily nicotine) increases the risk of various **cancers, COPD**, respiratory infections, atherosclerosis	Counseling, transdermal (patch) or mucosal (gum) **nicotine** to reduce cravings for cigarettes, hypnosis, **varenicline**, bupropion
Opioids	**Euphoria**, slurred speech, **pupillary constriction**, inattentiveness, decreased consciousness, respiratory depression	Depression, anxiety, **stomach cramps, nausea, vomiting**, diarrhea, myalgias	Constipation, increased risk of **bloodborne infection** with IV drug use	**Methadone therapy**; inpatient rehabilitative counseling; naltrexone may prevent euphoria with use; naloxone is opioid antagonist used for acute overdose with significant respiratory depression
Phencyclidine (PCP)	Euphoria, impulsiveness, **aggressive behavior, nystagmus (vertical** and horizontal), hyperreflexia	**Sudden violent behavior**, variable levels of consciousness	Psychosis, memory deficits, impaired cognitive function, inability to retrieve words	Isolated containment until after resolution of intoxication, benzodiazepines, antipsychotics, ascorbic acid

COPD, chronic obstructive pulmonary disease; GI, gastrointestinal; HTN, hypertension; IV, intravenous; LSD, lysergic acid diethylamide.

Psychiatric Disorders

Psychiatric Disorders

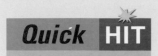

Most children with ADHD continue to the diagnostic criteria for ADHD in adulthood.

B. Attention deficit hyperactivity disorder (ADHD)

1. Disorder of **inattention** and **hyperactivity** in school-aged children that causes problems in multiple settings (e.g., both at home and at school)
2. **Risk factors** = two to four times more common in males than females
3. H/P
   a. **Inattention: decreased attention span, difficulty following instructions**, carelessness in tasks, easily losing items, forgetfulness, poor listening, easy distractibility, difficulty organizing activity, avoidance of tasks requiring prolonged focus
   b. **Hyperactivity and impulsivity**: fidgetiness, inability to remain seated at times when prolonged sitting is required, constantly "on the go," excessive talking, difficulty waiting turn to speak, interrupts others, answers questions before they are completed
   c. Diagnosis requires child to have **six** inattention symptoms **or six** hyperactivity or impulsivity symptoms that **limit ability to function** in social, educational, or organized settings. Several symptoms must have been evident before 12 years of age.
4. Treatment
   a. Behavioral therapy is often recommended first line, and may be combined with pharmacotherapy.
   b. Stimulants (e.g., methylphenidate, dexmethylphenidate, amphetamine, dextroamphetamine) or atomoxetine improve ability to focus and control behavior.
   c. α_2-Adrenergic agonists and TCAs may be used in refractory cases.
   d. Adjustments may need to be made in selecting an educational setting to optimize ability to learn and participate.

C. Tourette syndrome

1. Chronic tic disorder beginning in childhood; associated with ADHD and OCD
2. **H/P** = **multiple motor** (e.g., blinking, twitching, etc.) and **vocal** (e.g., sounds, words) tics that occur every day and worsen with stress; location, frequency, and severity of tics change over time; diagnosis requires presence of tics for >1 year and beginning before patient is 18 years of age
3. **Treatment** = behavioral therapy may reduce tics; low-dose fluphenazine, pimozide, or tetrabenazine may reduce tic occurrence; SSRIs and α_2-agonists are useful in treating comorbid behavioral disorders

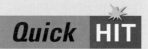

Coprolalia (vocal **tics** of repeated obscenities) is seen only in a **minority (40%)** of cases of Tourette syndrome.

D. Conduct disorder

1. Repetitive disruptive and antisocial behavior that violates others' rights and social norms
   a. May have onset during either childhood or adolescence
   b. Individuals over 18 years of age are more likely to meet criteria for antisocial personality disorder.
2. **H/P** = **aggressive behavior** toward people or animals, **destruction of property, deceitfulness** or theft, **violation of serious rules**
3. **Treatment** = psychotherapy involving family and parent management training; psychostimulants are helpful when comorbid ADHD is diagnosed; mood stabilizers may be used in severe cases

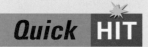

Oppositional defiant disorder is similar to conduct disorder in that patients exhibit aggressive, argumentative, or vindictive behavior, but illegal and destructive behavior does not occur.

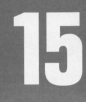

EPIDEMIOLOGY AND ETHICS

 I. Research Studies

A. Study requirements

1. Subjects in a study must be **representative of the population** that the study seeks to examine.
2. The study must contain a **sufficient number of subjects** to make it statistically significant.
3. Subjects must give **informed consent**, except under special circumstances approved by an institutional review board (IRB) (e.g., trauma patients).

TABLE 15-1	Study Designs Used in Clinical Research			
Study Type	**Description**	**Conclusions**	**Advantages**	**Disadvantages**
Case series	• Report of characteristics of a disease by examining multiple cases	Hypothesis for risk factors	• May be easy to complete • Provides insight into poorly understood conditions	Cannot be used to test hypotheses
Cross-sectional survey	• **Survey** of large number of people at one time to assess exposure and disease prevalence	Hypothesis for risk factors; disease prevalence	• Can be used as estimate for disease **prevalence** following exposure	Cannot be used to test hypotheses
Case-control study	• Retrospective comparison of patients with a **disease** with healthy controls; frequency of certain exposures in both groups is considered	**Odds ratio**	• Can examine **rare diseases** or those with **long course** in short amount of time • Can study multiple types of exposure • May examine small group size	Susceptible to **recall** and **selection bias**; cannot determine disease incidence
Cohort study	• Examines a group of subjects **exposed** to a given situation or factor • Can be **prospective** (exposed group identified and followed over time) or **retrospective** (examines exposed group in whom disease has already occurred)	**Relative risk**	• Able to examine **rare exposures** • Can study multiple effects of exposure	May be costly and time consuming; difficult to study rare diseases
Randomized clinical trial	• **Prospective comparison** of **experimental** treatment with **placebo** controls and **existing** therapies • **Double-blinded** to avoid bias • Patients **randomized** into study groups	Effectiveness of experimental treatment compared with controls and existing therapies	• **Gold standard** for testing therapies • Can be controlled for several confounders	Often **costly** and **time consuming**; patients may not be willing to undergo randomization
Meta-analysis	• **Pooling** of multiple studies examining a given disease or exposure	Depends on original study type	• Larger study size • Can resolve conflicts in literature	Unable to eliminate limiting factors in original studies

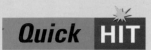

TABLE 15-2	Types of Bias in Clinical Studies	
Types of Bias	**Description**	**Consequences**
Enrollment (selection)	**Nonrandom** assignment of subjects to study groups	Results of study not applicable to general population
Investigator	Subjective interpretation of data by **investigator** deviates toward "desired" conclusions	Results of study incorrectly resemble proposed hypothesis
Lead-time	Screening test provides **earlier diagnosis** in studied group compared with controls but has **no effect on time of survival**	Time from diagnosis to outcome gives the false appearance of increased time of survival; time from disease occurrence to outcome actually remains the same regardless of screening
Length	Screening test **detects** several **slowly** progressive cases of a disease and **misses rapidly** progressive cases	Effectiveness of screening test is overstated
Observational	Subjects may respond to subjective questions in a different way than normal because **awareness** of the study changes their perception of the examined issue	Effectiveness of therapy is not accurately depicted by study group
Publication	Studies that show a difference between groups are **more likely to be published** than studies that do not show a difference	Data available for meta-analyses may not include studies that support the null hypothesis
Recall	Errors of memory within subjects because of **prior confounding experiences**	Patients with negative experiences are more likely to recall negative details
Self-selection	Patients with a certain **medical history** may be more likely to participate in a study related to their condition	Subjects are not representative of the general population and introduce confounding variables

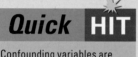

4. Proper **controls** should be included in studies that examine the efficacy of a given treatment.
5. The interests of the patient must take priority over the interests of the study (study must be approved by IRB), and researchers must follow data to determine if a study carries any risk to the subjects at any point during its course.
6. Subject confidentiality must be maintained, and subjects must consent to the release of personal information.

B. Study designs (*see Table 15-1*)

C. Bias (*see Table 15-2*)

 II. Biostatistics

A. Rates of disease
 1. Incidence
    a. Number of new cases that occurs at a given time within a population (i.e., likelihood of developing that condition in that period of time)
    b. Incidence =

$$\frac{(\text{\# of new cases of a disease in a given time})}{(\text{total population at risk})}$$

2. **Prevalence**
   a. Number of individuals with a certain condition at a given time
   b. Prevalence =

$$\frac{(\text{\# of existing cases of a disease})}{(\text{total population})}$$

3. **Case fatality rate**
   a. Percentage of people with a given disease who die within a certain amount of time
   b. Fatality rate =

$$\frac{(\text{people who die from a disease in a given time})}{(\text{\# of cases of disease during a given time})}$$

B. Risk of disease

1. **Relative risk (RR)**
   a. Probability of getting a disease in a group exposed to a specific risk factor compared to the probability of getting that disease in an unexposed group
   b. RR =

$$\frac{(\text{probability of disease in exposed population})}{(\text{probability of disease in unexposed population})} = \frac{A/(A+B)}{C/(C+D)}$$

(see Table 15-3)

   c. RR value
      (1) >1 suggests a **positive** relationship between exposure and disease
      (2) <1 suggests a **negative** relationship between exposure and disease
      (3) =1 suggests **no** relationship between exposure and disease

2. **Odds ratio (OR)**
   a. Odds of exposure among patients with a disease compared with odds of exposure among patients without a disease
   b. Estimate of relative risk if prevalence is low
   c. OR =

$$\frac{A/C}{B/D} = \frac{A \times D}{B \times C} = \frac{A/B}{C/D} \quad (\text{see Table 15-3})$$

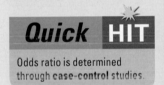

Quick HIT

Relative risk is determined through **cohort** studies.

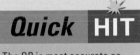

Quick HIT

Odds ratio is determined through **case-control** studies.

Quick HIT

The OR is most accurate as an estimate of RR in cases of **rare diseases**.

Epidemiology and Ethics

TABLE 15-3 Calculation of Disease Risk		Disease	
		Yes	**No**
Exposure	Yes	**A**	**B**
	No	**C**	**D**

Relative risk (RR) = $\dfrac{A/(A+B)}{C/(C+D)}$; **Odds ratio (OR)** = $\dfrac{A/C}{B/D} = \dfrac{A \times D}{B \times C} = \dfrac{A/B}{C/D}$

3. **Attributable risk (AR)**
   a. Difference in rates of disease between exposed and unexposed populations
   b. AR =
   (rate of disease in exposed population) – (rate of disease in unexposed population)

4. **Absolute risk reduction (ARR)**
   a. Difference in rate of disease when treated with a specific intervention
   b. ARR = (rate of disease in control group) – (rate of disease in intervention group)

5. **Number needed to treat (NNT)**
   a. Number of patients that have to be treated in order to prevent one negative outcome
   b. NNT = 1/ARR

C. Statistics of diagnostic tests

1. **Sensitivity**
   a. Probability that a screening test will be **positive** in **patients with a disease**
   b. Sensitivity =

   $$\frac{A}{A+C} \text{ (see Table 15-4)}$$

   c. Most acceptable screening tests are typically >80% sensitive.
   d. **False-negative findings** occur in patients with a disease and a negative test; approximated by (1 – sensitivity).

2. **Specificity**
   a. Probability that a test will be **negative** in **patients without a disease**
   b. Specificity =

   $$\frac{D}{B+D} \text{ (see Table 15-4)}$$

   c. Most acceptable confirmatory tests are typically >85% specific.
   d. **False-positive findings** occur in patients without a disease and a positive test; approximated by (1 – specificity).

3. **Positive predictive value (PPV)**
   a. Probability that a patient with a positive test has a disease
   b. PPV =

   $$\frac{A}{A+B} \text{ (see Table 15-4)}$$

4. **Negative predictive value (NPV)**
   a. Probability that a patient with a negative test does not have a disease
   b. NPV =

   $$\frac{D}{C+D} \text{ (see Table 15-4)}$$

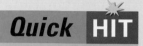

Quick HIT

Screening tests seek reliable detection of a disease in a patient without incorrectly diagnosing disease in people without the disease (ideally **both high sensitivity and high specificity**).

Quick HIT

Confirmatory tests are used to **validate** that a patient with a positive test truly has a disease.

Quick HIT

A disease with a
- **high** prevalence will be associated with a high **positive** predictive value in a screening test.
- **low** prevalence will be associated with a high **negative** predictive value in a screening test.

Epidemiology and Ethics

TABLE 15-4	Analysis of Diagnostic Tests		
		Disease	
		Yes	**No**
Test	Positive	**A**	**B**
	Negative	**C**	**D**

Sensitivity = $\frac{A}{A+C}$; Specificity = $\frac{D}{B+D}$; Positive predictive value (PPV) = $\frac{A}{A+B}$;

Negative predictive value (NPV) = $\frac{D}{C+D}$

5. **Likelihood ratios**
   a. Odds that a person with a disease will test positive compared to the odds that a nondiseased person will test positive (positive likelihood ratio) or odds that a nondiseased person will test negative compared with the odds that a diseased person will test negative (negative likelihood ratio)
   b. Measures performance of diagnostic tests while eliminating dependence on disease prevalence
   c. Positive likelihood ratio (PLR) =

   $$\frac{\text{(sensitivity)}}{\text{(1 – specificity)}}$$

d. Negative likelihood ratio (NLR) =

$$\frac{(1 - \text{sensitivity})}{(\text{specificity})}$$

6. **Accuracy**
   a. Performance of diagnostic tests considering only number of true results
   b. Accuracy =

   $$\frac{A + D}{A + B + C + D}$$

D. Types of error

1. **Null hypothesis**: states that no association exists between exposure and disease or treatment and response
2. **Type I error**: null hypothesis is rejected even though it is true (false-positive)
3. **Type II error**: null hypothesis is not rejected even though it is false (false-negative)
4. Risk of these errors decreases with increasing sample size (therefore increasing power).

E. Statistical significance

1. Statistically detectable difference between groups
2. Probability value (*p*-value)
   a. Chance of a type I error occurring for a given result
   b. If $p < 0.05$, the null hypothesis can be rejected (i.e., a significant relationship exists between groups).

F. Power

1. Ability of a study to detect an actual difference between two groups
2. Studies with insufficient power may state two groups are equal when they are actually significantly different (i.e., occurrence of a type II error).

III. Ethics

A. Rights of the patient

1. Confidentiality
   a. All information regarding the patient must be kept **private** between the **physician** and the **patient**.
   b. The Health Insurance Portability and Accountability Act (HIPAA)
      (1) All patient account handling, billing, and medical records must be designed to maintain patient confidentiality.
      (2) Exchange of patient information can occur only between care providers involved with the care of the patient in question.
   c. Confidentiality is **not mandated** when the patient
      (1) Allows the physician to share information with designated others (family, etc.)
      (2) Has a disease that is legally reportable (reported only to appropriate public officials)
      (3) Is considered to be **suicidal** or **homicidal**
      (4) Has suffered a gunshot or other type of penetrating wound from an assault
      (5) Is an adolescent with a condition that is potentially harmful to self or others
2. **Public reporting**
   a. Reporting of several diseases to a public health department is required by law (including **HIV**, **STDs**, hepatitis, Lyme disease, several foodborne illnesses, meningitis, rabies, and **tuberculosis**).
   b. Impaired ability to drive, **child abuse**, and **elder abuse** must be reported to authorities (exact legal requirements vary from state to state).
3. Informed consent
   a. **Before any procedure or therapy**, the patient must be made aware of the indications, risks, and potential benefits of a proposed treatment; alternative treatments and their risks and the risks of refusing treatment must also be described.

Quick HIT

The **null hypothesis** suggests that **no association** exists between exposure and disease or treatment and response. The **alternative hypothesis** suggests that **an association does exist**.

Quick HIT

Confidentiality should be maintained in **adolescents** seeking contraception, treatment for sexually transmitted diseases (**STDs**), or treatment for **pregnancy** (this point may need to be clarified with parents).

Quick HIT

The patient should be made aware that certain diseases or conditions must be reported.

b. Informed consent or parental consent for minors is not required for emergent therapy (i.e., **implied consent**).

c. If a patient is not capable of making a decision, a designated surrogate decision-maker is required for nonemergent care.

4. **Full disclosure**

a. Patients have the right to be made aware of their medical status, prognosis, treatment options, and medical errors in their care.

b. If a family requests that a physician withhold information from the patient, physicians must deny the request unless it is determined that disclosing information would significantly harm the patient.

B. Patient decision making

1. **Capacity**

a. "Capacity" means that the patient has the mental ability to make decisions regarding his or her medical care. A patient that lacks capacity might be declared "incompetent" by the legal/judicial system.

b. To be judged competent, a patient must

(1) Not be diagnosed as presently psychotic or intoxicated

(2) Have an **understanding** of his or her **medical situation**

(3) Must be capable of making decisions that are in agreement with his or her history of values

c. Medical decisions for non-emancipated minors (i.e., <18 years of age) are made by a minor's parents unless legally ruled not to be in the best interests of the child.

2. **Durable power of attorney**

a. Legal documentation that designates a **second party** (e.g., family member) **as a surrogate decision maker** for medical issues

b. Designated individual should be able to make decisions **consistent with the patient's values**.

c. Not valid in all U.S. states (e.g., NY)

3. **Living will**

a. Written document that details a patient's wishes in specific medical situations (e.g., resuscitation, ventilation, extraordinary maintenance of life)

b. May be less flexible than durable power of attorney

C. End-of-life issues

1. **Do-not-resuscitate (DNR) order**

a. A type of advanced directive document that details care in cases of coma, cardiac arrest, severe dementia, and terminal illness

b. DNR can refuse all nonpalliative therapies or can only restrict use of specific therapies (e.g., ventilation, cardiopulmonary resuscitation, feeding tubes, antibiotics, etc.).

2. **Life support**

a. Competent patients can request having supportive measures withdrawn at any time.

b. Wishes for life support (or withholding it) can be described in a living will or DNR.

c. Physicians can remove respiratory care in cases in which **no living will** exists and the patient is **incapable** of voicing a decision if the **family** and the **physician** believe that removal of care is **consistent** with **what the patient would want**.

3. **Physician-aided death**

a. Physician-assisted suicide occurs when a physician **supplies** a patient with a means of ending his or her life.

b. Euthanasia is the **active administration by a physician** of a lethal agent to a patient to end suffering from a condition.

c. Physician-assisted suicide is currently legal only in Oregon, and euthanasia is illegal in the entire United States.

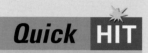

Quick **HIT**

A **competent** patient can change his or her mind regarding accepting therapy **at any time**.

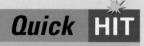

Quick **HIT**

Parents' decisions regarding their children can be legally **overruled** if they are considered **harmful** to the children.

Epidemiology and Ethics

4. Death
   a. **Brain death** is defined as the irreversible **absence** of all brain activity (including the brainstem) in a patient lasting >6 hr.
      (1) Absence of cephalic (i.e., cranial nerve) reflexes (e.g., gag, corneal, and caloric reflexes)
      (2) Apnea off of a ventilator for a duration considered sufficient to produce a normal hypercarbic drive
      (3) Absent brainstem-evoked responses, absent cerebral circulation on radiologic testing, or persistent isoelectric EEG
      (4) Patient appearance cannot be explained by a medical condition that mimics death
      (5) Absence of hypothermia or intoxication
   b. **Heart death** is considered the inability to restore a spontaneous heartbeat in an asystolic patient.
   c. Either brain death or heart death can be used to define formal patient death (both are not required).
   d. **Hypothermic** patients must be warmed to normal body temperature before death can be declared.
5. Organ donation
   a. Patients can declare themselves as organ donors before death (e.g., living will, driver's license).
   b. Hospitals receiving payments from Medicare are required to approach the family of the deceased regarding organ donation.
   c. Patients and families can define exactly what organs are to be donated.
   d. Organs may be judged unsuitable for donation in cases of widespread or uncured **neoplasm, sepsis,** compromised organ function, organ-specific infection or disease, hypothermia, HIV infection, age >80 years, hemoglobinopathy, or **prolonged ischemia.**

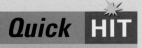

The absence of electroencephalogram (EEG) activity does **not** define brain death but may help prompt a brain death workup.

Quick HIT

Conditions that can mimic brain death include metabolic encephalopathy, hypothermia, intoxication, locked-in syndrome, and Guillain-Barré syndrome.

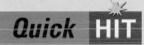

Physicians are not required to supply therapies that are irrational for the current condition or when the maximal therapy has already failed.

Epidemiology and Ethics

INDEX

NOTE: Page numbers followed by *f* indicate figures; *t* indicates tables.

A

AAA. *See* Abdominal aortic aneurysm
A-a gradient. *See* Alveolar-arterial gradient
Abacavir (ABC), 145*t*
Abciximab, 8*t*, 9, 139*t*
ABCs, 160
Abdomen, acute, 170–171, 171*t*
Abdominal aortic aneurysm (AAA), 26
Abdominal bleeding, 163
Abdominal trauma, 163
Abducens nerve (CN VI), 195
Abnormal uterine bleeding, 248
ABO blood groups, 166
Abortion, spontaneous, 270–271, 270*t*
Abruptio placenta, 274
Absolute risk reduction (ARR), 307
Abstinence, 244*t*
Abuse, 164–165
ACA. *See* Anterior cerebral artery
Acarbose, 112*t*
Acceleration-deceleration injuries, 160
Accidents and injury, 153–156
    bites and stings, 156, 156*t*
    burns, 153–154, 153*f*
    choking, 155
    drowning, 154–155
    heat emergencies, 155, 155*t*
    hypothermia, 155, 156*f*
Accuracy, 309
ACE-I. *See* Angiotensin-converting enzyme inhibitor
Acetaminophen poisoning, 157*t*
Acetazolamide, 91*t*, 198
Acetylcholinesterase, 194
Acetylsalicylic acid (ASA), for myocardial
    infarction, 8*t*, 9
Achalasia, 20, 61, 62*f*
Acid-base disorders, 99–100
    anion gap disturbances, 99, 100*t*, 100*f*
    mixed disturbances, 100
    renal tubular acidosis, 99, 99*t*
Acid-base disturbances, 99–100
Acid-base physiology, 99
Acidosis
    metabolic, 100*t*, 126
    renal tubular, 99, 99*t*
    respiratory, 100*f*, 100*t*
Acid poisoning, 157*t*
ACL. *See* Anterior cruciate ligament
Acne vulgaris, 225–226, 292*t*
Acoustic neuroma, 200–201
Acoustic schwannoma, 200–201
Acquired immunodeficiency syndrome (AIDS), 142,
    143–144*t*
Acral lentiginous, 236
Acromegaly, 120
ACTH. *See* Adrenocorticotropic hormone
Actinic keratosis, 234, 235*f*
Action potentials, 3, 3*f*
Acute abdomen, 170–171, 171*t*
Acute kidney injury (AKI), 97–98
Acute lymphocytic leukemia (ALL), 146–147, 148*f*
Acute myelogenous leukemia (AML), 148
Acute pericarditis, 20
Acute promyelocytic leukemia, 148*f*

Acute renal failure (ARF), 97–98
Acute respiratory distress syndrome (ARDS),
    40–41, 49
Addison disease, 122
Adenocarcinoma
    bladder, 105
    cervical, 254
    esophageal, 64–65, 64*f*
    gallbladder, 81–82
    lung, 44, 44*t*, 45*f*
Adenomatous polyposis coli (APC) gene, 76
Adenomyosis, 247
Adenosine, 14*t*
Adenosine reuptake inhibitors, 139*t*
ADHD. *See* Attention-deficit hyperactivity disorder
Adie pupil, 196*t*
Adjustment disorder, 298
Adolescents
    confidentiality with, 287, 309
    development of, 287, 287*t*
Adrenal disorders, 121–124
    adrenal insufficiency, 122–123
    congenital adrenal hyperplasia, 123–124, 123*f*
    Cushing syndrome, 121, 122*f*
    hyperaldosteronism, 121–122
    pheochromocytoma, 124
Adrenal function, 121, 121*t*
Adrenal insufficiency, 122–123
Adrenocorticotropic hormone (ACTH), 118, 119*f*,
    120*t*, 121
Adult onset diabetes, 109–111, 111*t*, 112*t*
A-Fetoprotein, 194
Afib. *See* Atrial fibrillation
Afterload, 2, 14
AICA. *See* Anterior inferior cerebellar artery
AIDS. *See* Acquired immunodeficiency syndrome
Albright hereditary osteodystrophy, 118
Albuterol, 42*t*
Alcohol, 303*t*
    related liver disease, 84
Aldosterone antagonists, for CHF, 15
A-line. *See* Arterial line
Alkali poisoning, 157*t*
Alkalosis
    metabolic, 100*f*, 100*t*, 126
    respiratory, 100*f*, 100*t*
ALL. *See* Acute lymphocytic leukemia
Allergic contact dermatitis, 229–230, 230*f*
Allopurinol, 210, 211
Alogliptin, 112*t*
17-α-Hydroxylase deficiency, 123, 123*f*
21-α-Hydroxylase deficiency, 123–124, 123*f*
α₁-Antitrypsin deficiency, 86
α-Blocker, for hypertension, 23*t*
α-Fetoprotein, maternal, 262*t*, 263, 263*t*
α-Glucosidase inhibitors, 112*t*
α-Thalassemia, 134
Alport syndrome, 96*t*
ALS. *See* Amyotrophic lateral sclerosis
Alveolar-arterial (A-a) gradient, 35, 35*t*
Alzheimer disease, 201
Amantadine, 187*t*
Amblyopia, 196*t*
Amenorrhea, 239*t*, 243, 245–247, 246*f*, 292*t*

Amiloride, 91*t*
Aminoglycosides, teratogenic effects of, 268*t*
Amiodarone, 14, 14*t*
AML. *See* Acute myelogenous leukemia
Amlodipine, 23*t*
Amniocentesis, 263*t*
Amniotic fluid deficiency, 271
Amphetamines, 303*t*
Amyloidosis, 97*t*
Amyotrophic lateral sclerosis (ALS), 176*t*, 187
Anal fissures, 75
Anaphylactic shock, 26*t*
Anaphylaxis, 137
Anaplastic thyroid carcinoma, 116*t*
Anemia, 126–133
    alcohol abuse and, 128*t*
    aplastic, 132–133
    of chronic disease, 128*t*, 130*t*, 132
    Diamond-Blackfan, 151–152
    Fanconi, 151
    folate-deficiency, 128*t*, 131
    hemolytic, 128, 128*t*, 129*t*
    hypovolemia, 128*t*
    iron-deficiency, 76, 128–130, 128*t*, 130*t*, 131*f*
    lead poisoning, 128*t*, 130–131, 130*t*, 131*f*
    liver disease and, 128*t*
    pernicious, 65
    sideroblastic, 128*t*, 130*t*, 133, 133*f*
    thalassemia, 128*t*, 130*t*
    vitamin B_{12} deficiency, 128*t*, 132, 132*f*
Anencephaly, 194
Angelman syndrome, 291*t*
Angina pectoris, 6
Angina, unstable, 6–7
Angiotensin-converting enzyme inhibitor (ACE-I), 23
    for CHF, 15, 16*f*
    for hypertension, 23*t*, 24*t*
    for myocardial infarction, 8*t*, 9
    teratogenic effects of, 265, 268*t*
Angiotensin receptor blockers (ARB)
    for hypertension, 23*t*, 24*t*
    teratogenic effects of, 265
Anion gap disturbances, 99, 100*t*, 100*f*
Ankle fracture, 205*t*
Ankylosing spondylitis, 214*t*, 217
Anorectal abscesses, 75
Anorexia nervosa, 300
Anovulation, 248
Anterior cerebral artery (ACA), 174*f*, 175*t*, 180*f*
Anterior communicating artery, 174*f*
Anterior cruciate ligament (ACL) tear, 204
Anterior inferior cerebellar artery (AICA), 174*f*, 175*t*
Anterior spinal artery, 174*f*
Antibiotic-resistant strains, 35
Anticholinergic poisoning, 157*t*
Anticoagulation
    deep vein thrombosis, 169*t*
    during pregnancy, 267
    pulmonary embolism, 169*t*
    systemic lupus erythematosus, 216
Anticonvulsants
    in pregnancy, 266
    seizures, 184
    trigeminal neuralgia, 179

Antidepressant medications, 295t
Antidiuretic hormone (ADH), 118
Antidotes, 157, 157t
Antilipid therapy, 180
Antimalarials, 141
Antimicrobial agents, 154
Antimuscarinic agents, 187t
Antiphospholipid syndrome, 140t
Antiplatelet therapy, 180, 181
Antipsychotics, 293, 294t, 296
Antiretroviral therapy, 145, 145t
Antisocial cluster, 301t
Antithrombotic drugs, 138, 139t
Antithymocyte globulin, 173t
Anxiety disorders, 296–297, 297t
    generalized, 297
    panic disorder, 296–297
    social, 297
    specific phobia, 297
Anxiolytic medications, 297t
Aortic dissection, 26–27
Aortic regurgitation, 16f, 17t
Aortic stenosis, 16f, 17t
APC gene. See Adenomatous polyposis coli gene
Apgar scoring system, 279, 279t
Aphasias, 184, 184t
Apixaban, 139t
Aplastic anemia, 132–133
Apnea, sleep, 51–52, 191
Appendicitis, 73, 171t
ARB. See Angiotensin receptor blockers
Arboviruses, 178
ARDS. See Acute respiratory distress syndrome
ARF. See Acute renal failure
Argatroban, 139t
Argyll Robertson pupil, 196t
Arnold-Chiari malformation type II, 193
Arrhythmias, 9–14
    atrial fibrillation, 12, 12f
    atrial flutter, 13, 13f
    bradycardia, 12
    heart block, 9, 10f
    medications for, 14t
    multifocal atrial tachycardia, 11, 12f
    paroxysmal supraventricular tachycardia, 9–11, 10f, 11f
    premature ventricular contraction, 13
    ventricular fibrillation, 14
    ventricular tachycardia, 13–14, 13f
Arterial aneurysm, 182
Arterial line (A-line), in ICU, 166
Arteriovenous malformations (AVM), 27
Arthritis. See also Osteoarthritis; Rheumatoid arthritis
    psoriatic, 214t, 217, 231
    septic, 211–212, 212t, 250
ASA. See Acetylsalicylic acid
Asbestosis, 47t
Ascending loop of Henle, 90f, 91
ASD. See Atrial septal defect
Asherman syndrome, 245
Aspiration of foreign body, 155
Aspirin (ASA), 139t
Asthma, 41, 42t, 43t
    maternal, 266
Astigmatism, 196t
Asystole, 158, 159f
Ataxia-telangiectasia, 288t
Atazanavir, 145t
Atelectasis, 52
Atenolol, 23t
Atherosclerosis, 4–5, 4f
    in diabetes, 113
Atherosclerotic cardiovascular disease (ASCVD), statin therapy for, 5, 5f
Athetosis, 190t
Atopic dermatitis, 231, 232f
Atrial fibrillation (Afib), 12, 12f

Atrial flutter, 13, 13f
Atrial septal defect (ASD), 30, 31f, 292t
Atrophic vaginitis, 253
Attention deficit hyperactivity disorder (ADHD), 292t, 304
Attributable risk (AR), 307
Audiovestibular disorders, 200–201
    acoustic neuroma, 200–201
    benign paroxysmal positional vertigo, 200
    Ménière disease, 200
    otitis externa, 200
    otitis media, 200
Autism spectrum disorder, 302
Autologous blood, 167t
Autonomic neuropathy, 113
Autosomal dominant polycystic kidney disease, 181
AVM. See Arteriovenous malformations
AV nodal reentry, 9, 10f
Avoidant cluster, 301t
AV reentry, 11, 11f
Axillary nerve injury, 204
Azathioprine, 173t
AZT. See Zidovudine

B

Bacillus Calmette-Guérin (BCG) vaccine, 37
Back pain, 206, 206f
Bacterial gastroenteritis, 57t
Bacterial meningitis, 177, 177t
Bariatric surgery, 52
Barium swallow
    for achalasia, 61
    for diffuse esophageal spasm, 61, 62f
    for diverticular disease, 74, 74f
    for dysphagia, 61
    for esophageal cancer, 64–65, 64f
    for gastric lesion, 66
    for Zenker diverticulum, 61, 63, 63f
Barlow maneuver, 219
Barrier methods of contraception, 244t, 251
Basal cell carcinoma, skin, 235, 236f
Basilar artery, 174f, 175t
B-cell Disorders, 288t
BCG vaccine. See Bacillus Calmette-Guérin
BCR-ABL gene, 149
Becker muscular dystrophy, 222
Beck triad, 20
Beclomethasone, 42t
Bell's palsy, 189, 212
Benign cystic teratoma, ovarian, 255t
Benign essential tremor, 190t
Benign ovarian tumors, 255–256, 255t
Benign paroxysmal positional vertigo (BPPV), 200
Benign prostatic hyperplasia (BPH), 106
Benzodiazepines, 297
    anxiolytic medications, 297t
    for epilepsy, 186t
    poisoning, 157t
    substance abuse, 303t
Berger disease, 96t
Berry aneurysms, 181
Berylliosis, 47t
11-β-Hydroxylase deficiency, 123f, 124
β-Blocker, 2, 14t, 297
    for CHF, 15
    for hypertension, 23t, 24t
    for myocardial infarction, 8t, 9
    poisoning with, 157t
β-Globin defects, 135
β-Thalassemia, 134
Bethesda classification, 254t
β-hCG pregnancy test, 246
Biguanides, 111, 112t
Bilateral renal artery stenosis, 24
Bilateral salpingo-oophorectomy, 254

Bile acid sequestrants, 6t
Biliary disorders, 80–84
    cholangitis, 81, 82f
    cholecystitis, acute, 80–81
    cholelithiasis, 80, 81f
    gallbladder cancer, 81–82
    hepatic bilirubin transport, 83–84, 83t
        Crigler-Najjar syndrome, 83–84, 83t
        Gilbert disease, 83, 83t
    primary biliary cirrhosis, 82
    primary sclerosing cholangitis, 82–83
Bilirubinemia, 83–84, 83t
Bilirubin transport disorders, hepatic, 83–84, 83t
Binge eating disorder, 300
Biostatistics, 306–309
    of diagnostic tests, 308–309, 308t
    error types in, 309
    power, 309
    rates of disease, 306–307
    risk of disease, 307–308, 307t
    statistical significance, 309
Bipolar disorder, 296
Birth canal trauma, 280
Birth defects, nutrients and, 261, 262t
Bishop scoring system, 278t
Bisoprolol, for CHF, 15
Bites
    and stings, 156, 156f
    venomous, 156, 156t
Bitolterol, 42t
Black widow spider bite, 156, 156t
Bladder disorders, 104–105
    bladder cancer, 105
    urinary incontinence, 104–105
    urinary tract infection, 104
Bladder cancer, 105
Bleeding
    abnormal uterine, 248
    gastrointestinal, 77–78, 77f
    postmenopausal, 253
    postpartum, 280
Blood loss, traumatic, 163
Blue bloaters, 41
Body dysmorphic disorder, 298
Bone abnormalities, 191
Bone infection
    osteomyelitis, 212
    septic joint and septic arthritis, 211–212, 212t
Bone marrow transplantation, 172t
Bone metastases, 218
Borderline cluster, 301t
Bouchard nodes, 213
Boutonniere deformities, 214
Bowel obstruction, 71, 72f, 73t
Bowman capsule, 90
Boxer fracture, 205t
BPH. See Benign prostatic hyperplasia
BPPV. See Benign paroxysmal positional vertigo
Brachial plexus, 208, 208f, 209t
Bradycardia, 12
    hypertension with, 161
Brain abscess, 178
Brain death, 158, 311
Braxton-Hicks contractions, 275
BRCA1/BRCA2 gene, 256, 259
Breast abscess, 256
Breast cancer, 257–259, 258t
    estrogen and, 240
Breast disorders, 256–259
    abscess, 256
    cancer, 257–259, 258t
    fibroadenoma, 257
    fibrocystic changes, 257
    intraductal papilloma, 257
Breast milk, 279
Breech presentation, 278, 278f
Bretylium, 14t

Broca aphasias, 184, 184t
Bromocriptine, 187t
Bronchiectasis, 42
Bronchiolitis, 54
Bronchitis
    acute, 37
    chronic, 41
Brown recluse spider bite, 156, 156t
Brown-Séquard syndrome, 176t
Brudzinski signs, 177
Buffalo hump, 121
Bulimia nervosa, 300
Bullous diseases, 233–234
    bullous pemphigoid, 233, 234f
    pemphigus vulgaris, 233, 233f
    porphyria cutanea tarda, 233–234
Bullous pemphigoid, 233, 234f
Bumetanide, 91t
Bupropion, 295t
Burns, 153–154, 153f
Burr cells, 128, 129–130f
Buspirone, 297t

C

CA-125, 256
CABG. See Coronary artery bypass graft
CAD. See Coronary artery disease
Caesarean section, 279
Café-au-lait macules, 191
Caffeine, 303t
CAH. See Congenital adrenal hyperplasia
Calcified gallbladder, 82
Calcitonin, 117, 117f
Calcium channel blockers, 14t
    for hypertension, 23t
    poisoning with, 157t
Calcium, in pregnancy, 262t
Calcium pyrophosphate dihydrate deposition disease
        (CPPD), 211, 211f
Canagliflozin, 112t
Cancer. See specific cancer
    surgery for, 150
Capacity, 310
Captopril, 23t
Carbamazepine, 186t
    teratogenic effects of, 268t
Carbidopa, 187t
Carbonic anhydrase, 90, 91t
Carbon monoxide poisoning, 126, 158
Carcinoid tumor, 75–76
Cardiac anatomy, 1, 1f
Cardiac arrest, 158, 158f, 159f
Cardiac cycle, 2f
Cardiac function, 3
Cardiac output (CO), 2
Cardiac risk, preoperative assessment of, 168
Cardiac tamponade, 20
Cardiac transplantation, 172t
Cardiogenic shock, 26t
    post-MI, 9
Cardiomyopathies, 18f, 19t
Cardiopulmonary resuscitation (CPR), 158f
Cardiovascular disorders, 1–32
    arrhythmias, 9–14
        atrial fibrillation, 12, 12f
        atrial flutter, 13, 13f
        bradycardia, 12
        heart block, 9, 10f
        medications for, 14t
        multifocal atrial tachycardia, 11, 12f
        paroxysmal supraventricular tachycardia,
            9–11, 10f, 11f
        premature ventricular contraction, 13
        ventricular fibrillation, 14
        ventricular tachycardia, 13–14, 13f
    cardiomyopathies, 18f, 19t

heart failure, 14–16
    congestive, 15, 16f
    diastolic dysfunction, 15
    systolic dysfunction, 15
hypertension, 22–25
    hypertensive urgency, 24–25
    primary, 22–23, 23t, 24t
    secondary, 24, 25t
ischemic heart disease, 4–9
    angina pectoris, 6
    atherosclerosis, 4–5, 4f
    coronary artery disease, 4
    dyslipidemia, 5, 6t
    myocardial hypoxia, 4
    myocardial infarction, 7–9, 7f, 8t
    unstable angina, 6–7
myocardial infections, 20–22, 21f, 22t
    endocarditis, 21–22, 22t
    myocarditis, 20–21
    rheumatic fever, acute, 21, 21f
pediatric, 29–32
    atrial septal defect, 30, 31f
    endocardial cushion defect, 31f, 32
    fetal circulation, 29–30, 29f
    patent ductus arteriosus, 30, 31f
    persistent truncus arteriosus, 31, 31f
    tetralogy of Fallot, 31f, 32
    transposition of great vessels, 31f, 32
    tricuspid atresia, 32
    ventricular septal defect, 30, 31f
pericardial diseases, 20
shock, 25, 26t
valvular diseases, 16f, 17t
vascular diseases, 26–29
    abdominal aortic aneurysm, 26
    aortic dissection, 26–27
    arteriovenous malformations, 27
    Churg-Strauss syndrome, 28
    deep vein thrombosis, 27
    eosinophilic granulomatosis with
        polyangiitis, 28
    Henoch-Schonlein purpura, 29
    Kawasaki disease, 28
    peripheral vascular disease, 27
    polyarteritis nodosa, 28
    Takayasu arteritis, 28
    temporal arteritis, 28
    varicosities, 27
    vasculitis, 28–29
Cardiovascular emergencies, 158–160
    acute stroke, 158, 160f
    cardiac arrest, 158, 158f, 159f
Carotid massage, 11
Carpal tunnel syndrome, 203, 203f
Carvedilol, for CHF, 15
Case-control study, 305t
Case fatality rate, 307
Case series, 305t
Cataracts, 197
Catheter ablation, 11
Cauda equina syndrome, 208
Caustics poisoning, 157t
CCR5 antagonist, 145t
Celiac disease, 67
Celiac sprue, 67, 68f
Cellulitis, 224, 224f
Central nervous system neoplasms
    metastatic, 190
    primary, 190
Cerebral hypoxia, 154
Cerebral palsy (CP), 190t, 194, 292t
Cerebral vasculature, 174, 174f, 175t
Cerebrovascular accident (CVA), 180–181,
        180f, 181f
Cerebrovascular and hemorrhagic diseases, 179–184
    aphasias, 184, 184t
    epidural hematoma, 182–183, 183f

parenchymal hemorrhage, 181–182
    stroke, 180–181, 180f, 181t
    subarachnoid hemorrhage, 182, 182f
    subdural hematoma, 183–184, 183f
    transient ischemic attack, 179–180
Cervical cancer, 254–255, 254t
Cervical cap, 244t
Cervical dysplasia, 254–255
Cervicitis, 250
CF. See Cystic fibrosis
Chagas disease, 20, 61
Chancroid, 252
Chandelier sign, 251
Charcot joints, 113
Charcot triad, 81
Chediak-Higashi syndrome, 289t
Chemotherapy, 150, 151t
    teratogenic effects of, 268t
Chest trauma, 162–163
CHF. See Congestive heart failure
Chickenpox, 227, 227t, 228f
Child abuse, 164, 283
Childhood. See Pediatric entries
Childhood health maintenance, 283, 285–286t
Childhood hydrocephalus, 193
Chlamydia trachomatis, 197
    infection, 250
    in pregnancy, 269t
Chlorthalidone, 91t
Choking, 155
Cholangitis, 81, 82f
    primary sclerosing, 82–83
Cholecystitis, acute, 80–81
Cholelithiasis, 80, 81f
Cholesterol, 5
    absorption inhibitors, 6t
Cholestyramine, 6t
Chorea, 190t
Choriocarcinoma, 281
Chorionic villi sampling, 263t
Chromosome abnormalities, 245
Chronic constrictive pericarditis, 20
Chronic granulomatous disease, 289t
Chronic kidney disease (CKD), 98
Chronic lymphocytic leukemia (CLL), 148–149, 149f
Chronic mucocutaneous candidiasis, 288t
Chronic myelogenous leukemia (CML), 149
Churg-Strauss syndrome, 28
Circle of Willis, 174, 174f, 175t
Cirrhosis, 84
CKD. See Chronic kidney disease
CK-MB. See Creatine kinase myocardial fraction
Clavicular fracture, 221
Claw hand, 209t
Clean catch urine sample, 104
CLL. See Chronic lymphocytic leukemia
Clopidogrel, 139t
    for myocardial infarction, 8t, 9
Closed angle glaucoma, 197–198
Clotting disorders, 137–141
    disseminated intravascular coagulation, 140–141
    hemophilia, 139–140
    thrombocytopenia, 138, 140t
    vitamin K deficiency, 139
    von Willebrand disease, 138
Clotting factors, 167t
Club foot, 220
Clusters, 301, 301t
CML. See Chronic myelogenous leukemia
CO. See Cardiac output
Coagulation cascade, 137, 138f
Coagulation concerns, in preoperative
        assessment, 169
Coal worker disease, 47t
Cocaine, 303t
    on pregnancy, 267t
    poisoning, 157t

Codman triangle, 218, 219f
Cohort study, 305t
Colesevelam, 6t
Colestipol, 6t
Collecting duct, 90f, 91
Collecting tubule, 90f, 91
Colles fracture, 205t
Colon cancer, 128
Colorectal cancer, 76–77, 76t, 77t
Colostrum, 279
Coma, 192, 192f
Common cold, 35
Common variable immunodeficiency, 288t
Compartment syndrome, 164, 204
Complement deficiencies, 289t
Complete breech, 278, 278f
Composite graft, 237t
Compulsions, 298
Condom, 244t
Conduct disorder, 304
Conduction aphasias, 184t
Confidentiality, 287, 309
Confirmatory tests, 308
Congenital adrenal hyperplasia (CAH), 123–124, 123f
Congenital disease assessment, 263t
Congenital immune disorders, 287, 288–289t
Congenital infections, 268, 269t
Congestive heart failure (CHF), 15, 16f
Conjunctivitis, 197
Constrictive pericarditis, 18
Contemplation, 302
Continuous positive airway pressure (CPAP), 52
Contraception, 243–245, 243–245t
    barrier methods of, 244t, 251
    hormonal methods of, 243–244t
    intrauterine devices of, 245t
    sexual practice methods of, 244t
    surgical methods of, 245t
Contraceptive sponge, 244t
Contractility, 2, 14
Contraction stress test, 275
Conversion disorder, 299
Coombs test, 128
COPD, right-sided failure from, 15
Copperhead snake bite, 156, 156t
Copper intrauterine device, 245t
Coprolalia, 304
Coral snake bite, 156, 156t
Coronary angiography, 5
Coronary arteries. See also specific arteries
    anatomy of, 1, 1f
    atherosclerosis of, 4
Coronary artery bypass graft (CABG), 7
Coronary artery disease (CAD), 4, 6
Coronary artery occlusion, 1
Coronary vessel occlusion, 7
Cor pulmonale, 15
Corpus luteum cyst, ovarian, 255t
Corticoadrenal insufficiency
    secondary, 122
    tertiary, 122
Corticospinal tract, 175f, 175t
Corticosteroids
    Cushing syndrome and, 121
    for transplant rejection, 173t
Corticotrophin-releasing hormone (CRH), 119f
Cosmetic surgery, 238
Cotton wool spots, 199
COX-2. See Cyclooxygenase-2
CP. See Cerebral palsy
CPAP. See Continuous positive airway pressure
CPPD. See Calcium pyrophosphate dihydrate deposition disease
CPR. See Cardiopulmonary resuscitation
Cradle cap, 231
Cranial nerves, 175, 176t

Creatine kinase myocardial fraction (CK-MB), 7
CREST syndrome, 214t, 217
Cretinism, 125, 292t
Cri du chat syndrome, 291t
Crigler-Najjar syndrome, 83–84, 83t
Critical care, 165–167
    hemodynamic stability, 166–167
        transfusions, 166–167, 167t
        vasoactive medications, 167, 167t
    ICU issues, 165–166
Crohn's disease, 71, 71t
Cross-sectional survey, 305t
Croup, 53, 53f, 292t
Cryoprecipitate, 167t
Cryptorchidism, 108
Curling ulcers, 66
Cushing syndrome, 121, 122f
Cushing ulcers, 66
CVA. See Cerebrovascular accident
Cyanide poisoning, 157t
Cyclooxygenase-2 (COX-2), for PUD, 66
Cyclosporine, 173t
Cyclothymic disorder, 296
Cystic fibrosis (CF), 55, 292t
    infertility and, 107
Cytomegalovirus, 269t

D
Dalteparin, 139t
Dandy-Walker malformations, 193
Dantrolene, 171
Dapagliflozin, 112t
Darunavir, 145t
DCIS. See Ductal carcinoma in situ
DDH. See Developmental dysplasia of hip
Death, 311
    brain, 158, 311
    heart, 311
    physician-aided, 310
Decision-making, patient, 310
Deep vein thrombosis (DVT), 27
    maternal, 267
Degenerative disc disease, 206–207, 207f, 207t
Degenerative neurologic disorders, 186–188
    amyotrophic lateral sclerosis, 187
    Huntington disease, 187–188
    multiple sclerosis, 188
    Parkinson disease, 186–187
    syringomyelia, 188
Deletion syndromes, 291, 291t
Delirium, 201–202
    compared with dementia, 202t
Delivery. See Labor and delivery
Deltoid malfunction, 204
Deltoid paralysis, 209t
Delusional disorder, 293
Delusions, 293
Dementia, 201
    Alzheimer disease, 201
    compared with delirium, 202t
    frontotemporal, 201
    with Lewy bodies, 201
Dependent cluster, 301t
Dermatitis
    allergic contact, 229–230, 230f
    atopic, 231, 232f
    seborrheic, 231
Dermatology, 224–238
    bullous diseases, 233–234
        bullous pemphigoid, 233, 234f
        pemphigus vulgaris, 233, 233f
        porphyria cutanea tarda, 233–234
    infections, 224–229
        acne vulgaris, 225–226
        cellulitis, 224, 224f
        fungal, 228, 229f, 229t

gangrene, 225
        herpes simplex virus, 226, 227f
        impetigo, 225, 226f
        molluscum contagiosum, 228
        necrotizing fasciitis, 225
        scabies, 228
        skin abscess, 224–225
        varicella, 227, 227t
        warts, 228
    inflammatory conditions, 229–233
        atopic dermatitis, 231, 232f
        erythema multiforme, 230
        erythema nodosum, 233
        hypersensitivity reactions, 229–230, 230f
        pityriasis rosea, 232–233, 232f
        psoriasis, 231–232, 232f
        seborrheic dermatitis, 231
        Stevens-Johnson syndrome, 230
        toxic epidermal necrolysis, 230–231, 231f
    neoplasms, 234–237
        actinic keratosis, 234, 235f
        basal cell carcinoma, 235, 236f
        melanoma, 235–237, 236f, 237f
        squamous cell carcinoma, 234, 235f
    plastic surgery, 237–238
        cosmetic surgery, 238
        grafts and flaps, 237, 237t
        reconstructive surgery, 238
Dermatomyositis, 214t, 216
Descending loop of Henle, 90f, 91
Developmental dysplasia of hip (DDH), 219–220, 292t
Developmental milestones, 283, 284t
Dexamethasone suppression test, 121
DI. See Diabetes insipidus
Diabetes insipidus (DI), 102
Diabetes mellitus (DM)
    complications of, 109, 111–113
    gestational, 264–265, 264f
    myocardial ischemia in, 6
    pregestational, 265
    in preoperative assessment, 169
    type I, 109, 110f, 110t, 111t
    type II, 109–111, 111t, 112t
Diabetic ketoacidosis (DKA), 109, 111–112
Diabetic nephropathy, 97t, 113
Diabetic neuropathy, 113
Diabetic retinopathy, 113, 198f
Dialysis, 98
Diamond-Blackfan anemia, 151–152
Diaphragm, 244t
Diarrhea, 69–70, 69f, 70f
Diastole, 1
Diastolic dysfunction, 15
Diazepam, teratogenic effects of, 268t
DIC. See Disseminated intravascular coagulation
Diethylstilbestrol, teratogenic effects of, 268t
Diffuse esophageal spasm, 61, 62f
Diffusing capacity of lungs (DLco), 33, 41
DiGeorge syndrome, 288t
Digoxin poisoning, 157t
Dihydropyridines, 23t
Dilated cardiomyopathy, 18f, 19, 19t
Diltiazem, 14t, 23t
Dipyridamole, 139t
Direct factor Xa inhibitors, 139t
Direct thrombin inhibitors, 139t
Disclosure, full, 310
Disseminated intravascular coagulation (DIC), 140–141
Distal convoluted tubule, 90f, 91
Diuretics, 91, 91t. See also Thiazides
    for hypertension, 23t
    loop, 91, 91t, 104
Diverticulitis, 75, 171t
Diverticulosis, 74, 74f
Dix-Hallpike maneuver, 200
Dizygotic twinning, 274

DKA. *See* Diabetic ketoacidosis
DM. *See* Diabetes mellitus
DNR. *See* Do not resuscitate
Dobutamine, 167*t*
Doctor-parent-child relationship, 283
Do not resuscitate (DNR), 159, 310
Donovan bodies, 253
Dopamine, 167*t*
Dorsal columns, 175*f*, 175*t*
Down syndrome. *See* Trisomy 21
Doxazosin, 23*t*
DPP-IV inhibitors, 112*t*
Dressler syndrome, 9
Drowning, 154–155
Drug-induced lupus, 214*t*
Drug use, maternal, 267–268, 267*t*, 268*t*
Dry gangrene, 225
Duchenne muscular dystrophy, 222–223
Ductal carcinoma in situ (DCIS), 258, 258*t*
Duke Classification of colorectal cancer, 76, 77*t*
Duke criteria, 22, 22*t*
Duodenal ulcers, 66, 66*t*
Durable power of attorney, 310
DVT. *See* Deep vein thrombosis
Dyslipidemia, 5, 6*t*
Dysmenorrhea, 247
Dyspareunia, 243
Dysphagia, 61
Dystonia, 190*t*
Dystrophin, 222

E
Eating disorders, 300
    anorexia nervosa, 300
    binge eating disorder, 300
    bulimia nervosa, 300
EBV. *See* Epstein-Barr virus
ECG. *See* Electrocardiogram
Echocardiography. *See also* Transesophageal
        echocardiogram
    exercise stress test with, 4
Eclampsia, 266
Ectopic pregnancy, 247, 270
    ruptured, 171*t*
Eczema, 231, 232*f*
Edrophonium, 189
EF. *See* Ejection fraction
Efavirenz (EFV), 145*t*
Ehlers-Danlos syndrome, 181
Eisenmenger syndrome, 30
Ejection fraction (EF), 14
Elder abuse, 165
Electric burn, 153
Electrocardiogram (ECG), 3
    action potentials and, 3, 3*f*
    of atrial fibrillation, 12, 12*f*
    of cardiac cycle, 2*f*
    general structure of, 3*f*
    of heart block, 9, 10*f*
    of hypothermia, 156*f*
    of MI, 6, 7*f*, 8*t*
    of multifocal atrial tachycardia, 11, 12*f*
    ST elevation on, 9, 20
    of ventricular tachycardia, 13, 13*f*
    of Wolff-Parkinson-White syndrome, 11, 11*f*
Electrolyte disorders, 101–104
    diabetes insipidus, 102
    hypercalcemia, 103
    hyperkalemia, 102–103
    hypernatremia, 101, 101*f*
    hypocalcemia, 104
    hypokalemia, 103, 104*f*
    hyponatremia, 102, 103*f*
    syndrome of inappropriate ADH secretion, 102
Elvitegravir, 145*t*
Embolic ischemic stroke, 180

Embryonic age, 260
Emergency contraception, 244*t*
Emergency medicine, 153–165
    abuse, 164–165
    accidents and injury, 153–156
        bites and stings, 156, 156*t*
        burns, 153–154, 153*f*
        choking, 155
        drowning, 154–155
        heat emergencies, 155, 155*t*
        hypothermia, 155, 156*f*
    cardiovascular, 158–160
    toxicology, 156–158, 157*t*
    traumatology, 160–164
        abdominal, 163
        assessment of, 160–161
        chest, 162–163
        extremity, 164
        genitourinary and pelvic, 163
        head, 161
        mechanisms of injury in, 160
        neck, 162, 162*f*
        during pregnancy, 164
        spinal cord, 161–162
Emphysema, 41–42
Emtricitabine, 145*t*
Enalapril, 23*t*
Encephalitis, 178
Encephalopathy, 227
Endocardial cushion defect, 31*f*, 32
Endocarditis, 21–22, 22*t*
Endocrine disorders, 109–125
    adrenal disorders, 121–124
        adrenal insufficiency, 122–123
        congenital adrenal hyperplasia,
            123–124, 123*f*
        Cushing syndrome, 121, 122*f*
        hyperaldosteronism, 121–122
        pheochromocytoma, 124
    glucose metabolism, 109–114
        diabetes complications, 111–113
        diabetes mellitus type I, 109, 110*f*, 110*t*, 111*t*
        diabetes mellitus type II, 109–111, 111*t*, 112*t*
        hypoglycemia, 113–114, 114*t*
        multiple endocrine neoplasia, 124, 124*t*
    parathyroid, 117–118
        hyperparathyroidism, 117–118, 124*t*
        hypoparathyroidism, 118
        pseudohypoparathyroidism, 118
    pediatric, 125
    pituitary and hypothalamic disorders, 118–121
        acromegaly, 120
        hyperprolactinemia, 118
        hypopituitarism, 120–121, 120*t*
    thyroid, 114–116
        Hashimoto thyroiditis, 116
        hyperthyroidism, 114, 115*t*
        thyroid carcinoma, 116, 116*t*
        thyroid storm, 114–115
End-of-life issues, 310–311
Endometrial cancer, 248, 253–254
Endometrioma, ovarian, 255*t*
Endometriosis, 247–248
Enfuvirtide, 145*t*
Enoxaparin, 139*t*
Enrollment bias, 306*t*
Enuresis, 108
Eosinophilia, 136
Eosinophilic granulomatosis with polyangiitis, 28
Epididymitis, 106–107
Epidural hematoma, 182–183, 183*f*
Epiglottitis, 53, 54*f*, 292*t*
Epilepsy, 193
    eclampsia compared with, 266
Epinephrine, 167*t*
    for anaphylaxis, 137
Eplerenone, 15, 91*t*

Epstein-Barr virus (EBV), 141
Eptifibatide, 139*t*
    for myocardial infarction, 8*t*, 9
Erb-Duchenne palsy, 209*t*
Error, 309
ERV. *See* Expiratory reserve volume
Erythema chronicum migrans, 212, 213*f*
Erythema multiforme, 230
Erythema nodosum, 233
Erythematous nodules, 233
Esmolol, 14*t*, 23*t*
Esophageal cancer, 64–65, 64*f*
Esophageal spasm, diffuse, 61, 62*f*
Estrogen, in menstrual cycle, 241, 242*t*
Estrogen-progesterone challenge, 246
Ethacrynic acid, 91*t*
Ethanol, on pregnancy, 267*t*
Ethics, 309–311
    end-of-life issues, 310–311
    patient decision-making, 310
    rights of patient, 309–310
Ethosuximide, 186*t*
Ethylene glycol
    alcohol abusers and, 156
    poisoning with, 157*t*
Etravirine, 145*t*
Ewing sarcoma, 218
Exenatide, 112*t*
Exercise, during pregnancy, 261
Exercise stress test, 4
    with echocardiography, 4
Expiratory reserve volume (ERV), 33*f*, 34*t*
Extremity trauma, 164
Exudates, 20
Eye function, 195, 196*f*, 196*t*
Ezetimibe, 6*t*

F
Facial nerve palsy, 189. *See also* Bell's palsy
Factitious disorder, 299–300
Failure to thrive, 89
Falsification, 299
Familial adenomatous polyposis (FAP), 76, 76*t*
Familial hypocalciuric hypercalcemia, 104
Fanconi anemia, 151
FAP. *See* Familial adenomatous polyposis
Fasciocutaneous flap, 237*t*
Fasciotomy, 164
Febrile seizures, 193
Femur fracture, 205*t*
Fenofibrate, 6*t*
Fertilization, 241*f*, 242
Fertilizer poisoning, 157*t*
Fetal circulation, 29–30, 29*f*
Fetal demise, intrauterine, 271
Fetal development, 260, 260*f*
Fetal distress, 275
Fetal lung maturity, 272
Fetal scalp blood sampling, 275
Fetal scalp monitoring, 275
Fever, postoperative, 169–170, 169*t*, 170*f*
FFP. *See* Fresh frozen plasma
Fibrates, 6*t*
Fibrin clot, 137, 138*f*
Fibroadenoma, 257
Fibrocystic changes, breast, 257
Fibromyalgia, 216–217
Fick principle, 2
Flame hemorrhages, 23
Flecainide, 14*t*
Fluids, in pregnancy, 262*t*
Flumazenil, 297
Flunisolide, 42*t*
Fluoroquinolones, 92
    teratogenic effects of, 268*t*
Focal segmental glomerular sclerosis, 97*t*

Focused abdominal sonography for trauma (FAST), 163
Folate-deficiency anemia, 128t, 131
Folate, in pregnancy, 262t
Follicle-stimulating hormone (FSH), 118, 119f, 120, 120t
  in menstrual cycle, 241–242, 242t
Follicular cyst, ovarian, 255t
Follicular phase, 241f, 242
Footling breech, 278, 278f
Forced expiratory flow rate (FEF), 33
Forced expiratory volume (FEV), 33
Foreign body, aspiration of, 155
Formoterol, 42t
45XO karyotype, 290, 290t
Fosamprenavir, 145t
Fractures, 204, 205t
Fragile X syndrome, 291–292
Frank breech, 278, 278f
Frank-Starling relationship, 14
FRC. See Functional reserve capacity
Fresh frozen plasma (FFP), 167t
Frontotemporal dementia, 201
Fs, 5, 80
FSH. See Follicle-stimulating hormone
Full disclosure, 310
Full integrated test, 263t
Full-thickness epidermal necrosis, 230, 231f
Full-thickness graft, 237t
Functional reserve capacity (FRC), 33f, 34t
Functional vital capacity (FVC), 33f, 34t
Fungal infections, 228, 229f, 229t
Fungal meningitis, 177, 177t
Furosemide, 91t
Fusion inhibitor, 145t
FVC. See Functional vital capacity

G

Gabapentin, 186t
Galeazzi fracture, 205t
Galeazzi sign, 219
Gallbladder
  calcified, 82
  cancer, 81–82
Gallstones, 80–81, 81f
  obstruction of cystic duct, 80
Gangrene, 225
Gardner syndrome, 76, 76t
Gastric cancer, 67
Gastric conditions, 65–67
  gastritis, 65–66, 65t
  hiatal hernia, 65
  peptic ulcer disease, 66, 66t
  Zollinger-Ellison syndrome, 66–67
Gastric ulcers, 66, 66t
Gastritis, 65–66, 65t
Gastroenteritis
  bacterial, 57t
  viral, 56
Gastroesophageal reflux disease (GERD), 63, 64t
Gastrointestinal bleeding, 77–78, 77f
Gastrointestinal disorders, 56–89
  biliary, 80–84
    cholangitis, 81, 82f
    cholecystitis, acute, 80–81
    cholelithiasis, 80, 81f
    gallbladder cancer, 81–82
    hepatic bilirubin transport, 83–84, 83t
    primary biliary cirrhosis, 82
    primary sclerosing cholangitis, 82–83
  gastric conditions, 65–67
    cancer, 67
    gastritis, 65–66, 65t
    hiatal hernia, 65
    peptic ulcer disease, 66, 66t
    Zollinger-Ellison syndrome, 66–67

hepatic, 84–86
  alcohol-related liver disease, 84
  cirrhosis, 84
  hemochromatosis, 85–86
  neoplasms, 86
  portal hypertension, 84–85, 85f
  Wilson disease, 86
  α_1-antitrypsin deficiency, 86
infections, 56–60, 57t, 58f, 58t, 59f, 59t, 60f, 60t
intestinal conditions, 67–78
  appendicitis, 73
  bowel obstruction, 71, 72f, 73t
  carcinoid tumor, 75–76
  colorectal cancer, 76–77, 76t, 77t
  diarrhea, 69–70, 69f, 70f
  diverticulitis, 75
  diverticulosis, 74, 74f
  GI bleeding, 77–78, 77f
  ileus, 73–74
  inflammatory bowel disease, 71, 71t
  irritable bowel syndrome, 70–71, 70t
  ischemic colitis, 71, 73
  malabsorption disorders, 67–69, 68f
  rectal conditions, 75
  volvulus, 74
oral and esophageal conditions, 61–65
  achalasia, 61, 62f
  diffuse esophageal spasm, 61, 62f
  dysphagia, 61
  esophageal cancer, 64–65, 64f
  gastroesophageal reflux disease, 63, 64t
  salivary gland disorders, 61
  Zenker diverticulum, 61, 63, 63f
pancreatic, 78–80
  cancer, 79–80
  pancreatitis, 78, 78t, 79t
  pseudocyst, 79
pediatric, 86–89
  failure to thrive, 89
  Hirschsprung disease, 87–88
  intussusception, 88
  Meckel diverticulum, 88
  necrotizing enterocolitis, 87
  neonatal jaundice, 88–89
  pyloric stenosis, 87, 88f
  tracheoesophageal fistula, 86–87, 87f
Gastrointestinal infections, 56–60
  gastroenteritis
    bacterial, 57t
    viral, 56
  hepatitis, 59f, 59t, 60f, 60t
  parasitic and protozoan, 58f, 58t
GCS. See Glasgow Coma Scale
Gemfibrozil, 6t
Gender reassignment, 238
Generalized anxiety disorder, 297
Genetic disorders, 289–292
  deletion syndromes, 291, 291t
  fragile X syndrome, 291–292
  of hemoglobin, 133–136
  sex chromosomes, 289–290, 290t
  trisomies, 290–291, 290t
Genital fluids, 226
Genital herpes, 252
Genitourinary disorders, 90–108
  acid-base disorders, 99–100
    acid-base physiology, 99
    anion gap disturbances, 99, 100f, 100t
    mixed disturbances, 100
    renal tubular acidosis, 99, 99t
  bladder and ureteral, 104–105
    bladder cancer, 105
    urinary incontinence, 104–105
    urinary tract infection, 104
  electrolyte disorders, 101–104
    diabetes insipidus, 102
    hypercalcemia, 103

hyperkalemia, 102–103
hypernatremia, 101, 101f
hypocalcemia, 104
hypokalemia, 103, 104f
hyponatremia, 102, 103f
syndrome of inappropriate ADH secretion, 102
glomerular diseases, 95–97
  nephritic syndrome, 95, 96t
  nephrotic syndrome, 95, 97t
kidney, 92–95
  hydronephrosis, 93–94, 93f
  interstitial nephropathy, 95
  nephrolithiasis, 92–93, 92t, 93t
  polycystic kidney disease, 94, 94f
  pyelonephritis, 92
  renal cell carcinoma, 94–95
male reproduction, 105–107
  benign prostatic hyperplasia, 106
  epididymitis, 106–107
  impotence, 107
  infertility, 107
  prostate cancer, 106
  prostatitis, 106
  testicular cancer, 107
  testicular torsion, 107
  urethritis, 105–106
pediatric, 108
  cryptorchidism, 108
  enuresis, 108
  posterior urethral valves, 108
  undescended testes, 108
  urethral displacement, 108
  wilms tumor, 108
renal failure, 97–98
  acute, 97–98
  chronic, 98
  dialysis for, 98
Genitourinary reconstruction, 238
Genitourinary trauma, 163
GERD. See Gastroesophageal reflux disease
Gestational age, 260
Gestational diabetes mellitus, 264–265, 264f
Gestational trophoblastic disease, 280–281
GH. See Growth hormone
Giant cell arteritis, 28
Gigantism, 120
Gilbert disease, 83, 83t
Glasgow Coma Scale (GCS), 161, 161t
Glaucoma, 197–198
Glimepiride, 112t
Glipizide, 112t
Global aphasias, 184t
Glomerular diseases, 95–97
  nephritic syndrome, 95, 96t
  nephrotic syndrome, 95, 97t
Glucagon, 109
Glucagonoma, 80
Glucocorticoid, 122
Glucose intolerance, new onset, 264
Glucose metabolism disorders, 109–114
  diabetes mellitus type I, 109, 110f, 110t, 111t
  diabetes mellitus type II, 109–111, 111t, 112t
  hypoglycemia, 113–114, 114t
Glucose metabolism, normal, 109
Glyburide, 112t
Gonadotropin-releasing hormone (GnRH), 119f
Gonorrhea. See Neisseria gonorrhoeae infection
Goodpasture syndrome, 47, 96t
Gout, 210–211, 210f
Gower maneuver, 223
GP IIb/IIIa inhibitor, for myocardial infarction, 8t, 9
GP IIb/IIIa receptors, 139t
Grafts, skin, 237, 237t
Graft vs. host disease, 173
Granuloma inguinale, 253
Granulomatosis with polyangiitis, 47–48, 96t
Grasp reflex, 284t

Growth hormone (GH), 118, 119f, 120, 120t
Growth hormone-releasing hormone (GHRH), 119f
Growth in children, 282–283
Guillain-Barré syndrome, 189
Gunshot wounds, 160
Gynecologic development, 239
    by age, 239, 239t
    of female breast, 239, 240t
    hormone and oogonia levels by age in, 239, 240f
    of pubic hair, 239, 240t
Gynecologic infections, 249–250
    toxic shock syndrome, 249–250
    vaginitis, 249, 249t, 250f
Gynecologic neoplasms, 253–256
    benign ovarian tumors, 255–256, 255t
    cervical cancer, 254–255, 254t
    endometrial cancer, 253–254
    ovarian cancer, 256
    uterine fibroids, 253

H

HAART. See Highly active antiretroviral treatment
Haemophilus influenzae, meningitis and, 177
Haemophilus influenzae type B (Hib) vaccine
    childhood, 283, 286t
    epiglottitis and, 53
Hairy cell leukemia, 149, 150f
Hallucinations, 293
Hallucinogens, 303t
    on pregnancy, 267t
Hashimoto thyroiditis, 116
hCG. See Human chorionic gonadotropin
HDL. See High-density lipoprotein
Headache, 179, 179t
Head circumference, in children, 282–283
Head trauma, 161
Health maintenance, in children, 283, 285–286t
Heart
    anatomy of, 1, 1f
    physiology of, 14–15
Heart block, 9, 10f
Heart death, 311
Heart failure, 14–16
    congestive, 15, 16f
    diastolic dysfunction, 15
    systolic dysfunction, 15
Heart rate (HR), 2
Heart transplantation, 172t
Heat exhaustion/stroke, 155, 155t
Heberden nodes, 213
Height, in children, 282
Heimlich maneuver, 155
HELLP syndrome, 140t, 266
Hemangioblastoma, 94
Hematochezia, 76, 77, 77f
Hematology, 126–152
    anaphylaxis, 137
    anemias, 126–133
        aplastic, 132–133
        of chronic disease, 130t, 132
        folate-deficiency, 128t, 131
        hemolytic, 128, 128t, 129t
        iron-deficiency, 128–130, 128t, 130t, 131f
        lead poisoning, 128t, 130–131, 130t, 131f
        vitamin B₁₂ deficiency, 128t, 132, 132f
    clotting disorders, 137–141
        disseminated intravascular coagulation, 140–141
        hemophilia, 139–140
        thrombocytopenia, 138, 140t
        vitamin K deficiency, 139
        von Willebrand disease, 138
    genetic disorders of hemoglobin, 133–136
        sickle cell disease, 135–136, 135f
        sideroblastic anemia, 128t, 130t, 133, 133f
        thalassemia, 130t, 133–135, 134f, 134t

infections, 141–146
    human immunodeficiency virus, 142–146, 143–144t, 144f, 145t
    malaria, 141, 142f
    mononucleosis, 141–142
    sepsis, 141
leukocyte disorders, 136–137
    anaphylaxis, 136
    eosinophilia, 136
    hypersensitivity reactions, 136–137
    lymphopenia without immune deficiency, 136
    neutropenia, 136
leukocyte hypersensitivity reactions, 136–137, 137t
neoplastic conditions, 146–150
    leukemia, 146–150, 148f, 149f, 150f
    lymphoma, 146, 147f, 147t
    multiple myeloma, 146
    polycythemia vera, 146
pediatric disorders, 151–152
    Diamond-Blackfan anemia, 151–152
    Fanconi anemia, 151
    neuroblastoma, 152
    rhabdomyosarcoma, 152
Hematoma
    epidural, 182–183, 183f
    subdural, 183–184, 183f
Hematuria, 93t
Hemiballismus, 190t
Hemochromatosis, 85–86
Hemodialysis, 98
Hemodynamically unstable patient with blunt trauma, 163
Hemodynamic stability, 166–167, 167t
    transfusions, 166–167, 167t
    vasoactive medications, 167, 167t
Hemoglobin A₁c, 109
Hemoglobin disorders, genetic, 133–136
    sickle cell disease, 135–136, 135f
    sideroblastic anemia, 128t, 130t, 133, 133f
    thalassemia, 130t, 133–135, 134f, 134t
Hemoglobin-oxygen dissociation curve, 126, 126f
Hemolytic anemia, 128, 128t, 129t
Hemolytic disease of newborn, 151, 292t
Hemophilia, 139–140
Hemorrhage
    headache and, 179
    parenchymal, 181–182
    retinal, 199
    subarachnoid, 94
Hemorrhoids, 75
Hemothorax, 51
Henoch-Schönlein purpura, 29
Heparin, 48
    low molecular weight, 48, 138, 139t
    for myocardial infarction, 8t
    poisoning with, 157t
    PTT monitoring of, 138
    teratogenic effects of, 268t
Heparin-induced thrombocytopenia (HIT), 140t
Hepatic bilirubin transport disorders, 83–84, 83t
Hepatic concerns, in preoperative assessment, 168–169
Hepatic disorders, 84–86
    alcohol-related liver disease, 84
    cirrhosis, 84
    hemochromatosis, 85–86
    neoplasms, 86
    portal hypertension, 84–85, 85f
    Wilson disease, 86
    α₁-antitrypsin deficiency, 86
Hepatic neoplasms, 86
Hepatic shunting, 85
Hepatic transplantation, 172t
Hepatitis, 59f, 59t, 60f, 60t, 84
    hepatitis A virus, 56, 59t
    hepatitis B virus, 56, 59f, 59t, 60t

hepatitis C virus, 56, 59t, 60f
hepatitis D virus, 59t
hepatitis E virus, 59t
    in pregnancy, 269t
Hepatocellular carcinoma, 86, 94
Herald patch, 232, 232f
Hereditary nonpolyposis colorectal cancer (HNPCC), 76t
Hernia, hiatal, 65
Herniation, 206
Herpes simplex virus (HSV), 226, 227f
    in pregnancy, 269t
Heterosexual precocious puberty, 240
HHNS. See Hyperosmolar hyperglycemic nonketotic syndrome
Hiatal hernia, 65
Hib. See Haemophilus influenzae type B
High-density lipoprotein (HDL), 5
Highly active antiretroviral treatment (HAART), 145, 145t
Hip dislocations, 204
Hip fracture, 205t
Hirschsprung disease, 87–88
Histrionic cluster, 301t
HIT. See Heparin-induced thrombocytopenia
HIV. See Human immunodeficiency virus
HMG-CoA reductase inhibitors, 6t
    for myocardial infarction, 8t, 9
HNPCC. See Hereditary nonpolyposis colorectal cancer
Hoarding disorder, 298
Hodgkin disease, 146, 147f
Homan sign, 27
Hormonal methods of contraception, 243–244t
Hormone replacement therapy, breast cancer and, 257, 259
Horner syndrome, 44, 179t, 196t
Hot flashes, 243
HPV. See Human papillomavirus
HR. See Heart rate
Hs, 7, 48
HSV. See Herpes simplex virus
HTN. See Hypertension
Human bite, 156, 156t
Human chorionic gonadotropin (hCG), in menstrual cycle, 241, 242t
Human immunodeficiency virus (HIV), 142–146
    antiviral medications for, 145, 145t
    opportunistic infections with, 142, 143–144t
    in pregnancy, 269t
    serologic profile of, 144, 144f
Human papillomavirus (HPV), 228, 252, 252f
Humerus fracture, 205t
Huntington disease, 187–188, 190t
Hydatidiform mole, 280
Hydralazine, 23t, 24t
Hydrocephalus
    childhood, 193
    normal pressure, 201
Hydrochlorothiazide, 91t
Hydronephrosis, 93–94, 93f
Hydroxychloroquine, 173t
Hyperactivity, 304
Hyperaldosteronism, 121–122
Hyperbilirubinemia, 88
Hypercalcemia, 103, 117
Hypercoagulability, 138
Hyperemesis gravidarum, 266
Hyper-IgE disease, 289t
Hyper IgM disease, 288t
Hyperkalemia, 102–103
Hyperkinetic disorders, 189, 190t
Hypernatremia, 101, 101f
Hyperopia, 196t
Hyperosmolar hyperglycemic nonketotic syndrome (HHNS), 112

Hyperparathyroidism, 117–118, 124t
Hyperprolactinemia, 118
Hypersensitivity reactions
 leukocyte, 136–137, 137t
 of skin, 229–230, 230f
Hypersomnia, 191
Hypertension (HTN), 22–25
 with bradycardia, 161
 hypertensive urgency, 24–25
 portal, 84–85, 85f
 primary, 22–23, 23t, 24t
 pulmonary, 48
 secondary, 24, 25t
Hypertensive emergency, 24
Hypertensive urgency, 24–25
Hyperthermia, 155
 malignant, 171
Hyperthyroidism, 114, 115t, 190t
Hypertrophic cardiomyopathy, 18f, 19t
Hypocalcemia, 104, 116
Hypoglycemia, 113–114, 114t
Hypokalemia, 103, 104f
Hypomania, 296
Hypomanic episode, 296
Hyponatremia, 102, 103f
Hypoparathyroidism, 118
Hypopituitarism, 120–121, 120t
Hypothalamic disorders, 118–121, 119f
Hypothermia, 155, 156f
Hypothyroidism, 116
Hypovolemic shock, 26t
Hypoxia, chronic, 146
Hysterectomy, 253

I

IBD. See Inflammatory bowel disease
IBS. See Irritable bowel syndrome
IC. See Inspiratory capacity
ICP. See Increased intracranial pressure
ICU. See Intensive care unit
Idiopathic pulmonary fibrosis (IPF), 46
IgA antibodies, in breast milk, 279
IgA deficiency, 288t
Ileus, 73–74
Illness anxiety disorder, 299
Immune disorders, pediatric, 287–289
 congenital, 287, 288–289t
Immune thrombocytopenia (ITP), 140t
Immunosuppressive drugs, for transplantation, 172, 173t
Impacted stones, 92
Impetigo, 225, 226f
Impotence, 107
Impulsivity, 304
Inattention, 304
Incidence, 306
Incomplete breech, 278, 278f
Increased intracranial pressure (ICP), 177
Incretin mimetics, 112t
Infections
 with burns, 154
 congenital, 268, 269t
 dermatology, 224–229, 224f, 226f, 227f, 227t, 228f, 229f, 229t
 ear, 200
 eye, 197
 gastrointestinal, 56–60, 57t, 58f, 58t, 59f, 59t, 60f, 60t
 gynecologic, 249–250, 249t, 250f
 musculoskeletal, 212t, 213f
 myocardial, 20–22, 21f, 22t
 neurologic, 177–179, 177t
 respiratory
  lower, 36f, 37–40
  upper, 35–37, 36f
 with transplantation, 172
 urinary tract, 104

Infertility
 male, 107
 with transplantation, 172
Inflamed conjunctiva, 197
Inflammation, eye, 197
Inflammatory bowel disease (IBD), 71, 71t
Inflammatory carcinoma, 258t
Inflammatory conditions of skin, 229–233
 atopic dermatitis, 231, 232f
 erythema multiforme, 230
 erythema nodosum, 233
 hypersensitivity reactions, 229–230, 230f
 pityriasis rosea, 232–233, 232f
 psoriasis, 231–232, 232f
 seborrheic dermatitis, 231
 Stevens-Johnson syndrome, 230
 toxic epidermal necrolysis, 230–231, 231f
Informed consent, 305, 309–310
Injury. See Accidents and injury
Inotropes, 167, 167t
INR. See International normalized ratio
Insecticide poisoning, 157t
Inspiratory capacity (IC), 33f, 34t
Inspiratory reserve volume (IRV), 33f, 34t
Insulin, 109
Insulinomas, 80
Insulin resistance, with acromegaly, 120
Insulin therapy, 110f, 111t
Integrase inhibitor, 145t
Intensive care unit (ICU), 165–166
Internal carotid artery, 174t
International normalized ratio (INR), 138
Internuclear ophthalmoplegia, 196
Interstitial lung diseases, 46–48, 47t
 Goodpasture syndrome, 47
 granulomatosis with polyangiitis, 47–48
 idiopathic pulmonary fibrosis (IPF), 46
 pneumoconioses, 46–47, 47t
 sarcoidosis, 46
Interstitial nephropathy, 95
Intertrigo, 229t
Intestinal conditions, 67–78
 appendicitis, 73, 171t
 bowel obstruction, 71, 72f, 73t
 carcinoid tumor, 75–76
 colorectal cancer, 76–77, 76t, 77t
 diarrhea, 69–70, 69f, 70f
 diverticulitis, 75
 diverticulosis, 74, 74f
 GI bleeding, 77–78, 77f
 ileus, 73–74
 inflammatory bowel disease, 71, 71t
 irritable bowel syndrome, 70–71, 70t
 ischemic colitis, 71, 73
 malabsorption disorders, 67–69, 68f
 rectal conditions, 75
 volvulus, 74
Intoxication, 302
Intraductal papilloma, 257
Intrauterine devices (IUDs), 245t
Intrauterine devices of contraception, 245t
Intrauterine fetal demise, 271
Intrauterine growth restriction (IUGR), 271
Intravaginal ring, 244t
Intravenous pyelogram (IVP), 163
Intubation, 52, 165
Intussusception, 88, 292t
Invasive ductal carcinoma, 258t
Invasive lobular carcinoma, 258t
Invasive monitoring, in ICU, 166
Investigator bias, 306t
IPF. See Idiopathic pulmonary fibrosis
Ipratropium, 42t
Irbesartan, 23t
Iron
 chelation, 135
 poisoning, 157t
 in pregnancy, 262t

Irritable bowel syndrome (IBS), 70–71, 70t
IRV. See Inspiratory reserve volume
Ischemic colitis, 71, 73
Ischemic heart disease, 4–9
 angina pectoris, 6
 atherosclerosis, 4–5, 4f
 coronary artery disease, 4
 dyslipidemia, 5, 6t
 myocardial hypoxia, 4
 myocardial infarction, 7–9, 7f, 8t
 reproducible angina, 4
 unstable angina, 6–7
Ischemic stroke
 embolic, 180
 thrombotic, 180
Isoniazid poisoning, 157t
Isopropyl alcohol poisoning, 157t
Isoproterenol, 167t
Isosexual precocious puberty, 240
Isotretinoin, 226
IUDs. See Intrauterine devices
IUGR. See Intrauterine growth restriction

J

Janeway lesions, 22
Jaundice
 neonatal, 88–89
 prolonged, 125
Job syndrome, 289t
Jones criteria, 21, 21f
JRA. See Juvenile idiopathic arthritis
Juvenile idiopathic arthritis (JRA), 222t
Juvenile onset diabetes, 109, 110f, 110t, 111t
Juvenile polyposis, 76t

K

Kawasaki disease, 28
Kayser-Fleischer rings, 86
Kerley B lines, 15
Kernicterus, 89
Kernig signs, 177
Kidney disorders, 92–95
 hydronephrosis, 93–94, 93f
 interstitial nephropathy, 95
 nephrolithiasis, 92–93, 92t, 93t
 polycystic kidney disease, 94, 94f
 pyelonephritis, 92
 renal cell carcinoma, 94–95
Kidney function, 90, 90f
Klinefelter syndrome, 290t
Klumpke palsy, 209t
Kussmaul sign, 20

L

Labetalol, 24t
Labor and delivery, 275–281
 assessment of fetal well-being, 275, 276f, 276t
 caesarean section, 279
 fetal heart rate in, 275, 276f, 276t
 induction of, 277, 278t
 malpresentation, 278, 278f
 normal puerperium and postpartum activity, 279, 279t
 postpartum bleeding, 280
 preterm, 272–273
 stages of, 277, 277t
Lactase dehydrogenase (LDH), 7
Lactation, 244t
Lactose intolerance, 69
Lambert-Eaton syndrome, 188
Lamivudine (3TC), 145t
Lamotrigine, 186t
Large cell carcinoma, lung, 44t, 45t
Laryngeal cancer, 46
Latent syphilis, 251

Lateral meniscus tear, 204
LCIS. *See* Lobular carcinoma in situ
LDH. *See* Lactate dehydrogenase
LDL. *See* Low-density lipoprotein
Lead poisoning anemia, 128t, 130–131, 130t, 131f, 157t
Lead-time bias, 306t
Left anterior descending artery, 1, 1f
Left ventricular hypertrophy (LVH), 15
Left ventricular pressure-volume loop, 2f
Legg-Calvé-Perthes disease, 220
Length bias, 306t
Lentigo maligna, 236
Leopold maneuvers, 263
Lepirudin, 139t
Leukemia, 146–150, 292t
    acute lymphocytic, 146–147, 148f
    acute myelogenous, 148
    acute promyelocytic, 148f
    chronic lymphocytic, 148–149, 149f
    chronic myelogenous, 149
    hairy cell, 149, 150f
Leukocoria, 195, 195f
Leukocyte adhesion deficiency, 289t
Leukocyte disorders, 136–137
    anaphylaxis, 136
    eosinophilia, 136
    hypersensitivity reactions, 136–137, 137t
    lymphopenia without immune deficiency, 136
    neutropenia, 136
Levetiracetam, 186t
Levodopa, 187t
Lewy bodies, dementia with, 201
LH. *See* Luteinizing hormone
Libman-Sacks endocarditis, 21
Lidocaine, 14t
Life support, 310
Ligament tears, 204
Likelihood ratios, 308–309
Linagliptin, 112t
Liraglutide, 112t
Lisch nodules, 191
Lisinopril, 23t
Lithium, teratogenic effects of, 268t
Liver metastases, 86
Liver transplantation, 172t
Living will, 310
LMN disease, 187
LMWH. *See* Low molecular weight heparin
Lobular carcinoma in situ (LCIS), 258, 258t
Loop diuretics, 91, 91t, 104
Lopinavir, 145t
Losartan, 23t
Loss of consciousness, 161
Lovastatin, 6t
Low-density lipoprotein (LDL), 5
Lower respiratory infections, 36f, 37–40
    bronchitis, acute, 37
    pneumonia, 37, 38t, 39f, 39t
    tuberculosis, 37–38, 40f, 40t
Low molecular weight heparin (LMWH), 48, 138, 139t, 169
Lumpectomy, 258
Lung cancer, 44–46, 44t, 45t
Lung transplantation, 172t
Lung volume measurement, 33, 33f, 34f, 34t
Lupus nephritis, 96t
Luteal phase, 241f, 242
Luteinizing hormone (LH), 118, 119f, 120t, 121
    in menstrual cycle, 241–242, 242t
LVH. *See* Left ventricular hypertrophy
Lyme disease, 212, 213f
Lymphogranuloma venereum, 252–253
Lymphoid cell line development, 126, 127f
Lymphoma, 146, 147f, 147t
Lymphopenia without immune deficiency, 136

M
Macular degeneration, 198
Major depressive disorder (MDD), 293, 294–295, 295t
Malabsorption disorders, 67–69, 68f
Malaria, 141, 142f
Male reproductive disorders, 105–107
    benign prostatic hyperplasia, 106
    epididymitis, 106–107
    impotence, 107
    infertility, 107
    prostate cancer, 106
    prostatitis, 106
    testicular cancer, 107
    testicular torsion, 107
    urethritis, 105–106
Malignant hyperthermia, 171
Malignant mesothelioma, 51
Malpresentation, fetal, 278, 278f
Mammal bite, 156, 156t
Mammogram, 257
Manic episode, 296
Mannitol, 91t
MAOIs. *See* Monoamine oxidase inhibitors
Maraviroc, 145t
Marcus Gunn pupil, 196t
Marijuana, 303t
    on pregnancy, 267t
Mastectomy, 258
MAT. *See* Multifocal atrial tachycardia
Maternal asthma, 266
Maternal deep venous thrombosis, 267
Maternal drug use, 267–268, 267t, 268t
Maternal nausea and vomiting, 266
Maternal physiology, 260, 261t
Maternal seizures, 266
MCA. *See* Middle cerebral artery
MCL. *See* Medial collateral ligament
MCTD. *See* Mixed connective tissue disease
MCV. *See* Mean corpuscular volume
Mean arterial pressure, 2
Mean corpuscular volume (MCV), 128, 128t
Mechanical ventilation, 52
Meckel diverticulum, 88
Meconium aspiration syndrome, 55
Medial collateral ligament (MCL) tear, 204
Medial longitudinal fasciculus (MLF), 195
Medroxyprogesterone acetate, 243t
Medullary carcinoma, 258t
Medullary thyroid cancer, 116t, 124t
Meglitinides, 112t
Melanocyte-stimulating hormone (MSH), 120t, 121
Melanocytic nevi, 236, 237f
Melanoma, 235–237, 236f, 237f
Membranoproliferative glomerulonephritis, 97t
Membranous nephropathy, 97t
MEN. *See* Multiple endocrine neoplasia
Menarche, 239
Ménière disease, 200
Meningitis
    bacterial, 177, 177t
    fungal, 177, 177t
    viral, 177t, 178
Meningocele, 193
Meniscus tears, 204
Menopause, 242–243
Menorrhagia, 253
Menstrual cycle, normal, 241–242, 241f, 242t
Menstrual disorders, 245–249
    abnormal uterine bleeding, 248
    amenorrhea, 239t, 245–247, 246f
    dysmenorrhea, 247
    endometriosis, 247–248
    polycystic ovary syndrome, 248–249
    premenstrual syndrome, 247
Menstrual irregularity, 243
Menstrual physiology, 239–243
    gynecologic development, 239, 239t, 240f, 240t
    menopause, 242–243

menstrual cycle, normal, 241–242, 241f, 242t
    precocious puberty, 240–241
Mercury poisoning, 157t
Mesenteric ischemia, 171t
Mesothelioma, malignant, 51
Meta-analysis, 305t
Metabolic acidosis, 100t, 126
Metabolic alkalosis, 100f, 100t, 126
Metabolic bone diseases
    gout, 210–211, 210f
    osteogenesis imperfecta, 210
    osteopetrosis, 209
    osteoporosis, 209
    Paget disease of bone, 210
    pseudogout, 211, 211f
Metal poisoning, 157t
Metastases
    bone, 218
    CNS, 190
    liver, 86
Metformin, 112t
Methanol poisoning, 157t
Methyldopa, 24t
Methylprednisolone, 42t
Metolazone, 91t
Metoprolol, 14t, 23t
    for CHF, 15
MI. *See* Myocardial infarction
Middle cerebral artery (MCA), 174f, 175t, 180, 180f
Middle meningeal artery, 182
Milestones, developmental, 283, 284t
Mineralocorticoid, 122
Minerals, absorption of, 68f
Minimal change disease, 97t
Minoxidil, 23t
Mirtazapine, 295t
Mitral regurgitation, 16f, 17t
Mitral stenosis, 16f, 17t
Mitral valve prolapse, 16f
Mixed connective tissue disease (MCTD), 214t, 217–218
MLF syndrome, 196t
Molluscum contagiosum, 228, 252
Monitoring, invasive, in ICU, 166
Monoamine oxidase inhibitors (MAOIs), 295t
Monoarthritis, 212
Mononucleosis, 141–142
Monozygotic twinning, 274
Monteggia fracture, 205t
Montelukast, 42t
Mood disorders, 294–296, 295t
    bipolar disorder, 296
    cyclothymic disorder, 296
    major depressive disorder, 294–295, 295t
    persistent depressive disorder, 295–296
Mood stabilizers, 296
Moon facies, 121
Moro reflex, 284t
Morphine, for myocardial infarction, 8t
Mosaicism, 290, 290t
Motor neurons, 175, 175f, 175t
Motor neuropathy, 113
Motor vehicle accidents, 160
MS. *See* Multiple sclerosis
MSH. *See* Melanocyte-stimulating hormone
Mucinous carcinoma, 258t
Mucinous cystadenoma, ovarian, 255t
Mucosal neuromas, 124t
Multifocal atrial tachycardia (MAT), 11, 12f
Multiple endocrine neoplasia (MEN), 124, 124t
Multiple gestations, 274
Multiple myeloma, 146
Multiple sclerosis (MS), 188
Münchausen syndrome, 299–300
Murmurs, 16f
Muromonab-D3 (OKT3), 173t
Murphy sign, 80
Muscle flap, 237t

Musculoskeletal disorders, 203–223
  carpal tunnel syndrome, 203, 203*f*
  compartment syndrome, 204
  fractures, 204, 205*t*
  hip dislocations, 204
  infection, 211–212
    Lyme disease, 212, 213*f*
    osteomyelitis, 212
    septic joint and septic arthritis,
      211–212, 212*t*
  ligament tears, 204
  meniscus tears, 204
  metabolic bone diseases, 209–211
    gout, 210–211, 210*f*
    osteogenesis imperfecta, 210
    osteopetrosis, 209
    osteoporosis, 209
    Paget disease of bone, 210
    pseudogout, 211, 211*f*
  neoplasms, 218–219
    bone metastases, 218
    Ewing sarcoma, 218
    osteochondroma, 219
    osteosarcoma, 218, 219*f*
  osteoarthritis, 213–214, 213*f*
  pediatric, 219–223
    clavicular fracture, 221
    club foot, 220
    developmental dysplasia of hip, 219–220
    Duchenne muscular dystrophy, 222–223
    juvenile idiopathic arthritis, 222, 222*t*
    Legg-Calvé-Perthes disease, 220
    nursemaid's elbow, 221
    Osgood-Schlatter disease, 220
    physeal fractures, 220, 221*t*
    rickets, 221
    scoliosis, 221–222
    slipped capital femoral epiphysis, 220
  rheumatologic diseases, 214–218
    ankylosing spondylitis, 214*t*, 217
    dermatomyositis, 214*t*, 216
    fibromyalgia, 216–217
    mixed connective tissue disease, 214*t*,
      217–218
    polymyalgia rheumatica, 216
    polymyositis, 214*t*, 216
    psoriatic arthritis, 214*t*, 217
    rheumatoid arthritis, 214–215, 214*t*
    scleroderma, 214*t*, 217
    Sjögren syndrome, 214*t*, 218
    systemic lupus erythematosus, 214*t*,
      215–216, 215*f*
  shoulder dislocations, 204
  spine, 206–208
    back pain, 206, 206*f*
    brachial plexus, 208, 208*f*, 209*t*
    cauda equina syndrome, 208
    degenerative disc disease, 206–207,
      207*f*, 207*t*
    spinal stenosis, 207–208
  sprains, 204
Myasthenia gravis, 188–189
Mycophenolic acid, 173*t*
Mycoplasma pneumoniae, 38*t*
Myeloid cell line development, 126, 127*f*
Myelomeningocele, 193
Myocardial hypoxia, 4
Myocardial infarction (MI), 7–9, 7*f*, 8*t*
  ECG of, 6, 7*f*, 8*t*
  ST-elevation, 9
Myocardial infections, 20–22, 21*f*, 22*t*
  endocarditis, 21–22, 22*t*
  myocarditis, 20–21
  rheumatic fever, acute, 21, 21*f*
Myocardial ischemia
  in DM, 6
  temporary, 6

Myocarditis, 20–21
Myomectomy, 253
Myopia, 196*t*

N

Naegele's rule, 260
Narcissistic cluster, 301*t*
Narcolepsy, 191
Nateglinide, 112*t*
Nausea and vomiting, maternal, 266
Neck trauma, 162, 162*f*
Necrotizing enterocolitis, 87
Necrotizing fasciitis, 225
Negatively birefringent crystals, 210, 210*f*
Negative predictive value (NPV), 308, 308*t*
Neglect, 164, 165
Negri bodies, 179
Neisseria gonorrhoeae infection, 197, 250
  in pregnancy, 269*t*
Neonatal jaundice, 88–89
Neoplasms. *See specific neoplasm*
Nephritic syndrome, 95, 96*t*
Nephrolithiasis, 92–93, 92*t*, 93*t*
Nephrotic syndrome, 95, 97*t*, 114
Nerve impingement, 206
Neural tube disorders, 193–194, 292*t*
Neuroblastoma, 152
Neurofibromas, 191
Neurofibromatosis type 1, 191
Neurogenic shock, 26*t*
Neuroleptics. *See* Antipsychotics
Neurologic disorders, 174–202
  cerebrovascular and hemorrhagic diseases,
      179–184
    aphasias, 184, 184*t*
    epidural hematoma, 182–183, 183*f*
    parenchymal hemorrhage, 181–182
    stroke, 180–181, 180*f*, 181*t*
    subarachnoid hemorrhage, 182, 182*f*
    subdural hematoma, 183–184, 183*f*
    transient ischemic attack, 179–180
  coma, 192, 192*f*
  degenerative, 186–188
    amyotrophic lateral sclerosis, 187
    Huntington disease, 187–188
    multiple sclerosis, 188
    Parkinson disease, 186–187
    syringomyelia, 188
  headache, 179, 179*t*
  infections, 177–179
    bacterial meningitis, 177, 177*t*
    brain abscess, 178
    encephalitis, 178
    poliomyelitis, 178
    rabies, 178–179
    viral meningitis, 177*t*, 178
  neoplasms, 190–191
    metastatic CNS, 190
    neurofibromatosis type 1, 191
    primary CNS, 190
  pediatric, 193–195
    cerebral palsy, 194
    childhood hydrocephalus, 193
    febrile seizures, 193
    neural tube disorders, 193–194
    retinoblastoma, 195, 195*f*
    Tay-Sachs disease, 193
  peripheral, 188–189, 190*t*
  seizure disorders, 184–186
    causes of, 184, 185*t*
    status epilepticus, 184, 186
    treatment of, 184, 186*t*
    types of, 184, 185*t*, 186*t*
  sleep, 191
  syncope, 191–192
Neurologic organization, 175*f*, 175–176, 175*t*, 176*t*

Neutropenia, 136
Niacin, 6*t*
Nicotine, 303*t*
Nifedipine, 23*t*, 24*t*
Nipple discharge, 257
Nitroglycerin
  for angina pectoris, 6
  for myocardial infarction, 8*t*, 9
Nitroprusside, 23*t*
Non-nucleoside reverse transcriptase
    inhibitors, 145*t*
Nonstress test, 275
Norepinephrine, 167*t*
Normal clotting function, 137–138, 138*f*
Nuclear exercise test, 4
Nucleoside reverse transcriptase inhibitors, 145*t*
Null hypothesis, 309
Nulliparity, 265
Number needed to treat (NNT), 308
Nursemaid's elbow, 221
Nutrients
  absorption of, 68*f*
  birth defects and, 261, 262*t*
Nutrition
  pregnancy needs, 261
  for prenatal care, 261, 262*t*

O

OA. *See* Osteoarthritis
Obesity
  DM type II and, 110
  osteoporosis and, 209
Observational bias, 306*t*
Obsessions, 298
Obsessive-compulsive cluster, 301*t*
Obsessive-compulsive disorders (OCD), 298
  body dysmorphic disorder, 298
  hoarding disorder, 298
Obstetrics, 260–281
  activity during, 261
  gestational trophoblastic disease, 280–281
  labor and delivery, 275–281
    assessment of fetal well-being, 275,
      276*f*, 276*t*
    caesarean section, 279
    induction of, 277, 278*t*
    malpresentation, 278, 278*f*
    normal puerperium and postpartum activity,
      279, 279*t*
    postpartum bleeding, 280
    stages of, 277, 277*t*
  maternal physiology in, 260, 261*t*
  medical complications of pregnancy, 264–269
    congenital infections, 268, 269*t*
    eclampsia, 266
    gestational diabetes mellitus, 264–265, 264*f*
    maternal asthma, 266
    maternal deep venous thrombosis, 267
    maternal drug use, 267–268, 267*t*, 268*t*
    maternal nausea and vomiting, 266
    maternal UTIs, 267
    preeclampsia, 265–266
    pregestational diabetes mellitus, 265
  nutritional needs in, 261
  obstetric complications of pregnancy, 270–274
    abruptio placenta, 274
    ectopic pregnancy, 270
    intrauterine fetal demise, 271
    intrauterine growth restriction, 271
    multiple gestations, 274
    oligohydramnios, 271–272
    placenta previa, 273–274, 273*f*
    polyhydramnios, 272
    premature rupture of membranes, 272
    preterm labor, 272–273
    spontaneous abortion, 270–271, 270*t*

pregnancy physiology in, 260, 260f, 261t
prenatal care in, 261–263
nutrition, 261, 262t
visits, 261–263, 262t, 263t
Obstructive airway diseases, 41–42
asthma, 41, 42t, 43t
bronchiectasis, 42
chronic bronchitis, 41
emphysema, 41–42
Occlusion of coronary vessels, 7
OCD. See Obsessive-compulsive disorder
OCPs. See Oral contraceptive pills
Oculomotor nerve (CN III), 195
Odds ratio (OR), 307, 307t
OKT3. See Muromonab-D3
Oligoarthritis, 212
Oligohydramnios, 271–272
Oligoovulation, 248
Oncology therapy, 150, 151t
pediatric disorders, 152
Open angle glaucoma, 197
Ophthalmology, 195–199
cataracts, 197
common vision abnormalities, 195, 196t
glaucoma, 197–198
inflammation and infection, 197
macular degeneration, 198
normal eye function, 195, 196f, 196t
retinal detachment, 198
retinal vessel occlusion, 198–199, 198f, 199f
Opioids, 303t
poisoning with, 157t
on pregnancy, 267t
Oppositional defiant disorder, 304
Optic nerve (CN II), 195
Oral and esophageal conditions, 61–65
achalasia, 61, 62f
diffuse esophageal spasm, 61, 62f
dysphagia, 61
esophageal cancer, 64–65, 64f
gastroesophageal reflux disease, 63, 64t
salivary gland disorders, 61
Zenker diverticulum, 61, 63, 63f
Oral contraceptive pills (OCPs), 243t
Organ donation, 311
Organophosphates, poisoning with, 157, 157t
Orthopaedics. See Musculoskeletal disorders
Ortolani maneuver, 219
Osgood-Schlatter disease, 220
Osler nodes, 22
Osmotic agents, 91t
Osteoarthritis (OA), 213–214, 213f
Osteochondroma, 219
Osteogenesis imperfecta, 210
Osteomalacia, 221
Osteomyelitis, 212
Osteopetrosis, 209
Osteoporosis, 209
estrogen and, 243
Osteosarcoma, 218, 219f
Otitis externa, 200
Otitis media, 200
Ovarian cancer, 256
Ovarian cysts, 248
Ovarian tumors, benign, 255–256, 255t
Overflow incontinence, 105
Oxcarbazepine, 186t
Oxytocin, 118

P

Packed RBCs, 167t
Paget disease, 258t
of bone, 210
Pancoast syndrome, 45
Pancreas endocrine tumors, 124t
Pancreas transplantation, 172t

Pancreatic cancer
endocrine, 80
exocrine, 79–80
Pancreatic disorders, 78–80
cancer, 79–80
pancreatitis, 78, 78t, 79t
pseudocyst, 79
Pancreatic pseudocyst, 79
Pancreatitis, 78, 78t, 79t, 171t
Panic disorder, 296–297
Pannus formation, 214
Papillary thyroid carcinoma, 116t
Pap smears, 254
Paraneoplastic syndromes
with hepatocellular carcinoma, 86
with lung cancer, 44, 44t
with SIADH, 102
Paranoid cluster, 301t
Parasitic infections, 58f, 58t
Parathyroid adenoma, 124t
Parathyroid disorders, 117–118
hyperparathyroidism, 117–118, 124t
hypoparathyroidism, 118
pseudohypoparathyroidism, 118
Parathyroid function, 117, 117f
Parathyroid hormone (PTH), 117, 117f
Parathyroid hyperplasia, 124t
Parenchymal hemorrhage, 181–182
Parkinson disease, 186–187, 190t
Parkland formula, 154
Paroxysmal supraventricular tachycardia (PSVT),
9–11, 10f, 11f
Partial thromboplastin time (PTT), 137
Partner abuse, 165
Parvovirus B19, 269t
Patent ductus arteriosus (PDA), 30, 31f, 292t
Pathognomonic injuries, 164
Patient decision-making, 310
Patient rights, 309–310
Pavlik harness, 220
PBC. See Primary biliary cirrhosis
PCA. See Posterior cerebral artery
PCOS. See Polycystic ovary syndrome
PCP. See Phencyclidine
PDA. See Patent ductus arteriosus; Posterior
descending artery
PE. See Pulmonary embolism
PEA. See Pulseless electrical activity
Pediatric development and health supervision, 282–287
in adolescence, 287, 287t
childhood health maintenance, 283, 285–286t
developmental milestones, 283, 284t
physical growth in, 282–283
Pediatric disorders
cardiovascular, 29–32
atrial septal defect, 30, 31f
endocardial cushion defect, 31f, 32
fetal circulation, 29–30, 29f
patent ductus arteriosus, 30, 31f
persistent truncus arteriosus, 31, 31f
tetralogy of Fallot, 31f, 32
transposition of great vessels, 31f, 32
tricuspid atresia, 32
ventricular septal defect, 30, 31f
endocrine, 125
gastrointestinal, 86–89
failure to thrive, 89
Hirschsprung disease, 87–88
intussusception, 88
Meckel diverticulum, 88
necrotizing enterocolitis, 87
neonatal jaundice, 88–89
pyloric stenosis, 87, 88f
tracheoesophageal fistula, 86–87, 87f
genetic, 289–292
deletion syndromes, 291, 291t
fragile X syndrome, 291–292

sex chromosomes, 289–290, 290t
trisomies, 290–291, 290t
genitourinary, 108
hematologic, 151–152
immune, 287–289
congenital, 287, 288–289t
musculoskeletal, 219–223
clavicular fracture, 221
club foot, 220
developmental dysplasia of hip, 219–220
Duchenne muscular dystrophy, 222–223
juvenile idiopathic arthritis, 222, 222t
Legg-Calvé-Perthes disease, 220
nursemaid's elbow, 221
Osgood-Schlatter disease, 220
physeal fractures, 220, 221t
rickets, 221
scoliosis, 221–222
slipped capital femoral epiphysis, 220
neurologic, 193–194
cerebral palsy, 194
childhood hydrocephalus, 193
febrile seizures, 193
neural tube disorders, 193–194
retinoblastoma, 195, 195f
Tay-Sachs disease, 193
oncology, 152
pulmonary, 53–55
bronchiolitis, 54
croup, 53, 53f
cystic fibrosis, 55
epiglottitis, 53, 54f
meconium aspiration syndrome, 55
respiratory distress syndrome of newborn,
54, 55f
Pediatric psychiatric disorders, 302, 304
attention deficit hyperactivity disorder
(ADHD), 304
autism spectrum disorder, 302
conduct disorder, 304
tourette syndrome, 304
Pelvic fracture, 205t
Pelvic inflammatory disease (PID), 171t, 251
Pelvic trauma, 163
Pemphigus vulgaris, 233, 233f
Penetrating injuries, 160, 163
Pentobarbital, 186t
Peptic ulcer disease (PUD), 66, 66t
Percutaneous transluminal coronary angioplasty
(PTCA), 7
Percutaneous umbilical blood sampling, 263t
Pericardial diseases, 20
Pericarditis
acute, 20
chronic constrictive, 20
Perimenopausal period, 242
Peripheral neurologic disorders, 188–189, 190t
Peripheral vascular disease (PVD), 27
Peritoneal dialysis, 98
Peritonitis, 92
spontaneous bacterial, 85
Peritonsillar abscess, 36
Pernicious anemia, 65
Persistent behaviour, deviates from cultural
norms, 301
Persistent depressive disorder, 295–296
Persistent truncus arteriosus, 31, 31f
Persistent vegetative state, 192
Personality disorders, 301, 301t
clusters, 301, 301t
persistent behaviour, deviates from cultural
norms, 301
Peutz-Jeghers syndrome, 76t
PFTs. See Pulmonary function tests
Phagocytic Cell Disorders, 289t
Phalen sign, 203
Pharmacologic stress testing, 4

Pharyngitis, 35
Phencyclidine, 303t
Phenobarbital, 186t
    teratogenic effects of, 268t
Phenylephrine, 167t
Phenytoin, 186t
    teratogenic effects of, 268t
Pheochromocytoma, 94, 124, 124t
Philadelphia chromosome, 149
Phobia, specific, 297
Physeal fractures, 220, 221t
Physician-aided death, 310
PICA. See Posterior inferior cerebellar artery
Pick disease, 201
PID. See Pelvic inflammatory disease
Pilocarpine, 198
Pilonidal disease, 75
Pink puffers, 41
Pioglitazone, 112t
Pirbuterol, 42t
Pituitary adenoma, 121, 124t
Pituitary disorders, 118–121
    acromegaly, 120
    hyperprolactinemia, 118
    hypopituitarism, 120–121, 120t
Pituitary function, 118, 119f
Pityriasis rosea, 232–233, 232f
Pityriasis versicolor, 229f, 229t
Placental abruption, 164
Placental tissue, retained, 280
Placenta previa, 273–274, 273f
Placing reflex, 284t
Plaque rupture, 6
Plastic surgery, 237–238
    cosmetic surgery, 238
    grafts and flaps, 237, 237t
    reconstructive surgery, 238
Platelets, 137, 167t
Pleural diseases, 49–51
    hemothorax, 51
    malignant mesothelioma, 51
    pleural effusion, 49, 49t
    pneumothorax, 50f, 50–51, 50t
    sleep apnea, 51–52
Pleural effusion, 49, 49t
PMDD. See Premenstrual dysphoric disorder
PMS. See Premenstrual syndrome
Pneumoconioses, 46–47, 47t
Pneumonia, 37, 38t, 39f, 39t
Pneumothorax (PTX), 50f, 50–51, 50t
Podagra, 210, 211
Poisons, 156–158, 157t
Poliomyelitis, 176t, 178
Polyarteritis nodosa, 28
Polycystic kidney disease, 94, 94f, 181
Polycystic ovary syndrome (PCOS), 248–249
Polycythemia vera, 146
Polyhydramnios, 272
Polymyalgia rheumatica, 28, 216
Polymyositis, 214t, 216
Porphyria cutanea tarda, 233–234
Portal hypertension, 84–85, 85f
Positively birefringent, rhomboid crystals, 211, 211f
Positive predictive value (PPV), 308, 308t
Posterior cerebral artery (PCA), 174f, 175t
Posterior communicating artery, 174f
Posterior descending artery (PDA), 1, 1f
Posterior inferior cerebellar artery (PICA), 174f, 175t
Posterior urethral valves, 108
Postinfectious glomerulonephritis, 96t
Postmenopausal bleeding, 253
Postoperative fever, 169–170, 169t, 170f
Postpartum activity, 279, 279t
Postpartum bleeding, 280
Posttraumatic stress disorder (PTSD), 299
Potassium channel blockers, 14t
Potassium-sparing aldosterone antagonists, 91t

Power, 309
Power of attorney, durable, 310
Prader-Willi syndrome, 291t
Pramlintide, 112t
Pravastatin, 6t
Prazosin, 23t
Precocious puberty, 240–241, 292t
Precontemplation, 302
Prednisone, 42t
Preeclampsia, 265–266
Pregestational diabetes mellitus, 265
Pregnancy
    activity during, 261
    congenital disease assessment, 263t
    maternal physiology in, 260, 261t
    medical complications of, 264–269
        congenital infections, 268, 269t
        eclampsia, 266
        gestational diabetes mellitus, 264–265, 264f
        maternal asthma, 266
        maternal deep venous thrombosis, 267
        maternal drug use, 267–268, 267t, 268t
        maternal nausea and vomiting, 266
        maternal UTIs, 267
        preeclampsia, 265–266
        pregestational diabetes mellitus, 265
    nutritional needs in, 261, 262t
    obstetric complications of
        abruptio placenta, 274
        intrauterine fetal demise, 271
        intrauterine growth restriction, 271
        multiple gestations, 274
        oligohydramnios, 271–272
        placenta previa, 273–274, 273f
        polyhydramnios, 272
        premature rupture of membranes, 272
        preterm labor, 272–273
    obstetric complications of pregnancy, 270–274
        ectopic pregnancy, 270
        spontaneous abortion, 270–271, 270t
    physiology of, 260, 260f, 261t
    ruptured ectopic, 171t
    screening labs during, 262t
    trauma during, 164
Preload, 2, 14
Premature rupture of membranes (PROM), 272
Premature ventricular contraction (PVC), 13
Premenstrual dysphoric disorder (PMDD), 247
Premenstrual syndrome (PMS), 247
Prenatal care, 261–263
    nutrition, 261, 262t
    visits, 261–263, 262t, 263t
Preoperative risk assessment, 168–169
Preterm labor, 272–273
Prevalence, 307
Primary biliary cirrhosis (PBC), 82
Primary hypertension, 22–23, 23t, 24t
Primary sclerosing cholangitis (PSC), 82–83
Primary syphilis, 251
Procainamide, 14t
Progesterone, in menstrual cycle, 242, 242t
Progestin challenge, 246
Progestin implant, 243t
Progestin-releasing IUD, 245t
Prolactin, 118, 119f, 120, 120t, 246
Prolactinoma, 118
Prolactin-releasing hormone (PRH), 119f
Prolonged jaundice, 125
PROM. See Premature rupture of membranes
Propafenone, 14t
Propanolol, 14t, 23t
Prostate cancer, 106
Prostatitis, 106
Protease inhibitors, 145t
Protein, in pregnancy, 262t
Prothrombin time (PT), 137
Protozoan infections, 58f, 58t

Proximal convoluted tubule, 90, 90f
Ps
    3, 124
    6, 27, 204
PSC. See Primary sclerosing cholangitis
Pseudogout, 211, 211f
Pseudohyperkalemia, 103
Pseudohypertrophy, 223
Pseudohyponatremia, 102
Pseudohypoparathyroidism, 118
Psoriasis, 231–232, 232f
Psoriatic arthritis, 214t, 217, 231
PSVT. See Paroxysmal supraventricular tachycardia
Psychiatric disorders, 293–304
    anxiety disorders, 296–297, 297t
        generalized, 297
        panic disorder, 296–297
        social, 297
        specific phobia, 297
    eating disorders, 300
        anorexia nervosa, 300
        binge eating disorder, 300
        bulimia nervosa, 300
    mood disorders, 294–296, 295t
        bipolar disorder, 296
        cyclothymic disorder, 296
        major depressive disorder, 294–295, 295t
        persistent depressive disorder, 295–296
    obsessive-compulsive disorders, 298
        body dysmorphic disorder, 298
        hoarding disorder, 298
    pediatric psychiatric disorders, 302, 304
        attention deficit hyperactivity disorder, 304
        autism spectrum disorder, 302
        conduct disorder, 304
        Tourette syndrome, 304
    personality disorders, 301, 301t
        clusters, 301, 301t
        persistent behaviour, deviates from cultural
            norms, 301
    psychotic disorders, 293–294, 294t
        antipsychotics, 293, 294t
        delusional disorder, 293
        hallucinations, 293
        schizoaffective disorder, 293
        schizophreniform disorder, 293
    somatic symptom disorders, 299–300
        conversion disorder, 299
        factitious disorder, 299–300
        illness anxiety disorder, 299
        Münchausen syndrome, 299–300
    stress and trauma-related disorders, 298–299
        adjustment disorder, 298
        posttraumatic stress disorder (PTSD), 299
    substance abuse, 302, 303t
Psychotic disorders, 293–294, 294t
    antipsychotics, 293, 294t
    delusional disorder, 293
    hallucinations, 293
    schizoaffective disorder, 293
    schizophreniform disorder, 293
PT. See Prothrombin time
PTCA. See Percutaneous transluminal coronary
    angioplasty
PTH. See Parathyroid hormone
PTSD. See Posttraumatic stress disorder
PTT. See Partial thromboplastin time
PTX. See Pneumothorax
Pubarche, 240
Publication bias, 306t
Public reporting, 309
PUD. See Peptic ulcer disease
Puerperium, 279, 279t
Pulmonary artery catheter, in ICU, 166
Pulmonary concerns
    in ICU, 165
    in preoperative assessment, 168

Index

Pulmonary disorders, 33–55
  acute respiratory distress syndrome, 40–41
  interstitial and other lung diseases, 46–48, 47t
    Goodpasture syndrome, 47
    granulomatosis with polyangiitis, 47–48
    idiopathic pulmonary fibrosis (IPF), 46
    pneumoconioses, 46–47, 47t
    sarcoidosis, 46
  obstructive airway diseases, 41–42
    asthma, 41, 42t, 43t
    bronchiectasis, 42
    chronic bronchitis, 41
    emphysema, 41–42
  pediatric, 53–55
    bronchiolitis, 54
    croup, 53, 53f
    cystic fibrosis, 55
    epiglottitis, 53, 54f
    meconium aspiration syndrome, 55
    respiratory distress syndrome of newborn,
      54, 55f
  pleural diseases, 49–51
    hemothorax, 51
    malignant mesothelioma, 51
    pleural effusion, 49, 49t
    pneumothorax, 50f, 50–51, 50t
  pulmonary surgical concerns, 52
    atelectasis, 52
    intubation, 52
    ventilation, 52
  respiratory infections, 35–40
    lower, 36f, 37–40
    upper, 35–37, 36f
  respiratory neoplasms, 43–46
    laryngeal cancer, 46
    lung cancer, 44–46, 44t, 45t
    solitary pulmonary nodule, 43, 43f, 44f
  sleep apnea, 51–52
Pulmonary edema, 49, 91, 154
Pulmonary embolism (PE), 48
Pulmonary function tests (PFTs), 33, 33f, 34f, 34t
Pulmonary hypertension, 48
Pulmonary nodule, solitary, 43, 43f, 44f
Pulmonary surgical concerns, 52
    atelectasis, 52
    intubation, 52
    ventilation, 52
Pulmonic regurgitation, 16f
Pulmonic stenosis, 16f
Pulseless electrical activity (PEA), 158, 158f, 159f
Pulse oximetry, in carbon monoxide poisoning, 158
Pulse pressure, 2
PVC. See Premature ventricular contraction
PVD. See Peripheral vascular disease
Pyelonephritis, 92
Pyloric stenosis, 87, 88f, 292t

Q
Quadruple screen, 263t
Quinidine, 14t

R
RA. See Rheumatoid arthritis
Rabies, 178–179
Radiation therapy, 150
Radioallergosorbent test (RAST), 137
Raltegravir, 145t
Randomized clinical trial, 305t
Ranson Criteria, 79t
Rapamycin, 173t
Rape, 165
Rapidly progressive glomerulonephritis (RPGN), 96t
RAST. See Radioallergosorbent test
Rates of disease, 306–307
Rattlesnake bite, 156, 156t

Raynaud phenomenon, 217
RBCs. See Red blood cells
Recall bias, 306t
Reconstructive surgery, 238
Rectal fistula, 75
Red blood cells (RBCs)
    declining count of, 182
    packed, 167t
    physiology of, 126–128, 126f, 127f, 128t
Refeeding syndrome, 300
Reflexes in children, 284t
Rejection, of transplantation, 172, 172t
Relative risk (RR), 307, 307t
Renal cell carcinoma, 94–95
Renal concerns, in preoperative assessment, 168
Renal failure, 97–98
    acute, 97–98
    chronic, 98
    dialysis for, 98
Renal function, normal, 90–91, 90f
Renal transplantation, 172t
Renal tubular acidosis, 99, 99t
Repaglinide, 112t
Reproducible angina, 4
Research studies
    bias in, 306, 306t
    study designs, 305t, 306
    study requirements, 305–306
Residual volume (RV), 33f, 34t
Respiratory acidosis, 100f, 100t
Respiratory alkalosis, 100f, 100t
Respiratory distress syndrome of newborn, 54,
    55f, 292t
Respiratory infections, 35–40
    lower, 36f, 37–40
      bronchitis, acute, 37
      pneumonia, 37, 38t, 39f, 39t
      tuberculosis, 37–38, 40f, 40t
    upper, 35–37, 36f
      common cold, 35
      pharyngitis, 35
      sinusitis, 36–37
      tonsillar infections, 36
      viral influenza, 36
Respiratory neoplasms, 43–46, 50
    laryngeal cancer, 46
    lung cancer, 44–46, 44t, 45t
    solitary pulmonary nodule, 43, 43f, 44f
Restrictive cardiomyopathy, 18, 18f, 19t
Retained placental tissue, 280
Retinal artery, 195
    occlusion, 198, 199f
Retinal detachment, 198
Retinal hemorrhages, 199
Retinal vein, 195, 196f, 196t
    occlusion, 198, 199f
Retinal vessel occlusion, 198–199, 198f, 199f
Retinitis, 227
Retinoblastoma, 195, 195f, 292t
Retinoids, teratogenic effects of, 268t
RET protooncogene, 124
Reye syndrome, 178, 193
Rhabdomyosarcoma, 152
Rh blood groups, 166
RHD. See Rheumatic heart disease
Rheumatic fever, acute, 21, 21f
Rheumatic heart disease (RHD), 21
Rheumatoid arthritis (RA), 214–215, 214t
Rheumatologic diseases, 214–218
    ankylosing spondylitis, 214t, 217
    dermatomyositis, 214t, 216
    fibromyalgia, 216–217
    mixed connective tissue disease, 214t, 217–218
    polymyalgia rheumatica, 216
    polymyositis, 214t, 216
    psoriatic arthritis, 214t, 217
    rheumatoid arthritis, 214–215, 214t

scleroderma, 214t, 217
    Sjögren syndrome, 214t, 218
    systemic lupus erythematosus, 214t,
      215–216, 215f
Rhinitis, viral, 35
Rhythm method, 244t
Rib fracture, 205t
Rickets, 221
Rights of patient, 309–310
Right ventricular hypertrophy (RVH), 15
Rilpivirine, 145t
Rinne test, 200
Risk of disease, 307–308, 307t
Ritonavir (RTV), 145, 145t
Rivaroxaban, 139t
Rooting reflex, 284t
Rosiglitazone, 112t
Roth spots, 22
RPGN. See Rapidly progressive glomerulonephritis
RTV. See Ritonavir
Rubella, 269t
Rubeola, 269t
Rule of 2s, 88
Ruptured ectopic pregnancy, 171t
RV. See Residual volume
RVH. See Right ventricular hypertrophy

S
SAH. See Subarachnoid hemorrhage
Salicylate poisoning, 157t
Salivary gland disorders, 61
Salmeterol, 42t
Salter-Harris Classification of Physeal Fractures, 221t
Sarcoidosis, 46
Saxagliptin, 112t
Scabies, 228
Scaphoid fracture, 205t
SCFE. See Slipped capital femoral epiphysis
Schistocytes, 128, 129f
Schizoaffective disorder, 293
Schizoid cluster, 301t
Schizophreniform disorder, 293
Schizotypal cluster, 301t
SCID. See Severe combined immunodeficiency
    syndrome
Scleroderma, 61, 214t, 217
Scoliosis, 221–222, 292t
Scorpion bite, 156, 156t
Screening
    pediatric, 285–286t
    during pregnancy, 262t
    tests, 308
Seborrheic dermatitis, 231
Secondary corticoadrenal insufficiency, 122
Secondary hypertension, 24, 25t
Secondary syphilis, 251
Seizures, 184–186
    causes of, 184, 185t
    febrile, 193
    maternal, 266
    status epilepticus, 184, 186
    treatment of, 184, 186t
    types of, 184, 185t, 186t
Selection bias, 306t
Selective serotonin–reuptake inhibitors (SSRIs),
    295t, 297
Selegiline, 187t
Self-breast examinations, 256
Self-isolation, 298
Self-selection bias, 306t
Sensitivity, 308, 308t
Sensory neurons, 175, 175f, 175t
Sensory neuropathy, foot infections with, 113
Sentinel lymph node biopsy, 258
Sepsis, 141
Septic arthritis, 211–212, 212t, 250

Septic embolization, 22
Septic joint, 211–212, 212t
Septic shock, 26t
Serotonin norepinephrine–reuptake inhibitors (SNRIs), 295t, 297
Serous cystadenoma, ovarian, 255t
Severe combined immunodeficiency syndrome (SCID), 288t
Sex chromosome disorders, 289–290, 290t
Sexual abuse, 165
Sexual intercourse, during pregnancy, 261
Sexually transmitted diseases (STDs), 250–253
    cervicitis, 250
    chancroid, 252
    genital herpes, 252
    granuloma inguinale, 253
    human papillomavirus, 252, 252f
    lymphogranuloma venereum, 252–253
    molluscum contagiosum, 252
    pelvic inflammatory disease, 251
    syphilis, 251–252
Sexual practice methods of contraception, 244t
SGLT-2 inhibitors, 112t
Shave biopsy, 235
Shingles, 227, 227t
Shock, 25, 26t
Shoulder dislocations, 204
SIADH. See Syndrome of inappropriate ADH secretion
Sicca syndrome, 218
Sickle cell disease, 135–136, 135f, 212
Sideroblastic anemia, 128t, 130t, 133, 133f
Silicosis, 47t
Simvastatin, 6t
Sinusitis, 36–37
Sitagliptin, 112t
Sjögren syndrome, 214t, 218
Skin abscess, 224–225
Skin grafts, 237, 237t
Skin sloughing, 230, 231f
SLE. See Systemic lupus erythematosus
Sleep apnea, 51–52, 191
Sleep disorders, 191
Slipped capital femoral epiphysis (SCFE), 220
Small bowel ischemic, 71, 73
Small cell carcinoma, lung, 44t, 45t
Smith fracture, 205t
Smoke inhalation, 154
Snake bite, 156, 156t
SNRIs. See Serotonin norepinephrine–reuptake inhibitors
Social anxiety disorder, 297
Sodium channel blockers, 14, 14t
Sodium urate crystals, 210
Solitary pulmonary nodule, 43, 43f, 44f
Somatic symptom disorders, 299–300
    conversion disorder, 299
    factitious disorder, 299–300
    illness anxiety disorder, 299
    Münchausen syndrome, 299–300
Sotalol, 14t
Specificity, 308, 308t
Spermicide, 244t
Spherocytes, 128, 129f
Spider bite, 156, 156t
Spina bifida occulta, 193
Spinal artery syndrome, 176t
Spinal cord
    lesions of, 175, 176t
    trauma of, 161–162
Spinal stenosis, 207–208
Spine disorders, 206–208
    back pain, 206, 206f
    brachial plexus, 208, 208f, 209t
    cauda equina syndrome, 208
    degenerative disc disease, 206–207, 207f, 207t
    spinal stenosis, 207–208
Spinothalamic tract, 175f, 175t

Spironolactone, 15, 91t
Splinter hemorrhages, 22
Split-thickness graft, 237t
Spontaneous abortion, 270–271, 270t
Spontaneous bacterial peritonitis, 85
Spousal abuse, 165. See also Partner abuse
Sprains, 204
Squamous cell carcinoma
    bladder, 105
    cervical, 254
    esophageal, 64–65, 64f
    lung, 44t, 45t
    skin, 234, 235f
Ss, 3, 53
SSRIs. See Selective serotonin–reuptake inhibitors
Stab wounds, 160
Stanford classification, 26
Staphylococcal infections, 141
Statin, for myocardial infarction, 8t, 9
Statistical significance, 309
Statistics. See Biostatistics
Status asthmaticus, 41
Status epilepticus, 184, 186
STDs. See Sexually transmitted diseases
ST-elevation MI (STEMI), 9
Sterilization, 245t
Stevens-Johnson syndrome, 230
Stimulants, on pregnancy, 267t
Stings, venomous, 156, 156f
St. John's wort, 295t
Stomach. See Gastric entries
Strabismus, 196t
Streptococcal infections, 35, 37
    in pregnancy, 269t
Stress and trauma-related disorders, 298–299
    adjustment disorder, 298
    posttraumatic stress disorder (PTSD), 299
Stress incontinence, 105
String sign, 87
Stroke, 180–181, 180f, 181t
    acute, 158, 160f
    ischemic
        embolic, 180
        thrombotic, 180
Stroke volume (SV), 2
Stromal cell tumor, ovarian, 255t
Subarachnoid hemorrhage (SAH), 94, 182, 182f
Subdural hematoma, 183–184, 183f
Subjects, for research study, 305
Substance abuse, 302, 303t
Sulfonamides, teratogenic effects of, 268t
Sulfonylurea poisoning, 157t
Sulfonylureas, 112t
Sunburst pattern, 218, 219f
Sunscreen, 234
Superior cerebellar artery, 174f
Superior vena cava syndrome, 45
Surgical concerns, 168–173
    postoperative fever, 169–170, 169t, 170f
    preoperative risk assessment, 168–169
    wounds and healing, 170
Surgical emergencies, 170–171
Surgical methods of contraception, 245t
SV. See Stroke volume
Swan-Ganz catheter, 49
    in ICU, 166
Swan neck deformities, 214
Symmetric polyarthropathy, 214
Syncope, 191–192
Syndrome of inappropriate ADH secretion (SIADH), 102
Synovial hypertrophy, 214
Syphilis, 251–252
    latent, 251
    in pregnancy, 269t
    primary, 251
    secondary, 251
    tertiary, 176t, 251

Syringomyelia, 176t, 188
Systemic lupus erythematosus (SLE), 214t, 215–216, 215f
Systole, 1
Systolic dysfunction, 15

T

Tabes dorsalis, 176t, 251
Tacrolimus, 173t
Takayasu arteritis, 28
Tanner stages, 239, 240t, 287t
Tardive dyskinesia, 294
Tay-Sachs disease, 193
TB. See Tuberculosis
3TC. See Lamivudine
TCAs. See Tricyclic antidepressants
T-cell Disorders, 288t
TEE. See Transesophageal echocardiogram
Temporal arteritis, 28, 216
TEN. See Toxic epidermal necrolysis
Tenofovir, 145t
Tension headache, 179
Tension pneumothorax, 50f, 50t, 51
Teratogens, 260
Terazosin, 23t
Tertiary corticoadrenal insufficiency, 122
Tertiary syphilis, 176t, 251
Testicular cancer, 107, 246
Testicular torsion, 107
Tetracycline, teratogenic effects of, 268t
Tetralogy of Fallot, 31f, 32, 292t
Thalassemia, 130t, 133–135, 134f, 134t
Thalidomide, 173t
    teratogenic effects of, 268t
Thelarche, 240
Theophylline, 42t
Thermal airway injury, 158
Thermal burns, 158
Thiazides, 91t, 104
    for hypertension, 23t, 24t
Thiazolidinediones, 112t
Thienopyridines, 139t
Thrombocytopenia, 138, 140t
Thromboembolic pulmonary conditions, 48–49
Thrombolytics, for myocardial infarction, 8t
Thrombolytic therapy, 181
Thrombophlebitis, 27
Thrombotic ischemic stroke, 180
Thrombotic thrombocytopenic purpura-hemolytic uremic syndrome (TTP-HUS), 140t
Thymoma, 189
Thyroid carcinoma, 116, 116t
Thyroid disorders, 114–116
    carcinoma, 116, 116t
    Hashimoto thyroiditis, 116
    hyperthyroidism, 114, 115t
    thyroid storm, 114–115
Thyroid function, 114, 115f
Thyroid-stimulating hormone (TSH), 118, 119f, 120, 120t
Thyroid storm, 114–115
Thyrotropin- releasing hormone (TRH), 119f
Thyroxine (T4), 119f
TIA. See Transient ischemic attack
Tiagabine, 186t
Tibial fracture, 205t
Ticlopidine, 139t
Tics, 190t
Tidal volume (TV), 33f, 34t
Timolol, 23t
Tinea, 229t
Tinea versicolor, 229f, 229t
Tinel sign, 203
Tirofiban, 139t
Tissue flaps, 237, 237t
TLC. See Total lung capacity
Tobacco, on pregnancy, 267t

Tocainide, 14t
Tonic neck reflex, 284t
Tonsillar infections, 36
Topiramate, 186t
TORCH infections, 268
Torsades de pointes, 13
Torsemide, 91t
Total lung capacity (TLC), 33f, 34t
Tourette syndrome, 190t, 304
Toxic epidermal necrolysis (TEN), 230–231, 231f
Toxicology, 156–158, 157t
Toxic shock syndrome, 249–250
Toxoplasmosis, 269t
tPA, for myocardial infarction, 8t, 9
Tracheoesophageal fistula, 86–87, 87f
Transdermal contraceptive patch, 244t
Transesophageal echocardiogram (TEE), for Afib, 12
Transfusion reactions, 166–167, 167t
Transient ischemic attack (TIA), 179–180
Transitional cell carcinoma, bladder, 105
Transplantation, 172–173
    common types of, 172, 172t
    graft vs. host disease, 173
    immunosuppressive drugs for, 172, 173t
    indications and selection for, 172
    infection risk in, 172
    rejection of, 172, 173t
Transposition of great vessels, 31f, 32
Transudates, 20
Trastuzumab, 259
Traumatology, 160–164
    abdominal, 163
    assessment of, 160–161
    chest, 162–163
    extremity, 164
    genitourinary and pelvic, 163
    head trauma, 161
    mechanisms of injury in, 160
    neck, 162, 162f
    during pregnancy, 164
    spinal cord, 161–162
Trazodone, 295t
Triamterene, 91t
Tricuspid atresia, 32
Tricuspid regurgitation, 16f
Tricyclic antidepressants (TCAs), 295t
    poisoning with, 157t
Trigeminal neuralgia, 179
Triiodothyronine (T3), 119f
Trisomies, 290–291, 290t
Trisomy 13, 263t, 290t
Trisomy 18, 262t, 263, 263t, 290t
Trisomy 21, 262t, 263, 263t, 290, 290t
Trochlear nerve (CN IV), 195
Tropical sprue, 67, 68f, 69
Troponin-I, 7
Ts, 5, 31
TSH. See Thyroid-stimulating hormone
TTP-HUS. See Thrombotic thrombocytopenic
        purpura-hemolytic uremic syndrome
Tuberculosis (TB), 37–38, 40f, 40t
Tubo-ovarian abscess, 251
Tubular carcinoma, 258t
Turcot syndrome, 76, 76t
Turner syndrome, 290t
TV. See Tidal volume
Twins, 274
Twin-twin transfusion syndrome, 274
Type I error, 309
Type II error, 309

U

Ulcerative colitis, 71, 71t
Ulcers, 66
UMN disease, 187
Uncal herniation, 177

Undescended testes, 108
Unhappy triad, 204
Unresponsive patient, 158f
Unstable angina, 6–7
Upper respiratory infections (URI), 35–37, 36f
    common cold, 35
    pharyngitis, 35
    sinusitis, 36–37
    tonsillar infections, 36
    viral influenza, 36
Urea, 91t
Ureteral disorders, 104–105
    bladder cancer, 105
    urinary incontinence, 104–105
    urinary tract infection, 104
Uretero-vesical junction, 92
Urethral displacement, 108
Urethral rupture, 163
Urethritis, 104, 105–106
URI. See Upper respiratory infections
Urinary incontinence, 104–105
Urinary tract infection (UTI), 104
    maternal, 267
Urine sample, clean catch, 104
Urokinase, for myocardial infarction, 8t
Uterine artery embolization, 253
Uterine atony, 280
Uterine bleeding, abnormal, 248
Uterine fibroids, 253
Uterine leiomyoma, 253
UTI. See Urinary tract infection
Uveitis, 197

V

Vaccinations, 286t. See also specific vaccines
Vaginitis, 249, 249t, 250f
Valproate, 186t
    teratogenic effects of, 268t
Valsalva maneuver, 11, 206
Valsartan, 23t
Valvular diseases, 16f, 17t
Varicella-zoster infection, 227, 227t, 288f
    in pregnancy, 269t
Varicosities, 27
Vascular diseases
    abdominal aortic aneurysm, 26
    aortic dissection, 26–27
    arteriovenous malformations, 27
    Churg-Strauss syndrome, 28
    deep vein thrombosis, 27
    eosinophilic granulomatosis with polyangiitis, 28
    Henoch-Schönlein purpura, 29
    Kawasaki disease, 28
    peripheral vascular disease, 27
    polyarteritis nodosa, 28
    Takayasu arteritis, 28
    temporal arteritis, 28
    varicosities, 27
    vascular and thromboembolic pulmonary condi-
        tions, 48–49
    vasculitis, 28–29
Vascular pulmonary conditions, 48–49
Vasculitis, 28–29
Vasoactive medications, 167, 167t
Vasodilators, 167, 167t
    for hypertension, 23t
Vasopressin, 167t
Vasopressors, 167, 167t
Vasospasm, 7
Vegetative state, persistent, 192
Velocardiofacial syndrome, 291t
Ventilation, 165
Ventilation, mechanical, 52
Ventricular fibrillation (Vfib), 14
    post-MI, 9
    treatment of, 158, 158f, 159f

Ventricular septal defect (VSD), 30, 31f, 292t
Ventricular tachycardia (Vtach), 13–14, 13f, 158f
    post-MI, 9
    treatment of, 158, 158f, 159f
Ventricular wall rupture, post-MI, 9
Verapamil, 14t, 23t
Vertebral artery, 174f
Vfib. See Ventricular fibrillation
VIPoma, 80
Viral gastroenteritis, 56
Viral influenza, 36
Viral meningitis, 177t, 178
Viral rhinitis, 35
Virchow triad, 27
Vitamin B₁₂ deficiency, 176t
    anemia, 128t, 132, 132f
Vitamin D, 117, 117f
1,25-(OH)₂ Vitamin D, 117, 117f
Vitamin K, 138
    deficiency, 139
Vitamins, absorption of, 68f
Volvulus, 74
von Recklinghausen disease, 191
von Willebrand disease, 138
VSD. See Ventricular septal defect
Vtach. See Ventricular tachycardia

W

Waiter's tip, 209t
Warfarin, 139t
    poisoning with, 157t
    PT monitoring of, 138
    teratogenic effects of, 267, 268t
    vitamin K and, 139
Warts, 288
Water moccasin bite, 156, 156t
Weber test, 200
Wegener granulomatosis, 47–48, 96t
Weight gain, in pregnancy, 261
Weight, in children, 282
Wernicke aphasias, 184, 184t
West Nile virus, 178
Wet gangrene, 225
Whipple disease, 69
Whipple's triad, 80
White matter lesions, 188
Whole blood transfusions, 167t
Williams syndrome, 291t
Wilms tumor, 108, 292t
Wilson disease, 86
Wiskott-Aldrich syndrome, 288t
Withdrawal method, 244t
Wolff-Parkinson-White (WPW) syndrome, 11, 11f
Wolf-Hirschhorn syndrome, 291t
Wound healing, 170
Wounds, 170
WPW syndrome. See Wolff-Parkinson-White
        syndrome
Wrist drop, 209t
Ws, 3, 201

X

X-linked agammaglobulinemia, 288t
XXX, 290t
XYY, 290, 290t

Z

Zafirlukast, 42t
Zenker diverticulum, 61, 63, 63f
Zidovudine (AZT), 145t
Zileuton, 42t
Zollinger-Ellison syndrome, 66–67
    endocrine pancreatic cancers with, 80
Zonisamide, 186t